Encyclopedia of Lung Diseases and Research

Volume II

Encyclopedia of
Lung Diseases and Research
Volume II

Edited by **Toby Botkin**

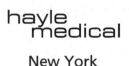

New York

Published by Hayle Medical,
30 West, 37th Street, Suite 612,
New York, NY 10018, USA
www.haylemedical.com

Encyclopedia of Lung Diseases and Research
Volume II
Edited by Toby Botkin

International Standard Book Number: 978-1-63241-168-6 (Hardback)

Printed in the United States of America.

Contents

Preface

The main aim of this book is to educate learners and enhance their research focus by presenting diverse topics covering this vast field. This is an advanced book which compiles significant studies by distinguished experts in the area of analysis. This book addresses successive solutions to the challenges arising in the area of application, along with it; the book provides scope for future developments.

The advancements in the field of molecular medicine are changing respiratory medicine significantly. This book consists of the knowledge and experience of renowned scientists and clinicians from around the world. It will benefit aspiring clinicians and scientists about the current developments in a variety of lung ailments that will enable them to understand respiration related disorders. The book discusses issues related to pediatric respiratory ailments and immune regulation. This book will be valuable to clinicians to keep up with the latest concepts, to enhance their diagnostic skills, and to understand the potential new therapeutic applications in lung diseases.

It was a great honour to edit this book, though there were challenges, as it involved a lot of communication and networking between me and the editorial team. However, the end result was this all-inclusive book covering diverse themes in the field.

Finally, it is important to acknowledge the efforts of the contributors for their excellent chapters, through which a wide variety of issues have been addressed. I would also like to thank my colleagues for their valuable feedback during the making of this book.

Editor

Part 1

Immunity and Infection

Current Status of the Mollicute (Mycoplasma) Lung Disease: Pathogenesis, Diagnostics, Treatment and Prevention

Silvia Giono-Cerezo[1,*], Guadalupe Estrada-Gutiérrez[2],
José Antonio Rivera-Tapia[3], Jorge Antonio Yáñez-Santos[3]
and Francisco Javier Díaz-García[4]
[1]*Departamento de Microbiología, Escuela Nacional de Ciencias Biológicas, IPN*
[2]*Departamento de Infectología, Instituto Nacional de Perinatología, México, D.F.,*
[3]*Benemérita Universidad Autónoma de Puebla, Puebla, México*
[4]*Departamento de Salud Pública, Facultad de Medicina, UNAM*
México

1. Introduction

The microorganisms referred as mycoplasmas ("mushroom form") are eubacteria included within the Class Mollicutes (from latin *mollis* ="soft", *cutis*= "skin"), which comprises the smallest self-replicating bacteria, showing distinctive features such as: a) lack of a rigid cell wall envelope, b) sterol incorporation into their own plasma membrane, and c) Reduced cellular (0.3 - 0.8 μm diameter) and genome sizes (0.58-2.20 Mb). Some genera use the UGA stop codon to encode tryptophan [Bove, 1993; Razin et al., 1998].

The term "mycoplasmas" will be used herein when referring to any species within the Class *Mollicutes*. Due to their reduced genome sizes, the mycoplasmas exhibit restricted metabolic and physiological pathways for replication and survival [Razin et al., 1998]. This makes evident why these bacteria display strict dependence to their hosts for acquisition of aminoacids, nucleotides, lipids and sterols as biosynthetic precursors. [Baseman & Tully, 1997; Razin et al., 1998].

Recognized human pathogenic mycoplasma species mostly belongs to the *Mycoplasma* and *Ureaplasma* genera (Table 1). Acute or fulminant diseases are rarely caused by these bacteria, instead they produce subclinical or covert infections that become chronic and/or persistent [Baseman & Tully, 1997; Razin et al., 1998]. Cell surface colonization and in some cases subsequent invasion and intracellular residence have been well documented for several *Mycoplasma* species which infect humans [Andreev et al., 1995; Baseman et al., 1995; Díaz-García et al., 2006; Giron et al., 1996; Jensen et al., 1994; Lo et al., 1993; Taylor-Robinson et al., 1991].

The primary habitats of the mycoplasmas infecting humans are the mucosal surfaces of the respiratory and genitourinary tracts [Cassell et al., 1994a; Taylor-Robinson, 1996]. Moreover,

---

* Corresponding Author

the mycoplasmas display host- and tissue-specific tropism, reflecting their nutritional demands and parasitic lifestyle [Razin et al., 1998]. Thus, *M. pneumoniae* is found principally in the respiratory tract, whereas *M. genitalium, Ureaplasma spp., M. hominis, M. fermentans* and *M. penetrans* are primarily urogenital residents, but exceptionally they can be isolated from other unusual tissues and organs, especially in immunocompromised patients or in patients undergoing solid organ transplantation [Waites & Talkington, 2004; Waites et al., 2005; Waites, 2008].

Mycoplasmal respiratory infections in humans can be ascribed mainly to *M. pneumoniae* and, in fetuses or newborns, to *Ureaplasma* species. *M. pneumoniae* is a well-known pathogen in atypical and community-acquired pneumonia, whereas *U. urealyticum* and *U. parvum* have been associated with vertically-transmitted intrauterine and neonatal pneumonia [Taylor-Robinson, 1996; Waites et al., 2005].

Species	Primary colonization sites		Substrate utilization		
	Oropharyngeal tract	Urogenital tract	Glucose	Arginine	Urea
Mycoplasma fermentans	✓	✓	✓	✓	✗
M. genitalium	✓	✓	✓	✗	✗
M. hominis	✓	✓	✗	✓	✗
M. penetrans	✗	✓	✓	✓	✗
M. pneumoniae	✓	✗	✓	✗	✗
Ureaplasma parvum	✓	✓	✗	✗	✓
U. urealyticum	✓	✓	✗	✗	✓

✓ Present; ✗ Absent
Modified from Taylor-Robinson, 1996.

Table 1. Mycoplasma species pathogenic for humans.

A worldwide rise in the frequency of *M. pneumoniae*-associated lower respiratory tract disease has been observed, from 6 - >30% in the 1990s, to 0 - 66.7% in 2010 [Reviewed by Loens et al., 2003, 2010]. Therefore the pathogenic role of *M. pneumoniae* in respiratory disease has been proved in persons of all ages, sometimes causing severe respiratory disease, and it may induce clinically significant manifestations in extrapulmonary sites by direct invasion and/or immunologic effects. Only in the USA, *M. pneumoniae* is responsible for more than 100,000 hospitalizations of adults each year [Waites & Talkington, 2004; Waites, 2008]. This close interplay between *M. pneumoniae* and the host's respiratory epithelium induces local damage and in turn elicits release of inflammatory mediators by the host. The magnitude of the later response appears to be related to the severity of disease [Waites, 2008].

Respiratory tract colonization with *Ureaplasma* spp., and rarely with *M. hominis,* in preterm infants has been associated with higher incidence of pneumonia, severe respiratory failure, bronchopulmonary dysplasia, and ultimately with death [Viscardi et al., 2002]. These bacteria can be transmitted from infected females to their fetus or newborn by three main different routes: a) Ascending intrauterine infection from vaginal colonization; b) Hematogenous spreading from placental infection, and c) Acquisition of the microorganism by the neonate during passage through an infected maternal birth canal. [Viscardi et al., 2002; Waites et al., 2005]. An inverse correlation between ureaplasmal vertical transmission rate and gestational age has been established, and this increases with duration of premature rupture of membranes. Improved molecular detection of colonizing *Ureaplasma* in respiratory tract specimens suggests a higher frequency of colonization in very low birth weight infants than that previously reported with culture-based studies (25–48% vs. 20%) [Viscardi & Hasday, 2009].

Infrequently, *M. fermentans* has been detected in adults who developed respiratory distress syndrome and/or from bronchoalveolar lavage in AIDS patients with pneumonia, highlighting the potential of this species to cause lower respiratory tract disease in susceptible hosts [Waites &Talkington, 2004].

2. Taxonomic characterization of Mollicutes

Modern mycoplasmal taxonomy relies on combined data from phenotypic traits and phylogeny based on the 16S rRNA gene sequences [Brown et al., 2007; International Committee on Systematics of Prokaryotes- Subcommittee on the taxonomy of Mollicutes (ICSP-STM), 2010]. Among the phenotypic characteristics, there are few useful metabolic markers including the ability to ferment glucose, the ability to hydrolyze urea and arginine, and dependence on cholesterol for growth and anaerobiosis. Despite the high rate of surface antigenic variation, serologic relatedness at the species level is still used in routine identification of mycoplasmas [Brown et al., 2007; ICSP-STM, 2010; Razin et al., 1998]. There are currently more than 200 species allocated into four orders, five families and eight genera within the class *Mollicutes* (Figure1), including the undefined *candidatus Phytoplasma* [Brown et al., 2007; ICSP-STM, 2010].

2.1 Phylogeny, genome content and molecular analysis

The Mollicutes 16S rRNA-based phylogenetic tree is monophyletic arising from a single branch of the *Clostridium ramosum* branch. The Mollicutes split into two major branches: the AAP branch, containing the *Acholeplasma*, *Anaeroplasma* and *Asteroleplasma* genera, and the *Candidatus Phytoplasma* phyla; the other is the SEM branch that includes the *Spiroplasma*, *Entomoplasma*, *Mesoplasma*, *Ureaplasma* and *Mycoplasma* genera [Johansson et al., 1998; Maniloff 1992; Razin et al., 1998). Interestingly, the genus *Mycoplasma* is polyphyletic, with species clustering within the Spiroplasma, Pneumoniae and Hominis phylogenetic groups [Behbahani et al., 1993; Johansson et al., 1998; Maniloff 1992]. Nevertheless, additional phylogenetic markers such as the elongation factor EF-Tu (*tuf*) gene, ribosomal protein genes, the 16S/23S rRNA intergenic sequences, etc, have been already used as complementary comparative data, thus there is no unique phylogenetic tree for *Mollicutes* [Razin et al., 1998].

The mycoplasmas may have evolved through regressive evolution from closely related Gram positive bacteria with low content of guanine plus cytosine (G+C), probably the Clostridia or *Erysipelothrix* [Bove, 1993; Brown et al., 2007; Razin et al., 1998]. The massive gene losses (i.e. genes involved in cell wall and aminoacid biosynthesis) had left mycoplasmas with a coding repertoire of 500 to 2000 genes [Sirand-Pugnet et al., 2007]. The G+C content in DNA of mycoplasmas varies from 23 to 40 mol%, while genome size range is 580–2200 Kbp, much smaller than those of most walled bacteria [Razin et al., 1998].

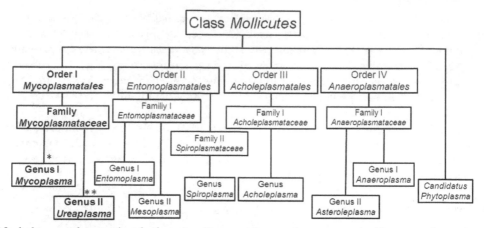

* Includes more than one hundred species. At present five species are recognized human pathogens.
** Includes seven species, two of them are pathogenic for humans.
Adapted from: Razin et al, 1998.

Fig. 1. Taxonomy of Class Mollicutes.

From a comparative analysis of the complete genome sequences from 17 mycoplasma species, Sirand-Pugnet et al., 2007, identified 729 clusters of orthologous groups of proteins (COGs) that represent 21 categories of diverse cellular functions. This analysis revealed that mycoplasmas shared a limited core genome (i.e. the essential translation machinery), while there is a wide diversity of COGs that are only found in one or a few species. Moreover, frequent chromosomal rearrangements occurring at specific loci involved in expression of surface proteins were also identified [Momynaliev & Govorun, 2001; Sirand-Pugnet et al., 2007].

3. Immune response

Host defense in respiratory mycoplasmosis is dependent on both innate and humoral immunity. In general terms, mycoplasmas reaching the lower respiratory tract may be opsonized by antibody and complement, and then activated macrophages begin phagocytosis and migration to the site of infection by chemotaxis. Finally, complement-mediated cytolysis may then play a role in limiting the growth of the mycoplasmas. However, immunity against mycoplasmal infection is typically short-lived, hence infection recurrence is common (Waites et al., 2007, 2008).

3.1 Innate and adaptive immune response

M. pneumoniae infection is able to activate the host innate immune system, so the inflammatory event elicited by accounts for the early signs and symptoms of the infection. After become opsonized, M. pneumoniae is susceptible to complement-mediated cytolysis, probably through both the alternative and classical pathways [Waites et al., 2007]. It has been suggested that innate immune recognition of M. pneumoniae has also a pivotal role for mucin expression in the airway, at both mRNA and protein levels, since blockage of the toll-like receptor (TLR)-2 signaling pathway results in marked reduction of mucin expression [Chu et al., 2005]. Moreover, M. pneumoniae is capable of interact with mast cells and surfactant protein (SP)-A, resulting in cytokine production and bacterial growth inhibition, respectively [Waites et al, 2007].

After primary encounter with *M. pneumoniae*, the immune system of an immunocompetent host responds by rapidly producing antibodies (mainly directed against the P1 adhesin and glycolipid antigens) that peak after 3 to 6 weeks, followed by a gradual decline over months to years [Waites & Talkington, 2004]. The onset of symptoms may coincide with demonstrable antibody titers due to prolonged incubation period. Acute infection can often be difficult observed by evidence of rising *M. pneumoniae*-specific IgM antibodies, especially in pediatric populations. [Waites, 2007, 2008]. IgA antibodies are produced early in the course of disease, rise quickly to peak levels, and decrease earlier than IgM or IgG [Waites & Talkington, 2004].

Adaptive immunity, characterized by both B and T lymphocyte responses, has a major impact on the progression of *M. pneumoniae* respiratory disease. Mycoplasmas activate the immune system by inducing non-specific proliferation of B- and T-lymphocyte populations (mitogenic stimulation), thereby inducing autoimmune responses with concurrent production of cytokines (Table 2). Immune responses that develop after infection often fail

Organism	Cells / Experimental system	Cytokine(s) released
M. pneumoniae	• Lung Alveolar type II pneumocytes	Interleukin (IL)-1β, tumour necrosis factor (TNF)-α, IL-8.
	• Nasal epithelial cells/peripheral blood macrophages	IL-2, IL-6, RANTES, intercellular adhesion molecule (ICAM)-1, transforming growth factor (TGF)-β1 and TNF-α
	• Peripheral blood mononuclear cells	IL-1β, IL-2/IL-2R, IL-6, Interferon (IF)-γ, and TNF-α.
	• Lung ephitelial carcinoma A549 cells	IL-1β, IL-8, and TNF-α.
	• *M. pneumoniae*-infected patients	IL-2/IL-2R, IL-4, IL-5, IL-6, IL-8, IL-12, IL-18, IF-γ, and TNF-α.
Ureaplasma spp.	• Neonatal fibroblasts	IL-6 and IL-8.
	• Peripheral blood/Cord blood monocytes	TNF-α, IL-8, IL-6, and IL-10.
	• THP-1-derived macrophages / Human lung fibroblasts	TNF-α, IL-6, ICAM-1, and vascular endothelial growth factor (VEGF).
	• THP-1 monocytes	IL-1α, TNF-α, and IL-8.

Data from Dakhama et al., 2003; Kazachkov et al., 2002; Li et al., 2000a; Manimtim et al., 2001; Peltier et al., 2008 ; Stancombe et al., 1993; Yang et al, 2004.

Table 2. Mycoplasma-induced cytokine secretion.

to eliminate the mycoplasma, indicating that adaptive immunity apparently has a limited effect on clearance of an established infection, thus leading to asymptomatic carriage for variable periods of time. Cytokine production and lymphocyte activation may either minimize disease through the enhancement of host defense mechanisms and subsequent elimination of the infecting organisms, or exacerbate disease through the development of immunologic hypersensitivity [Waites et al, 2007, 2008]. It has been suggested that there is no correlation between severity of pneumonia caused by *M. pneumoniae* and T-cell deficiencies, thus cell-mediated defense against respiratory mycoplasmosis appears to be rather limited [Cartner et al, 1998].

Molecular mimicry, survival within cells and phenotypic plasticity (antigenic variation) are the major mechanisms by which mycoplasmas evade the immune response [Chambaud et al, 1999; Razin et al., 1998; Rottem & Naot, 1998]. Furthermore, a transient impairment of T-lymphocyte function, or depletion of CD4+ T cells, can be induced by *M. pneumoniae* [Waites et al., 2007].

In the context of perinatal pneumonia, very low birth weight infants have relative deficiencies in mucosal barrier function and in both the innate and adaptive immune responses. These immature hosts may generate poor immune responses, including secretory IgA, serum complement components, defensins, fibronectin, and altered cytokine production. Impaired chemotaxis, phagocytosis, and microbial killing by neonatal immune cells highlight the vulnerability of preterm neonates to systemic infections, and partially explain the eventual systemic spread of bacteria [Waites et al., 2005].

3.2 Cell culture models

Mycoplasmas possess an impressive capability of maintaining a dynamic surface architecture that is antigenically and functionally versatile, contributing to their capability to adapt to a large range of habitats and cause diseases that are often chronic in nature [Rottem, 2003]. The probable role of mycoplasmas in chronic respiratory diseases has been studied *in vitro* using diverse cell culture models. Several of these models are focusing in the study of adherence, invasion and fusion as the strategies to induce damage to the host cells [Baseman et al., 1995; Razin, 1999; Rottem, 2003].

M. pneumoniae is the most extensively studied system with respect to adhesions and receptors [Rottem, 2003] because of its significance as pathogen for humans. Models in human lung cells analyzed by inmunofluorescence and confocal microscopy reveal that *M. pneumoniae* parasitize cells surface, enter the intracellular spaces and locate throughout the cytoplasmic and perinuclear regions within 2 hr postinfection [Baseman et al., 1995]. The microorganism can survive within the host cells for prolonged periods of time, well protected from the immune system and from de action of many antibiotics and may explain its pathogenic potential [Yavlovich et al., 2004]. Another *in vitro* studies show that this microorganism has a polar, tapered cell extension at one of the poles containing an electron-dense core in the cytoplasma. This structure, termed the tip organelle, functions both as an attachment organelle and as the leading end in gliding motility [Baseman et al., 1995; Razin, 1999; Rottem, 2003; Svenstrup et al., 2002]. Host-pathogen studies in an air-liquid culture of differentiated human airway epithelial cells revealed that the microorganism bounds initially to ciliated epithelial cells, but colonization become more evently distributed over the entire surface with time [Krunkosky et al., 2007]. We recently studied the adherence of *U. urealyticum* to a respiratory epithelial cell line, as a virulence factor for lung disease. We describe that *U. urealyticum* induce changes in cell morphology mediated probably by the loss of microvilli, and that the microorganism invades the cell forming vacuoles [Torres-Morquecho et al., 2010].

Since chronic lung disease is characterized by an early increased number of activated neutrophils and alveolar macrophages, with later architectural epithelial and endothelial cell damage [Li et al., 2002], all of these cells represent excellent targets for the study of mycoplasmal infections. As the key processes occurring in all respiratory diseases are the exacerbation of lung inflammation and injury, most of the *in vitro* models have been developed to study the inflammatory response mediated primarily by cytokines.

Different studies have demonstrated that the release of Interleukin (IL)-2, IL-6 RANTES, ICAM-1, TGF-β1 and TNF-α by human nasal epithelial cells and peripheral monocytes infected with *M. pneumoniae* could be implicated in the asthma exacerbation in children and may play a role in the pathogenesis of chronic asthma [Dakhama et al., 2003; Kazachkov et al., 2002; Krunkosky et al., 2007]. Additionally, it has been recently demonstrated that *M. pneumoniae* infection induces reactive oxygen species and DNA damage in human lung cells [Sun et al., 2008].

A number of studies show that *Ureaplasma urealyticum* induce the production of TNF-α, IL-8, IL-6 [Li et al., 2000a; Manimtim et al., 2001; Peltier et al., 2008], NF-κB and nitric oxide [Li et al., 2000b] by human macrophages and monocytes. Infection assays in macrophages performed in combination with LPS showed that *U. urealyticum* enhances the proinflammatory response to a second infection by blocking expression of counterregulatory cytokines (IL-6 and IL-10), predisposing the preterm infant to prolonged and dysregulated inflammation, lung injury, and impaired clearance of secondary infections [Manimtim et al., 2001]. Furthermore, *U. urealyticum* stimulates macrophages to produce vascular endothelial grow factor (VEGF) and intercellular adhesion molecule-1 (ICAM-1) *in vitro*, which are potentially associated with both early and later pathological changes in the lung during the development of chronic lung disease [Li et al., 2002a]. The same raise in proinflammatory cytokine release is observed when *U. urealyticum* interacts with neonatal pulmonary fibroblast [Stancombe et al., 1993], suggesting a role in the development of bronchopulmonary dysplasia. Finally, it has been demonstrated that *U. urealyticum* induces apoptosis in human lung epithelial cells and macrophages [Li et al., 2002b], involving in impairing lung structure observed in chronic lung disease.

4. Lung disease in humans

4.1 *Mycoplasma pneumoniae*

Respiratory infections due to *M. pneumoniae* can affect either the upper or the lower tract, or both simultaneously. This pathogen is responsible for up to 40% of cases of community-acquired pneumonia [Atkinson, et al., 2008]. Nearly 50% of the *M. pneumoniae*-infected patients show non-specific signs and symptoms, often similar to those produced by other respiratory pathogens such as *Chlamydophila pneumoniae*, *Streptococcus pneumoniae* and some viruses, and although these infections are usually mild or asymptomatic, they are not always self-limiting [Waites & Talkington, 2004; Waites et al., 2008].

Symptomatic disease emerges gradually within few days post-infection and persists for several weeks or months. Upper respiratory tract symptoms include sore throat, fever, cough, headache, coryza, myalgias, chills, earache and malaise. Clinical manifestations of lower respiratory tract infections generally include: non-productive cough which later turns productive with non-hemorrhagic sputum, dyspnoea, adenopathy, wheezing and, rarely, respiratory failure [Waites & Talkington, 2004; Waites et al., 2008].

4.1.1 Pathogenesis

Occurrence of airway disease initiates from the close interplay between the microorganism and the mucosal epithelium as a result of cytadherence, the main virulence factor of the bacterium, which is mediated through a polarized tip attachment organelle. This tip structure comprise the main protein adhesin, named P1, along with several other adhesins and accessory proteins (High Molecular Weight [HMW]-1, HMW-2, HMW-3, Protein [P]-90, P-40 and P-30) [Waites et al., 2008].

Unlike other bacterial lung pathogens (S. *pneumoniae*, *Pseudomonas aeruginosa* and *Haemophilus influenzae*) which bind specifically to glycolipids containing unsubstituted GalNAcβ1-4Gal residues, *M pneumoniae* attaches to host cells either through a sialic acid-free glycoprotein or sulfated glycolipids containing terminal $Gal(3SO_4)\_1$ residues. It is worthy to note that the apical microvillar border and cilia of the epithelium express the sialoglycoconjugate-type receptors, thus allowing the selective attachment of M. *pneumoniae* to the ciliated cells [Krivan et al., 1988, 1989; Roberts, D.D. et al, 1989; Olson & Gilbert, 1993; Rottem & Naot, 1998].

Cytadhered M. *pneumoniae* is able to cause damage through generation of reactive oxygen species (ROS), which act in concert with host's endogenous ROS to induce oxidative stress. Bacteria-derived superoxide anions act to inhibit catalase in host cells, thereby reducing the enzymatic breakdown of peroxides, rendering the host cell more susceptible to oxidative damage [Rottem & Naot, 1998; Waites et al., 2004]. Mycoplasmal species exert primarily deleterious effects on the host respiratory epithelium, such as ciliostasis and apoptosis, resulting in localized damage and an immune response which, although often robust, is poorly efficacious in terms of clearing the organism or preventing subsequent reinfections [Waites et al., 2004].

Recently, a M. *pneumoniae* protein homolog to the pertussis toxin S1 subunit was identified and it showed specific binding to surfactant protein A [Kannan et al., 2005] This protein also showed protein:ADPribosyltransferase activity, inducing vacuolation and ciliostasis in cultured host cells. This immunodominant protein has been named as community-acquired respiratory distress syndrome toxin (CARDS TX). Host-cell targets for CARDS TX remain unidentified at present, as does how the toxin's function might relate to its specific binding to surfactant protein A [Kannann & Baseman, 2006; Waites et al., 2004, 2008].

Cytopathic effects observed in M. *pneumoniae*-infected host cells include loss of ciliated epithelia, cell vacuolation, reduced oxygen consumption, reduced glucose utilization, diminished amino acid uptake and macromolecular synthesis, ultimately leading to exfoliation. Clinically, the above mentioned events in the lung tissues are noticeable by the persistent hacking cough [Waites et al., 2004, 2008].

Some clinical characteristics of M. *pneumoniae* infections are consistent with an intracellular location of the pathogen, mainly the establishment of latent or chronic infections, limited efficacy of some antimicrobials, necessity for prolonged treatment to eradicate infection in some instances and circumvention of the host immune response [Waites & Talkington, 2004]

4.1.2 Role in COPD and asthma

Chronic obstructive pulmonary disease (COPD) is an inflammatory disorder of the lungs that leads to blockage of the airways which eventually interferes with the exchange of oxygen and carbon dioxide, making breathing progressively more difficult. It is mainly associated with long-term smoking, but presence of persistent bacterial infections has been related to the etiology, pathogenesis and clinical course of COPD [Blasi, 2004; Sethi, 2000].

Well-known bacterial pathogens such as *Streptococcus pneumoniae, Haemophilus influenzae*, and *Moraxella catarrhalis* have been associated with acute exacerbations in COPD and asthma. [Guilbert & Denlinger, 2010; Sethi, 2000; Waites & Talkington, 2004]. Since late 1970's, several authors suggested a relationship between COPD and *M. pneumoniae* infection [Buscho *et al.*, 1978; Gump *et al.*, 1976; Smith *et al.*, 1980], but it was until late 1990's and early 2000's that several studies based on serology brought attention once more on this issue. [Lieberman et al., 2001, 2002; Mogulkoc *et al.*, 1999]. It is well known that mycoplasmas species pathogenic for humans have the ability to induce chronic disease states in which clearance of the bacteria is extremely difficult. [Rottem & Naot, 1998].

A growing body of evidence indicates that there is a link between *M pneumoniae* infection and COPD. In a Yemeni study, *M. pneumoniae* infection was demonstrated by culture and serologic methods in 20.4% (11/54) of COPD patients [Al-Moyed & Al-Shamahy, 2003]. In a group of 144 Dutch patients with CAP, 12.5 % were infected with *M. pneumoniae* and less than 40% of these *M. pneumoniae*-infected patients had COPD, even though specific serologic tests were mainly negative [Dorigo-Zetsma *et al.*, 2001]. In contrast, *M. pneumoniae* was the most frequent pathogen (22.7%, alone or in association with other microorganisms) among CAP patients that required hospitalization related to COPD, asthma and/or pulmonary fibrosis. [Caberlotto *et al.*, 2003].

A rather weak association between *M. pneumoniae* infection and acute asthma has been suggested on the basis of contradictory data about mycoplasma infection frequencies from several trials. Conversely, strong associations of this pathogen with chronic asthma have been established [Guilbert & Denlinger, 2010; Sutherland & Martin, 2007]. Evidence for this association includes the following: a) Higher prevalence of *M. pneumoniae* in asthmatics than in healthy subjects; b) Improved pulmonary function in mycoplasma-infected asthmatic patients after treatment with macrolide antibiotics; c) Demonstration of long-term airway dysfunction consistent with a persistent infection; and d) *M. pneumoniae*-induced production of inflammatory mediators (IgE, substance P and neurokinin 1, and IL-5) implicated in the pathogenesis of asthma [Waites & Talkington, 2004].

By means of murine models of chronic respiratory infection, it has been demonstrated *M. pneumoniae* can produce pneumonia, with consistent immunologic responses in term of specific IgM antibodies [Wubbel et al., 1998]. Other findings revealed post-infection time-dependent differential cytokine production, with increased expression of TNF-α, IL-1, IL-6, and IFN-γ in the acute phase, whereas IL-2 and IL-2 receptor gene expression was seen only during reinfection. [Pietsch et al., 1994].

Relationship between the timing of Mycoplasma infection, allergic sensitization, and subsequent pulmonary physiologic and immune response was assessed by Chu et al., 2003. Before ovalbumin sensitization, experimental *M. pneumoniae* infection resulted in reduced airway hyperresponsiveness (AHR), reduced lung inflammatory cell recruitment, and a predominantly Th1 response. In contrast, *M. pneumoniae* infection post-sensitization initially caused a transient reduction in AHR, followed by augmented AHR, and a Th2-dominant airway inflammatory process that potentiates organism survival in the lungs. Further characterization of the *M. pneumoniae* effects on ovoalbumin sensitized mice, long-term infection provoked collagen deposition in airway wall accompanied by augmented expression of TGF-β1 in the lungs [Chu et al., 2005].

4.2 *Mycoplasmas* in immunocompromised hosts

Association between immunodeficiency and mycoplasmal infections has been reported since the mid 1970s to the date. Mycoplasmas can disseminate from localized infections and cause invasive diseases, especially in hypogammaglobulinemic subjects. Significance of mycoplasma species other than *M. pneumoniae* or *Ureaplasma* spp. in respiratory diseases is a matter of controversy [Cassell et al., 1994a].

4.2.1 *Mycoplasma fermentans* associated to lung diseases

It has been well documented that *M. pneumoniae* produces respiratory disease in adults; it is also worthy of consideration as a cause of respiratory infections in persons of all age groups, though very few attempts have been made to determine whether it occurs in neonates and young infants [Waites et al., 2005]. However, due to their fastidious growth requirements and presumably less frequent occurrence than *Ureaplasma* spp. or *M. hominis*, much less is known about the epidemiology and disease associations of organisms such as *M. fermentans*, *M. genitalium*, and *M. penetrans* in humans. Waites and Talkington, 2005, recently reviewed the importance of *M. fermentans* in human diseases and provided more detail on the conditions described above as well as others [Waites et al., 2005].

The role of *M. fermentans* as a pathogen is unclear, it has been associated with the pathogenesis of rheumatoid arthritis [Williams et al., 1970]. However, the potential importance of *M. fermentans* in human diseases has recently been further demonstrated. Isolation of about 30 strains of *M. fermentans* from previously healthy non-AIDS patients who had a sudden onset of a severe and often fatal form of respiratory distress syndrome was recorded by R. Dular in Ottawa, Canada [unpublished, as cited by Hu et al., 1998]. Also they have reported the detection by PCR of *Mycoplasma fermentans* in the respiratory tract of children with pneumonia [Cassell et al., 1994b]. It has been demonstrated that a wild strain of *M. fermentans* isolated from the respiratory tract of an asthma patient was able to produce severe experimental respiratory disease in hamsters [Yáñez, 1997]. Román-Méndez et al., 2007, have showed that *Mycoplasma fermentans* persisted in the respiratory tract of hamsters during 120 days and all hamsters developed histological evidence of pulmonary inflammation. Lo et al., 1993, have reported the presence of infections due to *Mycoplasma fermentans* in patients with adult respiratory distress syndrome with or without systemic disease. *M. fermentans* can be detected in the upper and lower urogenital and respiratory tracts and bone marrow, and has been associated with a variety of systemic conditions in adults including inflammatory arthritis and pneumonia [Ainsworth et al., 2000a, 2001; Gilroy et al., 2001; Lo et al., 1989; Schaeverbeke et al.,1996; Taylor-Robinson, 1996; Tully, 1993; Waites & Talkington, 2005]

It has been recovered from the throats of 16% of children with community-acquired pneumonia, some of whom had no other etiologic agent identified, but the frequency of its occurrence in healthy children is not known. [Taylor-Robinson, 1996].

M. fermentans has also been detected in adults with an acute influenza-like illness who developed respiratory distress syndrome, and from bronchoalveolar lavage in AIDS patients with pneumonia, sometimes as the sole microbe, so it clearly has the potential to cause respiratory tract disease in susceptible hosts [Lo et al., 1993; Ainsworth et al., 2001]. This mycoplasma is also known to colonize mucosal surfaces in healthy persons, complicating efforts to understand its role in disease [Ainsworth et al., 2000b].

Mycoplasma fermentans, isolated decades ago from the urogenital tract, has been implicated in several disease conditions. Interest in this organism has recently increased because of its possible role in the pathogenesis of rheumatoid arthritis. Over the last decade, intensive studies have been carried out in order to understand the strategy employed by *M. fermentans* to interact with host cells and to avoid or subvert host protective measures [Rechnitzer et al., 2011].

Attention was focused on *M. fermentans* in the late 1980's because of reports that it may be important as a mediator or cofactor in the development of AIDS [Lo et al., 1989; Saillard et al., 1990]. The identification of mycoplasmal membrane components that participate in the adhesion of the parasite and the finding that some mycoplasmas can reside intracellularly [Rottem, 2003] open up new horizons in the study of the role of mycoplasma and host surface molecules in mycoplasma–host cell interactions [Rechnitzer et al., 2011].

Unlike *M. pneumoniae*, *M. fermentans* lacks a well-defined terminal attachment tip to mediate attachment and cell invasion. Since intracellular organisms are resistant to host defense mechanisms and to antibiotic treatment, this feature may account for the difficulty in eradicating mycoplasmas from cell cultures. A study by Yavlovich et al., 2001, demonstrated that *M. fermentans* binds plasminogen and converts it to plasmin, where upon mycoplasmal cell surface proteins are altered to promote its internalization. The role of plasminogen activation as a virulence factor and other aspects of *M. fermentans* pathogenesis, including the importance of membrane surface proteins that mediate cell fusion, cytadherence, and antigenic variation, are discussed by Rottem, 2003. The fusion of *M. fermentans* with eukaryotic host cells raises exciting questions on how microinjection of mycoplasmal components into eukaryotic cells affects host cells [Rottem, 2003].

The fusion process as well as the invasion of host cells by *M. fermentans* brings up an emerging theme in mycoplasma research, the subversion by *M. fermentans* of host cell functions mainly in signal-transduction pathways and cytoskeletal organization [As cited by Rechnitzer et al., 2011].

4.2.2 *Mycoplasma penetrans*, *Mycoplasma pirium* and Human Immunodeficiency Virus (HIV) disease

M. penetrans was first isolated from urine of homosexual men infected with (HIV), but not from healthy age-matched subjects. Subsequent studies suggested an association of this mycoplasma with Kaposi's sarcoma, but later findings did not confirm such association. This organism has been detected in HIV-negative persons, and despite its ability to invade epithelial cell, there is no conclusive evidence of any significant role in human disease [Yañez et al., 1999; Waites et al, 2005; Baseman & Tully, 1997].

Initial isolation of *M. pirum* from human peripheral blood lymphoid cells of HIV-positive patients, along with *M. penetrans* and *M. fermentans*, lead scientists to suggest a role as cofactor in acquire immunodeficiency syndrome (AIDS) progression. However, despite *M. pirum* was detected in rectal specimens of homosexual men and in urine of patients with AIDS, no conclusive evidence of its pathogenic role in human disease has been found. [Waites et al, 2005; Baseman & Tully, 1997]. Taking into account that *M. penetrans* and *M. pirum* have been associated with immune compromise, extragenital dissemination in infected patients, including respiratory disease, should be considered.

4.3 *Ureaplasma urealyticum* and *Ureaplasma parvum* in urogenital and respiratory tract infections

Although *U. urealyticum* and *U. parvum* are common commensals of the urogenital tract of humans, they are considered as important pathogens associated with infertility and nongonococcal urethritis in men, multiple obstetrical complications in women, and neonatal lung disease [Viscardi, 2010; Volgmann et al., 2005; Waites et al., 2005).

Genital ureaplasmas are natural residents of male urethra contaminating the semen during ejaculation. However, these microorganisms, particularly U. urealyticum, play and etiologic role in both genital infections and male infertility (Gdoura et al., 2008). Recent studies reveal that U. urealyticum strains are isolated more often in men with non-gonococcal urethritis than in healthy men (Deguchi et al., 2004; Maeda et al., 2004; Povlsen et al., 2002). Ureaplasmas are widespread among the male partners of infertile couples (Gdoura et al., 2007, 2008), and their presence is correlated with the alteration of some characteristics of semen, such as density, sperm motility, concentration, and probably morphology (Naessens et al., 1986; Reichart et al., 2000; Wang et al., 2006). The attachment to sperm and the induction of germ cell apoptosis have been proposed as mechanisms by which U. urealyticum affects sperm quality (Shang et al., 1999; Waites et al., 2005).

The infection of the female urinary tract with U. urealyticum is frequently overlooked. However, since a high isolation rate of this microorganism has been observed in urine and urethral samples from women with unexplained chronic urinary symptoms, treatment of the infection is now indicated (Baka et al., 2009; Potts et al., 2000).

Genital ureaplasmas can be found in vaginal flora in 40% of sexually inactive and 67% sexually active women (Viscardi, 2010). The infection is generally asymptomatic in nature, and is sexually transmitted between partners. Ureaplasmas can survive in the reproductive tract for many years, undetected, until the patient is specifically tested for the infection.

U. urealyticum is recovered from the lower genital tract of 70-80% of pregnant women (Carey et al., 1991; Volgmann, 2005), but vaginal carriage is not reliably predictive of preterm birth (Kafetzis et al., 2004; Povlsen et al., 2001). However, there is a consistent association when the infection is present in the amniotic fluid, chorioamnion or placenta (Eschenbach, 1993; Kundsin et al., 1996; Yoon et al., 2000, 2003). The secretion of phospholipases A and C has been suggested to be the means by which ureaplasmas may initiate preterm labor by liberating arachidonic acid and altering prostaglandin synthesis (De Silva & Quinn, 1986). In addition, recently we reported that the interaction between U. urealyticum, intrauterine leukocytes and fetal membranes results in the secretion of high amounts of IL-1b and prostaglandin E2, which could induce uterine contraction leading to preterm labor (Estrada et al., 2010). Isolation of U. urealyticum from chorioamnion has been consistently associated with histological chorioamnionitis and is inversely related to birth weight, even when adjusting for duration of labor, rupture of the fetal membranes, and the presence of other bacteria [Cassel et al., 1993; Waites et al., 2005].

There is accumulating epidemiologic and experimental evidence that intrauterine or postnatal infection with genital ureaplasmas is a significant risk factor for complications of extreme preterm birth such as bronchopulmonary dysplasia (BDP) and intraventricular hemorrhage [Kafetzis, et al., 2004; Viscardi, 2010]. Ureaplasma spp can be transmitted from an infected mother to the fetus or neonate by ascending intrauterine infection, hematogenous route involving umbilical vessels, or through passage of an infected maternal birth canal with resultant colonization of the skin, mucosal membranes or respiratory tract [Waites, 2005].

Among premature infants, respiratory tract colonization with genital ureaplasmas has been associated with pneumonia, chronic lung disease, infant wheezing, respiratory distress syndrome, acute respiratory insufficiency, and increased mortality [Cultrera et al., 2006;

Kafetzis et al., 2004]. For some infants, ureaplasmal infection triggers a vigorous response in the lungs involving the elevation of adhesion molecules, collagenases, proinflammatory cytokines and neutrophil activation and migration, which increase the risk of developing bronchopulmonary dysplasia characterized by delayed alveolarization, chronic inflammation, and fibrosis [Manimtim et al., 2001; Schelonka & Waites, 2007]. Additionally, free radical generation and oxidative injury induced by recruited neutrophils could contribute to lung damage [Buss et al., 2003]. Apoptosis of pneumocytes and pulmonary mesenchymal cells has been shown to occur as part of the pathogenesis of *U. urealyticum* [Li et al., 2002], while *U. parvum* lipoproteins activate NF-kB and induce TNF-α in macrophages, favoring the inflammatory response (Shimizu et al., 2008). Apparently, there is no trend in the prevalence of either species between infants with or without bronchopulmonary dysplasia [Katz et al., 2005].

5. Diagnostic procedures

Much of the mycoplasmal respiratory diseases, especially those caused by *M. pneumoniae*, are underdiagnosed because the laboratory diagnostic strategies are quite different than those for fast-growing bacteria. It is noteworthy that mycoplasmal etiology of respiratory diseases is considered only after failure of diagnosis of other common bacterial etiologies. In addition, there are few specialized or reference laboratories and skilled personnel [Cassell et al., 1994a; Waites et al., 2000].

5.1 Types of specimens, transport and collection
Detection or isolation of mycoplasmas in clinical specimens requires careful consideration of the type of specimen available and the organism (species) sought [Cassell et al., 1994a]. Specimens appropriate for laboratory diagnosis of respiratory mycoplasmal infections include: Bronchoalveolar lavage (BAL), sputum, pleural fluid, nasopharyngeal and throat swabs, endotracheal aspirates (ETA) and lung biopsies. Liquid specimens or tissues do not require special transport media if culture can be performed within 1 hour, otherwise specimens should be placed in transport media, such as SP-4 broth, 10B broth or 2SP broth. When swabbing is required, aluminum- or plastic-shafted calcium alginate or dacron swabs should be used, taking care to obtain as many cells as possible [Atkinson et al., 2008; Cassell et al., 1994a; Waites et al., 2002].
Other specimens such as blood, cerebrospinal fluid, pericardial fluid and synovial fluid must be considered when extrapulmonary disease is suspected, thus specimen collection should reflect the site of infection and/or the disease process. [Atkinson et al., 2008; Waites & Talkington, 2004].

5.2 Culture
Routine culture methods for isolation/detection of most mycoplasma species are time-consuming, thus emission of results may delay up to 5-6 weeks. Furthermore, there is no ideal formulation of culture media for all pathogenic species, mainly due to their different substrate and pH requirements [Waites et al., 2000]. Modified SP-4 media (broth and agar) [Lo et al., 1993], containing both glucose and arginine, can support the growth of all human pathogenic *Mycoplasma* species, including the fastidious *M. pneumoniae* and *M. genitalium*. A set of Shepard´s 10B broth and A8 agar can be used for cultivation of *Ureaplasma* species and *M. hominis*.

For cultivation, specimens in transport media should be thoroughly mixed, and then should be 10-fold serially diluted in broth (usually up to 10^{-6}) in order to overcome potential inhibitory substances, and to allow semiquantitative estimation of mycoplasmal load. Subcultures in agar media should be also performed. [Cassell et al., 1994a]. All inoculated media are incubated under microaerophilic atmosphere at 37°C.

Detection of *M. pneumoniae* in broth culture is based on its ability to ferment glucose, causing an acidic shift after 4 or more days, readily visualized by the presence of the phenol red pH indicator. Broths with any color change, and subsequent blind broth passages, should be subcultured to SP4 agar, incubated, and examined under the low-power objective of the light microscope in order to look for development of typical "fried egg"-like colonies of up to 100 μm in diameter (Figure 2). Examination of agar plates must be done on a daily basis during the first week, and thereafter every 3 to 4 days until completing 5 weeks or until growth is observed [Waites et al., 2000, 2004]. *M. genitalium, M. fermentans* and *M. penetrans* are also glucose-fermenting and formed colonies morphologically indistinguishable from those of *M. pneumoniae*, thus serologic-based definitive identification can be done by growth inhibition, metabolic inhibition, and mycoplamacidal tests [Cassel et al., 1993].

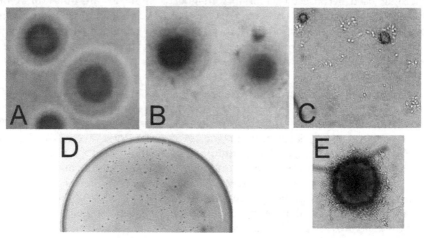

A) Typical "Fried-egg" appearance of *Mycoplasma* spp. colonies on SP-4 agar. B) Dienes-stained mycoplasma colonies. C) Tiny brown-colored ureaplasmal colonies on modified SP-4 agar. D) Macroscopic view of Dienes-stained mycoplasma colonies growth on SP-4 agar in 30 mm-diameter Petri dishes. E) Closer view of an ureaplasma colony.

Fig. 2. Morphology of mycoplasma colonies in culture.

Hidrolysis of urea by Ureaplasma and hidrolysis of arginine by *M. hominis* cause an alkaline shift, turning the colour of 10B broth from yellow to pink. Tiny brown or black irregular colonies of *Ureaplasma* species develop between 1 -5 days on A8 agar plates, due to urease production in the presence of manganese sulfate (Figure 2). Typical fried egg colonies are produced by *M. hominis* in this medium [Cassell et al., 1994a, Waites et al., 2000].

5.3 Immunodiagnosis by serological tests
As culture of *M. pneumoniae* is slow and insensitive, the laboratory diagnosis of *M. pneumoniae* infection has largely relied on serological testing. Seroconversion or rising

specific antibody titers are observed among *M. pneumoniae*-infected patients. This immunologic response can be measured by several tests, including: metabolic inhibition assay, complement fixation or enzyme-linked immunoassays (EIA). Serum samples are easy to collect and handle, but it is required paired acute- and convalescent-phase specimens. Commercial assay formats include indirect immunofluorescence, particle agglutination assay, and EIA [Atkinson et al., 2008, Cassell et al., 1994a; Waites & Talkington, 2004].

Prior to the widespread availability of commercialized antibody assays, presence of cold agglutinins (IgM antibodies that are produced 1 to 2 weeks after initial infection in about half of *M. pneumoniae*-infected subjects) was used to confirm primary atypical pneumonia (Waites & Talkington, 2004). Although there have been recent improvements, the sensitivity and specificity of antibody detection is still suboptimal. Nevertheless, the complex and time-consuming nature of many of the serological assays that have been used in the past have limited acceptance of serology for routine diagnostic testing. [Cassell et al., 1994a; Waites et al., 2000].

At present, besides research laboratories, no serologic tests assays for mycoplasmas other than *M. pneumoniae* have been standardized for diagnostic purposes in routine clinical microbiology laboratories nor made commercially available elsewhere. [Cassell et al., 1994a, Waites et al., 2005].

5.4 PCR and other molecular tests

Nucleic acid amplification techniques (NAATs) are more sensitive, and considerably more rapid than culture, showing a fair to good correlation with serology. PCR testing for species-specific mycoplasmal infection are suitable for both upper and lower respiratory samples. Interestingly, sample processing prior amplification must be optimized depending of the type of specimen to overcome the presence of PCR inhibitors (i.e., nasopharyngeal samples have higher rate of PCR inhibition than throat swabs). Differential sample preparation from the same specimen has been done when testing separate single-species PCRs on BAL [De Barbeyrac et al., 1993]. A culture-enhanced PCR approach has also been suggested to overcome the effect of inhibitors in the amplification process [Abele-Horne et al., 1998].

In early 2000s, Loens et al.(2003) stated that the development and application of new nucleic acid amplification techniques (NAATs) in diagnostic mycoplasmology required proper validation and standardization, and performance of different NAATs must be compared with each other in order to define the most sensitive and specific tests. The NAATs have demonstrated their potential to produce rapid, sensitive and specific results, and are now considered the methods of choice for direct detection of *M. pneumoniae, M. genitalium,* and *M. fermentans* [Cassell et al., 1994a]. There is a great variation in methods used from study to study, including variability of target gene sequences (P1, 16S RNA, ATPase, *tuf*), assay format (single, multiplex) or technologies (Real-time PCR, NASBA) [Loens et al., 2003a, 2010]. Also, different specimens have been used, such as sputum, nasopharyngeal or pharyngeal swabs, brochoalveolar lavages or pleural fluid, and then it is difficult to compare these data. A comprehensive review about the use of NAATs for the detection of *M. pneumoniae* in clinical samples was done by Loens et al., 2003b, 2010, and by Ieven, 2010. Table 3, shows a selection of primers sets developed in the 1990s for testing diverse clinical samples.

Organism	Primer sets		Sequence (5'→3')	Target	Amplicon size (bp)	Ref.
Mollicutes-specific	FW: RV:	GPO-1 MGSO	ACT CCT ACG GGA GGC AGC AGT A TGC ACC ATC TGT CAC TCT GTT AAC CTC	rDNA 16S	715	Van Kuppeveld et al., 1992
M. fermentans	FW: RV: IP:	RW005 RW004 RW006	GGT TAT TCG ATT TCT AAA TCG CCT GGA CTA TTG TCT AAA CAA TTT CCC GCT GTG GCC ATT CTC TTC TAC GTT	IS-like element	206	Wang et al., 1992
	FW: RV: IP:	Mf-1 Mf-2 GPO-1	GAA GCC TTT CTT CGC TGG AG ACA AAA TCA TTT CCT ATT CTG TC ACT CCT ACG GGA GGC AGC AGT A	rDNA 16s	272	Van Kuppeveld et al., 1992
M. genitalium	FW: RV: IP:	MGS-1 MGS-2 MGS-I	GAG CCT TTC TAA CCG CTG C GTG GGG TTG AAG GAT GAT TG AAG CAA CGT AGT AGC GTG AGC	MgPa adhesion gene	673	De Barbeyrac et al., 1993
	FW: RV: IP:	MGS-1 MGS-4 MGS-I	GAG CCT TTC TAA CCG CTG C GTT GTT ATC ATA CCT TCT GAT AAG CAA CGT AGT AGC GTG AGC	MgPa adhesion gene	371	De Barbeyrac et al., 1993
M. hominis	FW: RV: IP:	MYCHOMP MYCHOMN MYCHOMS	ATA CAT GCA TGT CGA GCG AG CAT CTT TTA GTG GCG CCT TAC CGC ATG GTG GAA CCG CAT GGT TCC GTT G	rDNA 16s	170	Grau et al., 1994
	FW: RV: IP:	Mh-1 Mh-2 GPO-1	TGA AAG GCG CTG TAA GGC GC GTC TGC AAT CAT TTC CTA TTG CAA A ACT CCT ACG GGA GGC AGC AGT A	rDNA 16s	281b	Van Kuppeveld et al., 1992
M. penetrans	FW: RV: IP:	MYCPENETP MYCPENETN MYCPENETS	CAT GCA AGT CGG ACG AAG CA AGC ATT TCC TCT TCT TAC AA CAT GAG AAA ATG TTT AAA GTC TGT TTG	rDNA 16s	407	Grau et al., 1994
M. pneumoniae	FW: RV: IP:	MP5-1 MP5-2 MP5-4	GAA GCT TAT GGT ACA GGT TGG ATT ACC ATC CTT GTT GTA AGG CGT AAG CTA TCA GCT ACA TGG AGG	Unknown gene	144	Bernet et al., 1989
	FW: RV: IP:	MP-P11 MP-P12 MP-I	TGC CAT CAA CCC GCG CTT AAC CCT TTG CAA CTG CTC ATA GTA CAA ACC GGG CAG ATC ACC TTT	P1 adhesin gene	466	De Barbeyrac et al., 1993
Ureaplasma spp.	FW: RV: IP:	U5 U4 U9	CAA TCT GCT CGT GAA GTA TTA C ACG ACG TCC ATA AGC AAC T GAG ATA ATG ATT ATA TGT CAG GAT CA	Urease genes	429	Blanchard et al., 1993
	FW: RV: IP:	Uu-1 Uu-2 UUSO	TAA ATG TCG GCT CGA ACG AG GCA GTA TCG CTA GAA AAG CAA C CAT CTA TTG CGA CGC TA	rDNA 16s	311	Van Kuppeveld et al., 1992
U. parvum U. urealyticum	FW: RV:	UMS-125 UMA-226-	GTA TTT GCA ATC TTT ATA TGT TTT CG CAG CTG ATG TAA GTG CAG CAT TAA ATT C	MBA gene	402,403 (Up) 443 (Uu)	Kong et al., 1999

bp, Base pairs; FW, Forward; RV, Reverse; IP, Internal probe.

Table 3. Selected primer sets used for detection of mycoplasmas in clinical specimens

6. Treatment and prevention

Due to absence of the cell wall envelope, mycoplasmas are insensitive to β-lactam antibiotics. However, antibiotics targeting protein synthesis or DNA modification molecules are highly effective against these bacteria. Macrolides, tetracyclines and fluoroquinolones eliminate mycoplasmas efficiently both *in vivo* and *in vitro* [Cassell et al., 1994a; Waites et al., 2000, 2008].

Mycoplasmal infections in the upper respiratory tract are usually self-limiting, so antibiotic treatment is not generally recommended, even though some clinicians recommend it to prevent the risk of recurrence of respiratory illness [Waites & Talkington, 2004]

The antimicrobial of choice for treating lower respiratory tract *M. pneumoniae* infections are the macrolides in both adults and children. Patients receiving macrolides of recent generation showed improved tolerance, require fewer doses and have shorter treatment duration than older compounds. However, empirical antimicrobial treatment for *M. pneumoniae*-infected ambulatory patients is more practical; hence if hospitalization is required and/or patient has underlying risk factor, antimicrobial susceptibility testing is recommended. Use of tetracycline and fluoroquinolones is restricted to treat adult patients and should not be used in children aged <8 years [Cassell et al., 1994a; Waites et al., 2000]. A potential problem in the antimicrobial management of *M. pneumoniae* infections is the emergence of macrolide resistance [Atkinson et al., 2008; Waites et al., 2008].

The recovery of *Ureaplasma spp* and/or *M. hominis* in pure or mixed cultures from clinical specimens of symptomatic patients, in absence of associated biota, should be considered sufficient to initiate antimicrobial therapy. These microorganisms are resistant to sulfonamides and trimethoprim, and often exhibit resistance to aminoglycosides and chloramphenicol. *Ureaplasma spp* is resistant to clindamycin and susceptible to erythromycin, whereas *M. hominis* shows the opposite susceptibility profile. While tetracyclines are the antibiotics of choice for treating ureaplasmal infections in adults, erythromycin therapy is recommended for neonates. In contrast, *M. hominis* infections other than central nervous system in children under 8 years of age can be treated with clindamycin [Cassell et al., 1994a; Waites et al., 2000, 2005].

Since strains from several mycoplasma species rapidly acquire resistance to antimicrobials, prevention of mycoplasmal infections via chemoprophylaxis is not recommended [Razin et al, 1998].

6.1 Mycoplasmal susceptibility testing

As antibiotic-resistant strains of mycoplasmas have appeared and become more common, antibiotic susceptibility testing for these microorganisms has become important. [Roberts, M.C., 1992]. However there are no official guidelines for performance, interpretation, or quality control of *in vitro* susceptibility tests for human mycoplasmas [Waites & Talkington, 2004].

The broth dilution method is the most widely used. Prior to test, pure cultures should be passage in appropriate broth and the color-changing units (CCU) or colony-forming units (CFU) quantitative method. For the assay, bacterial cultures should be adjusted to 1000 – 10000 CCU in 0.2 mL, followed by a 2-hour incubation at 37°C, to begin active growth. The broth microdilution assay involves the addition of 100-µL aliquots of adjusted cultures to wells 2 – 12, then 100 µL of broth containing the highest concentration of the antibiotics is added to wells 1 and 2, followed by 2-fold serial dilutions up to well 12 (concentration range 256-0.008 µg/mL). Positive and negative controls should be included. The initial minimal inhibitory concentration (MIC) is defined as the lowest dilution of antibiotic in which metabolism of the organism is inhibited, as evidenced by lack of color change in the media at the time the control organism well first shows color change. Presumptive MICs for ureaplasmas will be available at 16 to 24 h and those for *M. hominis* will be at 36 to 48 h but *M. pneumoniae* may require 5 days or more until evidence of grow in the control wells is evident [Cassell et al., 1994a; Waites et al., 2000].

There are commercial kits for mycoplasma susceptibility testing such as: Mycoplasma IST, Mycoplasma SIR, Mycofast "All In", and MYCOKIT ATB, although they are available only in Europe.

Reports of macrolide resistance in *M. pneumoniae* strains have been published since the past decade. These resistant strains were shown to possess gene mutations in the 23S rRNA. The impact of macrolide resistance on the clinical course of infections is still unclear, but PCR assays have been developed to detect some of these mutations in order to identify these resistant strains [Atkinson et al., 2008].

Tetracycline resistance among *Ureaplasma spp* and *M. hominis* isolates can be distinguished by broth- or agar-based methods since the resistant strains consistently have MICs of ≥ 8 µg/mL whereas susceptible strains have MICs of ≤ 2 µg/mL, with no overlapping between the two populations [Waites et al., 2000; Cassell et al., 1994a]. Tetracycline resistance among *M. hominis* and *Ureaplasma spp.* isolates has been associated with the presence of Tet M determinant which codes for production of a ribosome-binding protein that prevents tetracycline binding to ribosomes [Roberts, M.C., 2002].

6.2 Vaccines

The initial vaccine candidate for *M. pneumoniae* was formalin-inactivated bacteria, but their protective efficacy results were generally disappointing, since some immunized volunteers developed more severe illness after experimental challenge with live mycoplasmas. Development of live attenuated vaccines never made it to human use due to concern over residual virulence of the vaccine strain of *M. pneumoniae* [Waites et al., 2008]. Other vaccine candidates have included acellular protein and polysaccharide components and recombinant DNA. While the importance of the P1 adhesin in mediating *M. pneumoniae* cytadherence and initiation of disease cannot be denied, animal studies using P1 as a vaccine antigen have not demonstrated protective efficacy [Razin et al., 1998; Waites & Talkington, 2004].

As higher rates of surface antigenic variation among several human mycoplasmas have been described, whenever promising antigens are selected as vaccine candidates they are rapidly discarded. The three types of antigenic variation are: 1) Phase variation, a feature involving selective turning on/off of gene transcription; 2) Size variation as a result of variation in the number of tandem repeats near the 5' end; and 3) Differential masking of surface antigens by the lipid moiety of lipoproteins [Chambaud et al., 1999; Momynaliev & Govorun, 2001].

The availability of the full genome sequences of several human mycoplasmas, will allow better understanding of the structure and functionality of these bacteria, including virulence factors and immunogenic molecules.

7. Concluding remarks

It is undeniable the ability of *Mycoplasma pneumoniae* and *Ureaplasma* spp. to cause pneumonia. Other mycoplasma species are potential respiratory pathogens, especially in conjunction with immune compromise. There is strong evidence that mycoplasmal respiratory infections elicit inflammatory responses that can result chronic lung injury both in adults and neonates. Improvement of laboratory methods for research and diagnostic purposes in mycoplasmology has allowed establishing associations with pulmonary diseases such as COPD, asthma, and BPD. However additional work must be done for prevention, treatment strategies and vaccine development.

8. Acknowledgements

This work was supported by grants from:
Research Fellow System of SNI-CONACYT (SGC, GEG, JART, FJDG); EDI-COFAA grant by SEP-IPN, ICYT-DF (SGC); PRIDE C grant by DGAPA-UNAM (FJDG).

Corresponding author: Dra. Silvia Giono-Cerezo. Laboratorio de Bacteriología Médica, Departamento de Microbiología, ENCB-IPN. Carpio y Plan de Ayala S/N, Col. Casco de Sto. Tomás, C.P. 11340, México D.F.México. Phone: +52(55)57296300 ext. 62374.
Email: sgiono@yahoo.com

9. References

Abele-Horn, M., Busch, U., Nitschko, H., Jacobs, E., Bax, R., Pfaff, F., Schaffer, B., & Heesemann, J. (1998). Molecular Approaches to Diagnosis of Pulmonary Diseases Due to *Mycoplasma pneumoniae*. *Journal of Clinical Microbiology*, Vol. 36, No. 2 (February 1998), pp. 548–551, ISSN 0095-1137

Ainsworth, J.G., Clarke, J., Goldin, R., & Taylor-Robinson, D. (2000a). Disseminated *Mycoplasma fermentans* in AIDS Patients: Several Case Reports. *International Journal of STD & AIDS*, Vol. 11, No. 11 (November 2000), pp. 751-755, ISSN 0956-4624

Ainsworth, J.G., Hourshid, S., Webster, A.D., Gilroy, C.B., & Taylor-Robinson, D. (2000b). Detection of *Mycoplasma fermentans* in Healthy Students and Patients with Congenital Immunodeficiency. *Journal of Infection*, Vol. 40, No. 2 (March 2000), pp. 138-140, ISSN 0163-4453

Ainsworth, J.G., Easterbrook, P.J., Clarke, J., Gilroy, C.B., & Taylor-Robinson, D. (2001). An Association of Disseminated *Mycoplasma fermentans* in HIV-1 Positive Patients with Non-Hodgkin's Lymphoma. *International Journal of STD & AIDS*, Vol. 12, No. 8 (August 2001), pp. 499-504, ISSN 0956-4624

Al-Moyed, K.A., & Al-Shamahy, H.A. (2003). *Mycoplasma pneumoniae* Infection in Yemen: Incidence, Presentation and Antibiotic Susceptibility. *Eastern Mediterranean Health Journal*, Vol. 9, No. 3 (May 2003), pp. 279-290, ISSN 1020-3397

Andreev, J., Borovsky, Z., Rosenshine, I., & Rottem, S. (1995). Invasion of HeLa Cells by *Mycoplasma penetrans* and the Induction of Tyrosine Phosphorylation of a 145 kDa Host Cell Protein. *FEMS Microbiology Letters*, Vol. 132, No. 3 (October 1995), pp. 189-194. ISSN 0378-1097

Atkinson, T.P., Balish, M.F., & Waites, K.B. (2008). Epidemiology, Clinical Manifestations, Pathogenesis and Laboratory Detection of *Mycoplasma pneumoniae* Infections. *FEMS Microbiology Reviews*, Vol. 32 No. 6 (November 2008), pp. 956–973, ISSN 0168-6445

Baka, S., Kouskouni, E., Antonopoulou, S., Sioutis, D., Papakonstantinou, M., Hassiakos, D., Logothetis, E., & Liapis, A. (2009). Prevalence of *Ureaplasma urealyticum* and *Mycoplasma hominis* in Women with Chronic Urinary Symptoms. *Urology*, Vol.74. No.1 (July 2009), pp. 62-66, ISSN: 0090-4295.

Baseman, J.B., Lange, M., Criscimagna, N.L., Giron, J.A., & Thomas, C.A. (1995). Interplay Between *Mycoplasmas* and Host Target Cells. *Microbial Pathogenesis, Vol. 19*, No. 2 (August 1995), pp. 105-116, ISSN 0882-4010

Baseman, J.B., & Tully, J.G. (1997). *Mycoplasmas*: Sophisticated Reemerging and Burdened by Their Notoriety. *Emerging Infectious Diseases*, Vol. 3, No. 1 (January-March 1997), pp. 21-32, ISSN 1080-6040

Bernet, C., Garret, M., de Barbeyrac, B., Bebear, C., & Bonnet, J. (1989). Detection of *Mycoplasma pneumoniae* by Using Polymerase Chain Reaction. *Journal of Clinical Microbiology*, Vol. 27, No. (1989), pp. 2492-2496, ISSN 0095-1137

Blasi, F. (2004). Atypical Pathogens and Respiratory Tract Infections. *European Respiratory Journal*, Vol. 24, No. 1 (July 2004), pp. 171–181, ISSN 0903-1936

Bové, J.M. (1993). Molecular features of *Mollicutes*. *Clinical Infectious Diseases*, Vol. 17, Supplement 1 (August 1993), pp. S10-S31, ISSN 1058-4838

Brown, D.R., Whitcomb, R.F., & Bradbury, J.M. (2007). Revised Minimal Standards for Description of New Species of the Class *Mollicutes* (Division Tenericutes). *International Journal of Systematic and Evolutionary Microbiology*, Vol. 57, No. 11 (November 2007), pp. 2703–2719. ISSN 1466-5026

Buscho, R.O., Saxtan, D., Shultz, P.S., Finch, E., & Mufson, M.A. (1978). Infections with Viruses and *Mycoplasma pneumoniae* During Exacerbations of Chronic Bronchitis. *Journal of Infectious Diseases*, Vol. 137, No. 4 (April 1978), pp. 377–383, ISSN 0022-1899

Buss, I.H., Senthilmohan, R., Darlow, B.A., Mogridge, N., Kettle, A.J., & Winterbourn, C.C. (2003). 3-Chlorotyrosine as a Marker of Protein Damage by Myeloperoxidase in Tracheal Aspirates from Preterm Infants: Association with Adverse Respiratory Outcome. *Pediatric Research*, Vol. 53, No. 3 (March 2003), pp. 455-462. ISSN: 0031-3998

Caberlotto, O.J., Cadario, M.E., Garay, J.E., Copacastro, C.A., Cabot, A., & Savy, V.L. (2003). Community-Acquired Pneumonia in Patients in 2 Hospital Populations. *Medicina (B Aires)* Vol. 63, No. 1 (January-February 2003), pp. 1-8, ISSN 0025-7680

Carey, J.C., Blackwelder, W.C., Nugent, R.P., Matteson, M.A., Rao, A.V., Eschenbach, D.A., Lee, M.L., Rettig, P.J., Regan, J.A., & Geromanos, K.L. (1991). Antepartum Cultures for *Ureaplasma urealyticum* are not Useful in Predicting Pregnancy Outcome. The Vaginal Infections and Prematurity Study Group. *American Journal of Obstetrics and Gynecology*, Vol. 164, No. 3 (March 1991), pp.728-733. ISSN: 0002-9378.

Cartner, S.C., Lindsey, J. R., Gibbs-Erwin, J., Cassell, G.H., & Simecka. J.W. (1998). Roles of Innate and Adaptive Immunity in Respiratory Mycoplasmosis. *Infection and Immunity*, Vol. 66, No. 8 (August1998), pp. 3485–3491, ISSN 0019-9567

Cassell, G.H.; Waites, K.B.; Watson, H.L.; Crouse, D.T. & Harasawa, R. (1993). *Ureaplasma urealyticum* Intrauterine Infection: Role in Prematurity and Disease in Newborns. *Clinical Microbiology Reviews*, Vol.6. No.1. (January-March 1993), pp.69-87, ISSN 0893-8512.

Cassell, G.H., Blanchard, A., Duffy, L., Crabb, D., & Waites, K.B. (1994a). *Mycoplasmas*, In: *Clinical and Pathogenic Microbiology*, B.J. Howard, J.F. Keiser, A.S. Weissfeld, T.F. Smith, & R.C. Tilton (Eds), pp. 491-502, Mosby, ISBN 978-0801664267, Boston, USA.

Cassell, G.H., Yáñez, A., Duffy, L. B., Moyer, J., Cedillo, L., Hammerschlag, M.R., Rank, R.G., & Glass, J.I. (1994b). Detection of *Mycoplasma fermentans* in the Respiratory Tract of Children with Pneumonia. 10th International Congress of the International Organization for Mycoplasmology (IOM), Bordeaux, France, July 1994. In *IOM Letters* Vol. 3, p. 456, ISSN 1023-1226

Chambaud, I., Wróblewski, H., & Blanchard, A. (1999). Interactions Between Mycoplasma Lipoproteins and the Host Immune System. *Trends in Microbiology*, Vol. 7, No. 12 (December 1999), pp. 493-499, ISSN 0966-842X

Chu, H.W., Honour, J.M., Rawlinson, C.A., et al. (2003). Effects of Respiratory *Mycoplasma pneumoniae* Infection On Allergen-Induced Bronchial Hyperresponsiveness and Lung Inflammation in Mice. *Infection and Immunity*, 2003; Vol. 71, No 3 (March 2003), pp. 1520-1526, ISSN 0019-9567

Chu H.W., Jeyaseelan S., Rino J.G., Voelker D.R., Wexler R.B., Campbell K., Harbeck R.J., & Martin, R.J. (2005a). TLR2 Signaling Is Critical for *Mycoplasma pneumoniae*-Induced Airway Mucin Expression. *Journal of Immunology*, Vol. 174, No. 9 (May 2005), pp. 5713–5719, ISSN 0022-1767

Chu, H. W., Rino, J. G., Wexler, R.B., Campbell, K., Harbeck, R. J., & Martin, R. J. (2005b) *Mycoplasma pneumoniae* Infection Increases Airway Collagen Deposition in a Murine Model of Allergic Airway Inflammation. *American Journal of Physiology, Lung Cellular and Molecular Physiology*, Vol. 289, No. 1 (July 2005), pp. L125-L133, ISSN 1040-0605

Cultrera, R., Seraceni, S., Germani, R., & Contini, C. (2006). Molecular Evidence of *Ureaplasma urealyticum* and *Ureaplasma parvum* Colonization in Preterm Infants During Respiratory Distress Syndrome. *BMC Infectious Diseases*, Vol.21. No. 6 (November 2006), pp. 166, ISSN 1471-2334

Dakhama, A., Kraft, M.,Martin, R.J., & Gelfand, E.W. (2003). Induction of Regulated Upon Activation, Normal T cells Expressed and Secreted (RANTES) and Transforming Growth Factor-Beta 1 in Airway Epithelial Cells by *Mycoplasma pneumoniae*. *American Journal of Respiratory Cellular and Molecular Biology*, Vol. 29, No. 3 (September 2003), pp. 344-351, ISSN 1044-1549

De Barbeyrac, B., Bernet-Poggi, C., Febrer, F., Renaudin, H., Dupon, M., & Bebear, C. (1993). Detection of *Mycoplasma pneumoniae* and *Mycoplasma genitalium* in Clinical Samples by Polymerase Chain Reaction. *Clinical Infectious Diseases*, Vol. 17, Suppl 1 (August 1993), S83-S89, ISSN 1058-4838

De Silva, N.S., & Quinn, P.A. (1986). Endogenous Activity of Phospholipases A and C in *Ureaplasma urealyticum*. *Journal of Clinical Microbiology*. Vol. 23, No. 2 (February 1986), pp. 354-359, ISSN 0095-1137

Deguchi, T., Yoshida, T., Miyazawa, T., Yasuda, M., Tamaki, M., Ishiko, H., & Maeda, S. (2004). Association of *Ureaplasma urealyticum* (Biovar 2) with Nongonococcal Urethritis. *Sexually Transmitted Diseases*, Vol.31. No.3 (March 2004), pp. 192-195. ISSN 0148-5717.

Díaz-García, F.J., Herrera-Mendoza, A.P., Giono-Cerezo, S., & Guerra-Infante, F. (2006). *Mycoplasma hominis* Attaches to and Locates Intracellularly On Human Spermatozoa. *Human Reproduction*, Vol. 21, No. 6 (June 2006), pp. 1591-1598, ISSN 0268-1161

Dorigo-Zetsma, J.W., Verkooyen, R.P., van Helden, H.P., van der Nat, H., & van den Bosch, J.M. (2001). Molecular Detection of *Mycoplasma pneumoniae* in Adults with Community-Acquired Pneumonia Requiring Hospitalization. *Journal of Clinical Microbiology*, Vol. 39, No. 3 (March 2001), pp. 1184-1186, ISSN: 0095-1137

Eschenbach, D.A. (1993). *Ureaplasma urealyticum* and Premature Birth. *Clinical Infectious Diseases*. Vol. 17 Suppl. 1 (August 1993), pp. S100-S106, ISSN 1058-4838

Estrada-Gutierrez, G., Gomez-Lopez, N., Zaga-Clavellina, V., Giono-Cerezo, S., Espejel-Nuñez A., Gonzalez-Jimenez, M.A., Espino y Sosa, S., Olson, D.M., & Vadillo-Ortega, F. (2010). Interaction Between Pathogenic Bacteria and Intrauterine

Leukocytes Triggers Alternative Molecular Signaling Cascades Leading to Labor in Women. *Infection and Immunity,*.Vol.78. No.11. pp.4792-4799. ISSN: 0019-9567.

Gdoura, R., Kchaou, W., Chaari, C., Znazen, A., Keskes, L., Rebai, T., & Hammami, A. (2007). *Ureaplasma urealyticum, Ureaplasma parvum, Mycoplasma hominis* and *Mycoplasma genitalium* Infections and Semen Quality of Infertile Men. *BMC Infectious Diseases.* Vol.7. pp.129. ISSN 1471-2334.

Gdoura, R., Kchaou, W., Ammar-Keskes, L., Chakroun, N., Sellemi, A., Znazen, A., Rebai, T., & Hammami, A. (2008). Assessment of *Chlamydia trachomatis, Ureaplasma urealyticum, Ureaplasma parvum, Mycoplasma hominis,* and *Mycoplasma genitalium* in Semen and First Void Urine Specimens of Asymptomatic Male Partners of Infertile Couples. *Journal of Andrology.* Vol.29. No.2. pp. 198-206. ISSN:0196-3635.

Gilroy, C. B., Keat, A., & Taylor-Robinson, D. (2001). The Prevalence of *Mycoplasma fermentans* in Patients with Inflammatory Arthritides. *Rheumatology (Oxford),* Vol. 40, No. 12 (December 2001), pp. 1355-1358, ISSN 1462-0324

Girón, J.A., Lange, M., & Baseman, J. B. (1996). Adherence, Fibronectin Binding, and Induction of Cytoskeleton Reorganization in Cultured Human Cells by *Mycoplasma penetrans. Infection and Immunity,* Vol. 64, No. 1 (January 1996), pp. 197-208, ISSN 0019-9567

Guilbert T.W., & Denlinger, L.C. (2010). Role of Infection in the Development and Exacerbation of Asthma. *Expert Reviews in Respiratory Medicine,* Vol. 4, No. 1 (February 2010), pp. 71–83, ISSN 1747-6348

Gump, D.W., Phillips, C.A., Forsyth, B.R., McIntosh, K., Lamborn, K.R., & Stouch, W.H. (1976). Role of Infection in Chronic Bronchitis. *American Review of Respiratory Disease,* Vol. 113, (April 1976), pp. 465–474, ISSN 0003-0805

Hu, W.S., Hayes, M.M., Wang, R.Y., Shih, J.W., & Lo, S-H. (1998) High-Frequency DNA Rearrangements in the Chromosomes of Clinically Isolated *Mycoplasma fermentans. Current Microbiology,* Vol. 37, No. 1 (July1998), pp. 1–5, ISSN 0343-8651

Ieven, M. (2007). Currently Used Nucleic Acid Amplification Tests for the Detection of Viruses and Atypicals in Acute Respiratory Infections. *Journal of Clinical Virology,* Vol. 40, No. 4 (December 2007), pp. 259-276, ISSN 1386-6532

International Committee on Systematics of Prokaryotes- Subcommittee on the taxonomy of Mollicutes (ICSP-STM). (2011). *International Journal of Systematic and Evolutionary Microbiology,* Vol. 61, No. 3 (March 2011), pp. 695–697, ISSN 1466-5026.

Jensen, J.S., Blom, J., & Lind, K. (1994). Intracellular Location of *Mycoplasma genitalium* in Cultured Vero Cells as Demonstrated by Electron Microscopy. *International Journal of Experimental Pathology, Vol. 75,* No. 2 (April 1994), pp. 91-98, ISSN ISSN 0959-9673

Johansson K. E., Heldtander, M. U. K., & Petterson, B. Characterization of Mycoplasmas by PCR and Sequence Analysis with Universal 16S rDNA Primers, p. 145-165. In: Miles R & Nicholas R, *Mycoplasma protocols.* Humana Press.1998. ISBN 0-89603-525-5, Totowa, NJ, USA.

Kafetzis, D.A.; Skevaki, C.L.; Skouteri, V.; Gavrili, S.; Peppa, K.; Kostalos, C.; Petrochilou, V. & Michalas, S. (2004). Maternal Genital Colonization with *Ureaplasma urealyticum* Promotes Preterm Delivery: Association of the Respiratory Colonization of Premature Infants with Chronic Lung Disease and Increased Mortality. *Clinical Infectious Diseases.* Vol.39. No.8. pp.1113-1122. ISSN: 1058-4838.

Kannan, T.R., & Baseman, J.B. (2006). ADP-Ribosylating and Vacuolating Cytotoxin of *Mycoplasma pneumoniae* Represents Unique Virulence Determinant Among Bacterial Pathogens. *Proceedings of the National Academy of Sciences of U.S.A.*, Vol. 103, No. 17 (April 2006), pp.6724-6729. ISSN 0027-8424

Kannan, T.R., Provenzano, D., Wright, J.R., & Baseman, J.B. (2005). Identification and Characterization of Human Surfactant Protein A Binding Protein of *Mycoplasma pneumoniae*. *Infection and Immunity*, Vol. 73, No. 5 (May 2005), pp. 2828-2834, ISSN 0019-9567

Katz, B.; Patel, P.; Duffy, L.; Schelonka, R.L.; Dimmitt, R.A. & Waites, K.B. (2005). Characterization of Ureaplasmas Isolated from Preterm Infants with and without Bronchopulmonary Dysplasia. *Journal of Clinical Microbiology*. Vol.43. No.9. pp.4852-4854. ISSN: 0095-1137.

Kazachkov, M.Y.; Hu, P.C.; Carson, J.L.; Murphy, P.C.; Henderson, F.W., & Noah, T.L. (2002). Release of Cytokines by Human Nasal Epithelial Cells and Peripheral Blood Mononuclear Cells Infected with *Mycoplasma pneumoniae*. *Experimental biology and medicine (Maywood)*, Vol. 227, No. 5 (May 2002), pp. 330-335, ISSN: 1525-1373

Krivan, H. C., Roberts, D. D., & Ginsburg, V. (1988) Many Pulmonary Pathogenic Bacteria Bind Specifically to the Carbohydrate Sequence GalNAc Beta 1-4Gal Found in Some Glycolipids. *Proceedings of the National Academy of Sciences of U.S.A.*, Vol. 85, No. 16 (August 1988), pp. 6157-6161, ISSN 0027-8424

Krivan, H.C.; Olson, LD; Barile, MF, Ginsberg, V & Roberts, D (1989). Adhesion of *Mycoplasma pneumoniae* to Sulfated Glycolipids and Inhibition by Dextran Sulfate. *Journal of Biological Chemistry*, Vol. 264, No. pp. 9283-9288, ISSN 0021-9258

Krunkosky, T.M.; Jordan, J.L.; Chambers, E., & Krause, D.C. (2007). *Mycoplasma pneumoniae* Host-Pathogen Studies in an Air-Liquid Culture of Differentiated Human Airway Epithelial Cells. *Microbial Pathogenesis*, Vol. 42, No. 2-3 (February-March 2007), pp. 98-103, ISSN 0882-4010

Kundsin, R.B., Leviton, A., Allred, E.N., & Poulin, S.A. (1996). *Ureaplasma urealyticum* Infection of the Placenta in Pregnancies that Ended Prematurely. *Obstetrics and Gynecology*, Vol. 87, No. 1 (January 1996), pp.122-127, ISSN: 0029-7844.

Li, Y.H.; Brauner, A.; Jensen, J.S. & Tullus, K. (2002). Induction of Human Macrophage Vascular Endothelial Growth Factor and Intercellular Adhesion Molecule-1 by *Ureaplasma urealyticum* and Downregulation by Steroids. *Biol Neonate*. Vol.82. No.1. pp.22-28. ISSN: 0006-3126

Li, Y.H.; Brauner, A.; Jonsson, B.; van der Ploeg, I.; S√∂der, O.; Holst, M., & Jensen, J.S. (2000). Lagercrantz H, Tullus K. *Ureaplasma urealyticum*-Induced Production of Proinflammatory Cytokines by Macrophages. *Pediatric Research*, Vol. 48, No. 1 (July 2000) pp.114-119. ISSN: 0031-3998

Li, Y.H., Chen, M., Brauner, A., Zheng, C., Jensen, J.S., & Tullus, K. (2002). *Ureaplasma urealyticum* Induces Apoptosis in Human Lung Epithelial Cells and Macrophages. *Biology of the Neonate*, Vol. 82, No. 3, pp. 166-173. ISSN: 0006-3126.

Li, Y.H.; Yan, Z.Q.; Jensen, J.S.; Tullus, K., & Brauner, A. (2000). Activation of nuclear factor kappaB and induction of inducible nitric oxide synthase by *Ureaplasma urealyticum* in macrophages. *Infection and Immunity*, Vol. 68, No. 12 (December 2000), pp. 7087-7093, ISSN 0019-9567

Lieberman, D., Ben-Yaakov, M., Lazarovich, Z., Hoffman, S., Ohana, B., Friedman, M.G., Dvoskin, B., Leinonen, M., & Boldur, I. (2001). Infectious Etiologies in Acute Exacerbation of COPD. *Diagnostic Microbiology and Infectious Diseases*, Vol. 40, No. 3 (July 2001), pp. 95–102, ISSN 0732-8893

Lieberman, D., Ben-Yaakov, M., Shmarkov, O., Gelfer, Y., Varshavsky, R., Ohana, B., Lazarovich, Z., & Boldur, I. (2002). Serological Evidence of *Mycoplasma pneumoniae* Infection in Acute Exacerbation of COPD. *Diagnostic Microbiology and Infectious Diseases*, Vol. 44, No. 1 (September 2002), pp.1–6, ISSN 0732-8893

Lo, S.C., Wear, D.J., Green, S.L., Jones, P-G., & Legier, J.F. (1993). Adult Respiratory Distress Syndrome With or Without Systemic Disease Associated With Infections Due to *Mycoplasma fermentans*. *Clinical Infectious Diseases*, Vol. 17, Suppl. 1 (August 1993), pp. S259-S263, ISSN 1058-4838

Lo, S.C., Dawson, M.S., Wong, D.M., Newton 3rd, P.B., Sonoda, M.A., Engler, W.F., Wang, R.Y., Shih, J.W., Alter, H.J., & Wear, D.J. (1989) Identification of *Mycoplasma incognitus* Infection in Patients with AIDS: an Immunohistochemical, *in situ* Hybridization and Ultrastructural Study. *American Journal of Tropical Medicine, and Hygiene*, Vol. 41, No. 5 (November 1989), pp. 601-616, ISSN 0002-9637

Lo, S-C; Hayes, MM & Kotani, H (1993). Adhesion Onto and Invasion Into Mammalian Cells by *Mycoplasma penetrans* - A Newly Isolated Mycoplasma From Patients with AIDS. *Modern Pathology, Vol. 6*, No. 3 (May 1993), pp. 276-280, ISSN 0893-3952

Loens, K., Goossens, H., & Ieven. M. (2010). Acute Respiratory Infection Due to *Mycoplasma pneumoniae*: Current Status of Diagnostic Methods. *European Journal of Clinical Microbiology and Infectious Diseases*, Vol. 29, No. 9 (September 2010), pp. 1055–1069, ISSN 0934-9723

Loens, K., Ieven, M., Ursi, D., Beck, T., Overdijk, M., Sillekens, P., & Goossens, H. (2003a). Detection of *Mycoplasma pneumoniae* by Real-Time Nucleic Acid Sequence-Based Amplification. *Journal of Clinical Microbiology*, Vol. 41, No. 9 (September 2003), pp. 4448-4450, ISSN ISSN: 0095-1137

Loens, K., Ursi, D., Goossens, H., & Ieven, M. (2003b). Molecular Diagnosis of *Mycoplasma pneumoniae* Respiratory Tract Infections. *Journal of Clinical Microbiology*, 2003 Vol. 41, No. 11(November 2003), pp. 4915-4923; ISSN ISSN: 0095-1137

Macfarlane, J., Holmes, W., Gard, P., Macfarlane, R., Rose, D., Weston, V., Leinonen, M., Saikku, P., & Myint, S. (2001). Prospective study of the Incidence, Aetiology and Outcome of Adult Lower Respiratory Tract Illness in the Community. *Thorax*, Vol. 56, No. 2 (February 2001), pp. 109-114, ISSN 0040-6376

Maeda, S., Deguchi, T., Ishiko, H., Matsumoto, T., Naito, S., Kumon, H., Tsukamoto, T., Onodera, S., & Kamidono, S. (2004). Detection of *Mycoplasma genitalium, Mycoplasma hominis, Ureaplasma parvum* (Biovar 1) and *Ureaplasma urealyticum* (Biovar 2) in Patients with Non-gonococcal Urethritis Using Polymerase Chain Reaction-Microtiter Plate Hybridization. *International Journal of Urology*, Vol.11. No.9. pp.750-754. ISSN: 0919-8172.

Maniloff, J. (1992). Phylogeny of Mycoplasmas. In: *Mycoplasmas: Molecular biology and Pathogenesis*, J. Maniloff, R.N. McElhaney, L.R. Finch & J.B. Baseman (Eds.), pp. 549-559, American Society for Microbiology, ISBN1-55581-050-0, U.S.A.

Manimtim, W.M., Hasday, J.D., Hester, L., Fairchild, K.D., Lovchik, J.C., & Viscardi, R.M. (2001). *Ureaplasma urealyticum* Modulates Endotoxin-Induced Cytokine Release by

Human Monocytes Derived from Preterm and Term Newborns and Adults. *Infection and Immunity*, Vol. 69, No. 6 (June 2001), pp. 3906-3915, ISSN: 0019-9567.

Mogulkoc, N., Karakurt, S., Isalska, B., Bayindir, U., Celikel, T., Korten, V., & Colpan, N. 1999. Acute Purulent Exacerbation of Chronic Obstructive Pulmonary Disease and *Chlamydia pneumoniae* Infection. *American Journal of Respiratory Critical Care Medicine*, Vol. 160, No. 1 (July 1999), pp. 349-353, ISSN 1073-449X

Momynaliev, K.T., & Govorun, V.M. (2001). Mechanisms of genetic instability in Mollicutes (mycoplasmas). *Russian Journal of Genetics;* Vol. 37, No. 9 (2001), pp. 979-992, ISSN 1022-7954

Naessens, A.; Foulon, W.; Debrucker, P.; Devroey, P. & Lauwers, S. (1986). Recovery of Microorganisms in Semen and Relationship to Semen Evaluation. *Fertility and Sterility*. Vol.45. No.1. pp.101-105. ISSN: 0015-0282.

Olson, LD & Gilbert, AA (1993). Characteristics of *Mycoplasma hominis* adhesion. *Journal of Bacteriology*, Vol. 175, No. 10 (October 1993), pp. 3224-3227, ISSN 0021-9193

Peltier, M.R.; Tee, S.C., & Smulian, J.C. (2008). Effect of Progesterone on Proinflammatory Cytokine Production by Monocytes Stimulated with Pathogens Associated with Preterm Birth. *American Journal of Reproductive Immunology*, Vol. 60, No.4, pp. 346-353, ISSN 1046-7408

Pietsch, K., Ehlers, S., & Jacobs, E. (1994). Cytokine Gene Expression in the Lungs of BALB/c Mice During Primary and Secondary Intranasal Infection with *Mycoplasma pneumoniae*. *Microbiology*, Vol. 140, (August 1994), pp. 2043-2048, ISSN 1350-0872

Potts, J.M.; Ward, A.M. & Rackley, R.R. (2000). Association of Chronic Urinary Symptoms in Women and *Ureaplasma urealyticum*. *Urology*, Vol. 55, No. 4, pp. 486-489, ISSN 0090-4295

Povlsen, K.; Bjå ̦rnelius, E.; Lidbrink, P. & Lind, I. (2002). Relationship of *Ureaplasma urealyticum* Biovar 2 to Nongonococcal Urethritis. *European Journal of Clinical Microbiology and Infectious Diseases,*Vol. 21, No. 2, pp.97-101, ISSN: 0934-9723

Povlsen, K.; Thorsen, P. & Lind, I. (2001). Relationship of *Ureaplasma urealyticum* Biovars to the Presence or Absence of Bacterial Vaginosis in Pregnant Women and to the Time of Delivery. *European Journal of Clinical Microbiology and Infectious Diseases*, Vol. 20, No. 1, pp. 65-67, ISSN: 0934-9723.

Razin, S. (1999). Adherence of Pathogenic Mycoplasmas to Host Cells. *Bioscience Reports*, Vol. 19, No.5 (October 1999), pp.367-372, ISSN 0144-8463

Razin, S; Yoguev, D., & Naot, Y. (1998). Molecular Biology and Pathogenicity of Mycoplasmas. *Microbiology and Molecular Biology Reviews*, Vol. 62, No. 4 (December 1998), pp. 1094-1156, ISSN 1092-2172

Rechnitzer, H., Brzuszkiewicz, E., Strittmatter, A., Liesegang, H., Lysnyansky, I., Daniel, R., Gottschalk, G., & Rottem, S. (2011). Genomic Features and Insights Into the Biology of *Mycoplasma fermentans*. *Microbiology*, Vol. 157, pp. 760-773. ISSN: 1350-0872

Roberts, D.D., Olson, L.D., Barile, M.F., Ginsburg, V., & Krivan, H.C. (1989). Sialic Acid-Dependent Adhesion of *Mycoplasma pneumoniae* to Purified Glycoproteins. *Journal of Biological Chemistry*, Vol. 5, No. 264 (June 1989), pp. 9289-9293, ISSN 0021-9258

Roberts, M.C. (1992). Antibiotic Resistance. In: *Mycoplasmas: Molecular biology and Pathogenesis*, J. Maniloff, R.N. McElhaney, L.R. Finch & J.B. Baseman (Eds.), pp. 513-523, American Society for Microbiology, ISBN1-55581-050-0, U.S.A.

Román-Méndez, C., Santellán-Olea, M.R., Cedillo, L., & Rivera-Tapia, J.A.. (2007). Alteraciones histológicas a nivel pulmonar inducidas por *Mycoplasma fermentans*. *Revista Mexicana de Patología Clínica*, Vol. 54, No 1, pp. 40-46.

Rottem, S., & Naot, Y. (1998). Subversion and Exploitation of Host Cells by Mycoplasmas. *Trends in Microbiology*, Vol 6, No. 11 (November 1998), pp. 436-440, ISSN 0966-842X

Rottem, S. (2003). Interaction of Mycoplasmas with Host Cells. *Physiology Reviews*, Vol. 83, No.2 (Apr 2003), pp. 417-432, ISSN 0031-9333

Saillard, C., Carle, P., Bove, J.M., Bebear, C., Lo, S.C., Shih, J.W., Wang, R.Y., Rose, D.L., & Tully, J.G. (1990). Genetic and Serologic Relatedness Between *Mycoplasma fermentans* Strains and a Mycoplasma Recently Identified in Tissues of AIDS and Non-AIDS Patients. *Research in Virolology*, Vol. 141, No. 3 (May-June 1990), pp. 385-395, ISSN 0923-2516

Schaeverbeke, T., Gilroy, C.B., Bebear, C., Dehais, J., & Taylor-Robinson, D. (1996). *Mycoplasma fermentans*, but not *M penetrans*, detected by PCR assays in synovium from patients with rheumatoid arthritis and other rheumatic disorders. *Journal of Clinical Pathology*, Vol. 49, pp. 824-828, ISSN 0021-9746

Schelonka, R.L., & Waites, K.B. (2007). Ureaplasma Infection and Neonatal Lung Disease. *Seminars in Perinatology*, Vol. 31, No.1, pp. 2-9, ISSN: 0146-0005.

Sethi S. 2000. Bacterial Infection and the Pathogenesis of COPD. *Chest*, Vol. 117, No. 5, Suppl. 1 (May 2000), pp. 286-291, ISSN 0012-3692

Shang, X.J., Huang, Y.F., Xiong C.L., Xu, J.P., Yin, L. & Wan, C.C. (1999). *Ureaplasma urealyticum* Infection and Apoptosis of Spermatogenic Cells. *Asian J Androl*. Vol.1. No.3. pp.127-129. ISSN: 1008-682X.

Shimizu, T.; Kida, Y. & Kuwano, K. (2008). *Ureaplasma parvum* Lipoproteins, Including MB Antigen, Activate NF-{kappa}B through TLR1, TLR2 and TLR6. *Microbiology*. Vol.154. No.5. pp.1318-1325. ISSN: 1350-0872.

Sirand-Pugnet, P., Citti. C., Barré, A., & Blanchard, A. (2007), Evolution of Mollicutes: Down a Bumpy Road with Twists and Turns. *Research in Microbiology* 158 (2007) 754-766. ISSN 0923-2508

Smith, C. B., Kanner, R.E., Golden, C.A., Klauber, M.R., & Renzetti Jr., A.D. (1980). Effect of Viral Infections on Pulmonary Function in Patients with Chronic Obstructive Pulmonary Diseases. *Journal of Infectious Diseases*, Vol. 141, No. 3 (March 1980), pp. 271–280, ISSN 0022-1899

Stancombe, B.B.; Walsh, W.F.; Derdak, S.; Dixon, P., & Hensley, D. (1993). Induction of Human Neonatal Pulmonary Fibroblast Cytokines by Hyperoxia and *Ureaplasma urealyticum*. *Clinical Infectious Diseases*, Vol. 17, Suppl 1 (August 1993), pp. S154-S157, ISSN 1058-4838

Sun, G.; Xu, X.; Wang, Y.; Shen, X.; Chen, Z., & Yang, J. (2008). *Mycoplasma pneumoniae* Infection Induces Reactive Oxygen Species and DNA Damage in A549 Human Lung Carcinoma Cells. *Infection and Immunity*, Vol. 76, No. 10 (October 2008), pp. 4405-4413, ISSN 0019-9567

Svenstrup, H.F.; Nielsen, P.K.; Drasbek, M.; Birkelund, S. & Christiansen, G. (2002). Adhesion and Inhibition Assay of *Mycoplasma genitalium* and *M. pneumoniae* by Immunofluorescence Microscopy. *Journal of Medical Microbiology*, Vol. 51, No. 5 (May 2002), pp. 361-373, ISSN 0022-2615

Taylor-Robinson, D., Davies, H. A., Sarathchandra, P., & Furr, P. M. (1991). Intracellular Location of Mycoplasmas in Cultured Cells Demonstrated by Immunocytochemistry and Electron Microscopy. International Journal of Experimental Pathology, Vol. 72:, pp. 705-714. ISSN 0959-9673

Taylor-Robinson, D. (1996). Infections Due to Species of Mycoplasma and Ureaplasma: an Update. Clinical Infectious Diseases, 23: 671-684. ISSN 1058-4838

Torres-Morquecho, A., Rivera-Tapia, A., González-Velazquez, F., Torres, J., Chávez-Munguia, B., Cedillo-Ramírez, L., & Giono-Cerezo, S. (2010). Adherence and Damage to Epithelial Cells of Human Lung by Ureaplasma urealyticum strains biotype 1 and 2. African Journal of Microbiology Research, Vol. 4, No. 6 (March 2010), pp. 480-491, ISSN 1996-0808

Tully, J. G. 1993. Current Status of the Mollicute Flora of Humans. Clinical Infectious Diseases, Vol. 17, Suppl. 1(August 1993), pp. S2-S9, ISSN 1058-4838

Van Kuppeveld, F.J.M., Van Der Logt, J.T.M., Angulo, A.F., van Zoest ,M.J., Quint, W.G., Niesters, H.G., Galama, J.M., & Melchers, W.J. (1992). Genus- and Species-Specific Identification of Mycoplasmas by 16S rRNA Amplification. Applied and Environmental Microbiology, Vol. 58, No. 8 (August 1992), pp. 2606-2615, ISSN 0099-2240

Viscardi, R.M. (2010). Ureaplasma Species: Role in Diseases of Prematurity. Clinics in Perinatology, Vol.37. No.2 (June 2010). pp.393-409, ISSN 0095-5108.

Viscardi, R.M., Manimtim, W.M., Sun, C.-C.J., Duffy, L., & Cassell, G.H. (2002). Lung Pathology in Premature Infants with Ureaplasma urealyticum Infection. Pediatric and Developmental Pathology, Vol. 5, No. 2 (March-April 2002), pp. 141-150, ISSN 1093-5266

Volgmann, T.; Ohlinger, R. & Panzig, B. (2005). Ureaplasma urealyticum-Harmless Commensal or Underestimated Enemy of Human Reproduction? A review. Archives of Gynecology and Obstetrics, Vol. 273, No.3 (December 2005), pp. 133-139, ISSN: 0932-0067.

Waites, K.B., Bebear, C.M., Robertson, J.A., Talkington, D.F., & Kenny, G.E. Laboratory Diagnosis of Mycoplasmal Infections. Cumitech 34. (2000). Coordinating ed. FS Nolte. Washington: American Society for Microbiology.

Waites, K.B., & Talkington, D.F. (2004). Mycoplasma pneumoniae and Its Role as a Human Pathogen. Clinical Microbiology Reviews, Vol. 17, No. 4 (October 2004), pp. 697–728, ISSN 0893-8512

Waites, K.B., & Talkington, D.F. (2005). New Developments in Human Diseases Due to Mycoplasmas. In: Mycoplasmas: pathogenesis, molecular biology, and emerging strategies for control, A. Blanchard & G. Browning (ed.), p. 289-354, Horizon Scientific Press, ISBN 0849398614, Norwich, United Kingdom.

Waites, K.B., Katz, B., & Schelonka, R. (2005). Mycoplasmas and Ureaplasmas as Neonatal Pathogens. Clinical Microbiology Reviews, Vol. 18, No. 4 (October 2005), pp. 757–789, ISSN 0893-8512

Waites, K.B., Simecka, J.W., Talkington, D.F., & Atkinson, T.P. (2007). Pathogenesis of Mycoplasma pneumoniae Infections: Adaptive Immunity, Innate Immunity, Cell Biology, and Virulence Factors. In: Community-Acquired Pneumonia, N. Suttorp, T. Welte,& R. Marre (Eds.), pp. 183-198, Birkhäuser Verlag Basel, ISBN 3-7643-7562-0, Switzerland

Waites K. B., Balish M. F., & Atkinson T. P. New Insights Into the Pathogenesis and Detection of *Mycoplasma pneumoniae* Infections. *Future Microbiology*, Vol. 3, No. 6 (2008): pp. 635–648. ISSN 1746-0913

Wang, R.Y., Hu, W.S., Dawson, M.S., Shih, J.W., & Lo, S.C. (1992). Selective Detection of *Mycoplasma fermentans* by Polymerase Chain Reaction and By Using a Nucleotide Sequence Within the Insertion Sequence-Like Element. *Journal of Clinical Microbiology*, Vol. 30, No. 1 (January 1992), pp. 245-248, ISSN: 0095-1137

Wang, Y.; Liang, C.L.; Wu, J.Q.; Xu, C.; Qin, S.X. & Gao, E.S. (2006). Do *Ureaplasma urealyticum* Infections in the Genital Tract Affect Semen Quality? *Asian Journal of Andrology*, Vol. 8, No. 5, pp. 562-568, ISSN: 1008-682X.

Williams, M. H., Brostoff, J. & Roitt, I. M. (1970). Possible Role of *Mycoplasma fermentans* in Pathogenesis of Rheumatoid Arthritis. *Lancet, Vol.* 2, No. 7667 (August 8 1970), pp. 277–280, ISSN 0140-6736

Wubbel, L., Jafri, H. S., Olsen, K., et al *Mycoplasma pneumoniae* Pneumonia in a Mouse Model. *Journal of Infectious Diseases*, 1998;178,1526-1529, ISSN 0022-1899

Yang, J., Hooper, W.C., Phillips, D.J., & Talkington, D.F. (2004). Cytokines in *Mycoplasma pneumoniae* Infections. *Cytokine and Growth Factor Reviews*, Vol. 15, No. 2-3 (April-June 2004), pp. 157-168, ISSN1359-6101

Yáñez, A. 1997. Some aspects of the pathogenicity of *Mycoplasma fermentans* in the Respiratory Tract of Hamsters and Rabbit's Joints. Doctoral dissertation. National School of Biological Sciences, National Polytechnic Institute, Mexico.

Yáñez, A., Cedillo, L., Neyrolles, O., Alonso, E., Prévost, M.C., Rojas, J., Watson, H.L., Blanchard, A,, & Cassell, G.H. (1999). *Mycoplasma penetrans* Bacteremia and Primary Antiphospholipid Syndrome. *Emerging Infectious Diseases*, Vol. 5, No. 1 (January-February 1999), pp. 164-167, ISSN: 1080-6059

Yavlovich, A., A. A. Higazi, and S. Rottem. 2001. Plasminogen Binding and Activation by *Mycoplasma fermentans*. *Infection and Immunity*, Vol. 69, No. 4 (April 2001), pp. 1977-1982, ISSN 0019-9567

Yavlovich, A.; Tarshis, M., & Rottem, S. (2004). Internalization and Intracellular Survival of *Mycoplasma pneumoniae* by Non-Phagocytic Cells. *FEMS Microbiology Letters*, Vol. 233, No. 2 (April 2004), pp. 241-246, ISSN: 1574-6968

Yoon, B.H.; Romero, R.; Kim, M.; Kim, E.C.; Kim, T.; Park, J.S. & Jun, J.K. (2000). Clinical Implications of Detection of *Ureaplasma urealyticum* in the Amniotic Cavity with the Polymerase Chain Reaction. *American Journal of Obstetrics and Gynecology*, Vol.183, No.5 (November 2000), pp. 1130-1137, ISSN: 0002-9378.

Yoon, B.H.; Romero, R.; Lim, J.H.; Shim, S.S.; Hong, J.S.; Shim, J.Y. & Jun, J.K. (2003). The Clinical Significance of Detecting *Ureaplasma urealyticum* by the Polymerase Chain Reaction in the Amniotic Fluid of Patients with Preterm Labor. *American Journal of Obstetrics and Gynecology*. Vol. 189, Vol. 4 (October 2003), pp. 919-924, ISSN: 0002-9378.

2

Interleukin-17 and T Helper 17 Cells in Mucosal Immunity of the Lung

M.S. Paats, P.Th.W. van Hal, C.C. Baan, H.C. Hoogsteden,
M.M. van der Eerden and R.W. Hendriks
Erasmus Medical Center, Rotterdam
The Netherlands

1. Introduction

In all mammals, including humans, the immune system is responsible for the protection against potentially hazardous pathogens, such as bacteria, viruses, parasites and fungi. In this remarkably effective defense system leukocytes, which mediate both innate and adaptive immune responses, play a central role.

The innate immune system comprises granulocytes (neutrophils, eosinophils and basophils), natural killer (NK) cells, mast cells and macrophages. These cells are the first line of defense and provide the immediate response against pathogens. Neutrophils and macrophages can eliminate a pathogen directly by phagocytosis. Moreover, their pattern-recognition receptors, recognizing structurally conserved molecules derived from microbes such as bacterial lipopolysaccharides, unmethylated CpG, or viral double-stranded RNA, allow them to respond to a wide variety of microbial invaders, e.g. by producing cytokines that activate T lymphocytes of the adaptive immune system.

Acquired or adaptive immunity is characterized by a slower but highly specific immune response. Three major cell types are involved in adaptive immunity: antigen presenting cells (APCs), T lymphocytes and B lymphocytes. Dendritic cells (DCs) are the most potent APCs. They act as messengers between the innate and the adaptive immune system by taking up, processing and presenting antigens to T lymphocytes. In response to presented antigens, T lymphocytes may react in different ways: CD4+ T helper cells produce various cytokines that direct the immune response, whereas CD8+ cytotoxic T cells produce toxic granules that induce death of infected cells. B cells are able to respond to pathogens by terminal differentiation into plasma cells after which they produce large quantities of antibodies. Modulation of B cell function and antibody production by CD4+ T cells is an important step in coordinating immune responses. Upon activation, B cells can migrate to germinal centers, which are specialized structures in secondary lymphoid organs, where they interact with T cells and DCs. Costimulatory signals from T cells then facilitate selection of B cells with high affinity for immunoglobulins and control class switching of the immunoglobulin (Ig) to IgG, IgA and IgE.

Following pathogen elimination, lymphocytes leave a lasting legacy of the antigens they have come across represented by memory cells. As a result, lymphocytes are able to mount a faster and stronger immune response in future encounters with the same antigen. Defective T cell function can increase susceptibility to infections, allergies and autoimmune diseases. T lymphocytes can however also be manipulated to either eradicate tumor or control graft rejection after organ transplantation. Therefore, in addition to basic biological interest, knowledge on T cell biology is important to the understanding of the etiology of a wide variety of diseases and may improve current therapies.

During activation in a particular cytokine milieu, naïve CD4+ T cells can differentiate into one of the several subsets of T helper (Th) cells. Already in 1986, Mosmann and Coffman introduced the concept of distinct types of T helper cells, which was based on the distinct cytokines profiles that T cells produce when they are stimulated to differentiate (Mosmann and Coffman 1989). They described two types of Th lymphocytes, type 1 helper T cells (Th1 cells) and type 2 helper T cells (Th2 cells). Th1 cells produce large quantities of interferon (IFN)γ, induce delayed hypersensitivity reactions, activate macrophages, and are essential for the defense against intracellular pathogens. Th2 cells produce mainly interleukin (IL)-4 and are important in inducing IgE production, recruiting eosinophils to sites of inflammation, and helping to clear parasitic infections. Cytokines produced by cells of the innate immune system govern the differentiation of these T helper cells. IFNγ and IL-12 drive naive T cells into the Th1 pathway, whereas IL-4 initiates the differentiation of naive T cells into Th2 cells. At a molecular level, the differentiation of Th1 and Th2 cells requires specific transcription factors: T-bet for Th1 cells (Szabo et al. 2000) and GATA3 for Th2 cells (Zheng and Flavell 1997) (Figure 1). An additional T helper subset was recently identified which restrains excessive effector T cell responses and therefore accounts for the maintenance of immune homeostasis and prevention of immunopathology. These cells are called regulatory T (Treg) cells and are naturally present in the immune system as a functionally distinct CD4+ T cell expressing the forkhead transcription factor FoxP3 and producing the cytokines IL-10 and transforming growth factor (TGF)-β. The differentiation of naïve T cells towards this lineage is driven by IL-2 and TGF-β (Weaver and Hatton 2009) (Figure 1). T follicular helper (Tfh) cells are yet another CD4+ T cell population (Nurieva et al. 2008; Vogelzang et al. 2008). They are important for the formation of germinal centers. Once these germinal centers are formed, Tfh cells are needed to maintain and regulate B cell differentiation into plasma cells and memory B cells. The signals that specifically instruct the differentiation of human Tfh cells remain unclear, but IL-12 and IL-21 seem to be required. Tfh cells express Bcl6 as their master transcription factor and may produce IL-21 and IL-4 (Yusuf et al. 2010; Ma et al. 2009; Crotty 2011) (Figure 1).

Interestingly, in recent years T cells were shown to produce proinflammatory cytokines that could not be classified according to this Th1-Th2 scheme. IL-17 is the most prominent amongst these cytokines, and T cells that preferentially produce IL-17 but not IFNγ or IL-4 were named Th17 cells. The discovery of this new subset of helper T cells that selectively produces IL-17 has provided better and exciting insights into immunoregulation, host defense and the pathogenesis of autoimmune diseases. In particular, it now appears that Th17 cells do not only play a key role in chronic inflammatory lung disorders, but also mediate protective immunity against various pathogens at respiratory mucosal sites.

2. Interleukin 17 and T helper 17 cells

IL-17 (also denoted IL-17A) was cloned in 1993 and initially called CTLA-8 (Rouvier et al. 1993). In 1995, it was renamed as IL-17, its receptor was cloned and it was identified as a cytokine expressed by T cells, exerting effects on epithelial, endothelial, and fibroblast cells (Yao et al. 1995). IL-17 has diverse biological functions, but the best characterized functions

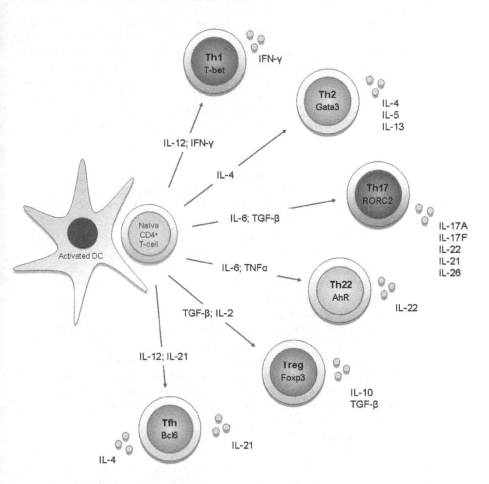

Fig. 1. Overview of human CD4+ effector T cell differentiation.
Upon activation in a particular cytokine milieu, naïve CD4+ T cells may differentiate into one of several lineages of T helper (Th) cells, including Th1, Th2, Th17, and Treg cells. These separate lineages are characterized by their distinct cytokine production pattern. The differentiation pathways are mainly based on the induction of transcription factors that serve as master regulators of specific lineages. However, cytokine production by Th cells seems to be more flexible than previously believed and recently new cells, such as Th22 and Tfh cells have been described. Whether these new subsets represent distinct lineages remains to be elucidated.

relate to its proinflammatory effects. Specifically, IL-17 recruits neutrophils via effects on granulopoiesis (Schwarzenberger et al. 1998; Fossiez et al. 1996) and CXC chemokine induction, including CXCL8/IL-8 (Laan et al. 1999). Furthermore, it acts on macrophages to promote their recruitment and survival and stimulates the production of proinflammatory cytokines and anti-microbial peptides, particularly β-defensins, from a variety of immune and non-immune cells (Kolls and Linden 2004; Weaver et al. 2007; Ouyang, Kolls, and

Zheng 2008; Crome, Wang, and Levings 2010). By now we know that the IL-17 family includes 6 family members: IL-17A, IL-17B, IL-17C, IL-17D, IL-17E and IL-17F. IL-17A and IL-17F are the most closely related isoforms, sharing 55% homology with each other. Because of their structural and functional similarities and the fact that they are both produced by Th17 cells, IL-17A and IL-17F have been most thoroughly studied and characterized. Although it was known for more than 15 years that IL-17 is a product of activated CD4+ T cells, it was not until 2005 that the Th17 cell was described as a distinct CD4+ T-cell subset, critically responsible for the production of IL-17 in the context of autoimmunity (Harrington et al. 2005).

2.1 Phenotype and differentiation of Th17 cells

IL-17A is the hallmark cytokine for Th17 cells. Nevertheless, these cells also produce other cytokines, such as IL-21, IL-22, tumor necrosis factor (TNF)-α, other members of the IL-17 family and, specifically in humans, IL-26 (Dong 2008). As with Th1 and Th2 cells, no single surface marker is specific for Th17 cells. However, human Th17 cells are thought to preferentially express CD161 on the cell surface (Cosmi et al. 2008). Additionally, the selective expression of chemokine receptors in subsets of human memory T cells has been useful in defining lineages with different effector functions and migratory capacity (Sallusto, Mackay, and Lanzavecchia 2000). It has been shown that human Th17 cells express the chemokine receptor CCR6 and its ligand CCL20 (Dong 2008; Wilson et al. 2007). Coexpression of CCR4 and CCR6 further defines human T cells that produce IL-17 but not IFNγ (Acosta-Rodriguez, Rivino et al. 2007). In contrast, expression of CCR6 and CXCR3 identifies a more heterogeneous effector T cell population that produces both IFNγ and IL-17 (Acosta-Rodriguez, Rivino et al. 2007). These patterns of chemokine receptors appear to be biologically significant, as memory Th17 cells specific for *Candida albicans* are mainly CCR6+CCR4+ positive, whereas those that recognize *Mycobacterium tuberculosis* antigens are present in the CCR6+CXCR3+ subgroup producing both IFNγ and IL-17 (Acosta-Rodriguez, Rivino et al. 2007; Annunziato et al. 2007).

The combination of cytokines that stimulate differentiation of Th17 cells has been subject of much debate. Initial studies on human T cell differentiation indicated that T cell activation in the presence of IL-1β, IL-6 and/or IL-23 was sufficient to induce Th17 cells, and that TGF-β inhibited this process (Acosta-Rodriguez, Napolitani et al. 2007; Chen et al. 2007; Crome, Wang, and Levings 2010; Wilson et al. 2007). In subsequent studies, however, TGF-β was reported to be important for the development of human IL-17 producing cells (Manel, Unutmaz, and Littman 2008; Volpe et al. 2008; Yang, Anderson et al. 2008). This discrepancy could be explained by more recent reports showing that the requirement for TGF-β in the differentiation process is indirect and relates to suppression of Th1 differentiation (Crome, Wang, and Levings 2010; Santarlasci et al. 2009). In the current view, the combination of IL-1β and IL-6 is essential for proper human Th17 cell differentiation whereas IL-23 is important for both expansion and survival of lineage-committed Th17 cells (Wilson et al. 2007). In addition to cytokine-driven Th17 lineage commitment, it has also been shown that prostaglandin E2 (PGE2), which is a mediator of tissue inflammation, directly promotes differentiation, expansion and proinflammatory function of human and mouse Th17 cells (Yao et al. 2009). In humans, PGE2 induces up-regulation of the IL-23 and IL-1 receptors (IL-23R and IL-1R, respectively) and by synergism with IL-1β, IL-6 and IL-23 (Boniface et al. 2009).

The observation that Th17 cells are a distinct lineage of cells with a unique cytokine and chemokine/chemokine receptor profile, led to the discovery of RORγt in mice (Ivanov et al. 2006). RORγt encodes the retinoid orphan nuclear receptor, and this transcription factor is required for the differentiation of Th17 cells. In the human system it has also been shown that forced over-expression of RORC2 (the human equivalent of RORγt) in human naïve T cells induces a Th17-like phenotype, by inducing IL-17A, IL-17F, IL-26 and CCR6 expression and down-regulating IFNγ secretion (Manel, Unutmaz, and Littman 2008; Crome et al. 2009) (Figure 1). Activation of RORγt also causes expression of the IL23R, indicating that IL-23 acts on T cells that are already committed to the Th17 lineage. Exposure of developing Th17 cells to IL-23 not only enhances the expression of IL-17 but also induces IL-22 and suppresses IL-10 and IFNγ (McGeachy et al. 2007). Yet, RORC2 alone can induce IL-17 production in only 20% of the T cell population (Chen and O'Shea 2008) indicating that it acts in cooperation with other transcription factors for full commitment of precursors to the Th17 lineage. In addition to RORC2, the most specific and master transcription factor, at least four other transcription factors are linked to the human Th17 cell fate. These include signal transducer and activator of transcription-3 (STAT3), interferon regulatory factor-4 (IRF4), runt box transcription factor-1 (Runx1), and the aryl hydrocarbon receptor (AhR) (Chen and O'Shea 2008). Together they form a sophisticated network with positive and negative feedback loops. In addition, Th17 cells are inhibited by IL-2 (produced by Treg cells), IFNγ (produced by Th1 cells), and IL-4 (produced by Th2 cells) but also by other negative regulators such as retinoic acid (Elias et al. 2008).

Although this scheme of T helper cell differentiation might seem complex (Figure 1), it is in fact an oversimplification. Recent studies on T helper cell differentiation have revealed more plasticity in cytokine production than predicted by conventional models of T helper cell lineage commitment. Activated memory T cells preserve plasticity to alter their cytokine program according to the stimuli they receive. A cytokine restricted to one T helper subset can therefore be secreted by another subset under changing stimulation conditions. This feature is also observed in human Th17 cells (Chen and O'Shea 2008). Acquisition of IFNγ-producing potential by Th17 cells, particularly the simultaneous production of IFNγ and IL-17, is common (Chen et al. 2007; Wilson et al. 2007) (see Figure 2). Additionally, Th17 cells can even stop producing IL-17 and become selective IFNγ producers resulting in a complete subset switch (O'Shea and Paul 2010). Although Th1 cells do not become IL-17 producers, under particular circumstances they can make IL-13 (Hayashi et al. 2007). Th17 cells produce IL-22, but cells that make IL-22 and not IL-17 ("Th22 cells") have recently been identified as well (Duhen et al. 2009; Trifari et al. 2009). Simultaneous production of IL-22 and IFNγ has also been described (O'Shea and Paul 2010). This plasticity even concerns master regulators: FoxP3 expression within Treg cells is heterogeneous and transient and former.

Treg cells have the capacity to produce proinflammatory cytokines such as IL-17 (Bluestone et al. 2009).

Moreover, also multiple master regulators can be expressed, such as Gata3 and FoxP3 in Tregs (Mantel et al. 2007), or a combination of RORC2 and FoxP3 (mixed Th17-Treg) (O'Shea and Paul 2010). Therefore, expression of master regulators should not be simplified as mutually exclusive but rather as a gradient of transcription factors (O'Shea and Paul 2010). It remains to be shown whether there are preferential directions for plasticity or whether effector T cells can change in any direction from every starting point (Bluestone et al. 2009). Plasticity could be an answer to the evolution of pathogens, allowing a proper response to new threats.

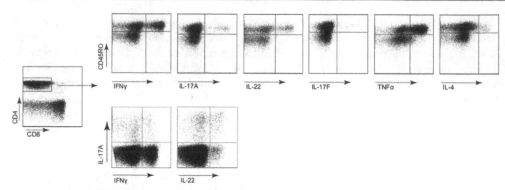

Fig. 2. Flow cytometric analysis of cytokine production by CD4+ T helper cells.
With the use of a technique called flow cytometry, it is possible to depict the cytokine
producing potential of individual cells. In this experiment peripheral blood mononuclear
cell (PBMC) suspensions were stained with monoclonal antibodies specific for CD3, CD4,
CD8, and the indicated cytokines. Live CD4+ CD3+ T cells were gated and analyzed for the
presence of the indicated cytokines in combination with the CD45R0 marker for memory T
cells. Results are shown as dot plots and illustrate that CD4+ T helper cells are capable of
producing all of the tested cytokines (top row, right upper quadrants). Moreover, CD4+ T
helper cells have the potential to be simultaneously positive for IL-17 and IFNγ, and IL-17A
and IL-22 respectively (bottom row, right upper quadrants).

2.2 IL-17 producing cells other than Th17 cells
Th17 cells are not the exclusive producers of IL-17 nor is this production their only function.
Other cell populations capable of producing IL-17 include both adaptive and innate immune
cells.
Within the adaptive arm of the immune system, a subset of CD8+ cytotoxic T cells is also
capable of producing IL-17. Studies have shown that these cells develop under conditions
that are similar to those required by Th17 cells, but different from those required by IFNγ
producing CD8+ T cells (Kondo et al. 2009). However, adaptive immune responses cannot
explain the early IL-17-mediated immune responses that have crucial roles during stress
responses and host defense. Early responses are induced within hours following tissue
injury or exposure to pathogens (Ferretti et al. 2003; Happel et al. 2003; Zheng et al. 2008),
which is not enough time to allow for Th17 differentiation, indicating that innate immune
cells play a crucial role in these early responses. The key feature of this innate IL-17 response
is the early neutrophil recruitment. This results in a more efficient resolution of infection, in
the maintenance of mucosal barrier integrity, but also in the potential induction of
autoimmunity (2). Recent studies have shown that γδ T cells are important innate-like IL-17-
producing cells during infectious diseases and autoimmune inflammation (Aujla, Dubin,
and Kolls 2007; Sutton et al. 2009; Ito et al. 2009). Additionally, innate(-like) IL-17-producing
cells described in literature include CD3+ invariant natural killer T (iNKT) cells, lymphoid
tissue inducer (LTi)-like cells, natural killer (NK) cells and myeloid cells (Cella et al. 2009;
Cua and Tato 2010; Michel et al. 2007).
The γδ T cell subset is an innate-like immune cell population that has an important role at
the mucosal barrier. These cells do not express the classical αβ T cell receptor (TCR) but a γδ
TCR instead. They bind to epitopes in much the same way as antibodies do and provide a

rapidly available source of IL-17 (Sutton et al. 2009). Like γδ T cells, iNKT cells play a pivotal role in immunity as they provide a rapid response, with the capacity to critically amplify and regulate adaptive immune responses (Godfrey et al. 2004). Initially, they have been divided into subsets that produce either IL-4 or IFNγ, but recently a new IL-17-producing subset that develops in the thymus has been described. This subset seems already committed to making IL-17 (Michel et al. 2008). The LTi cell represents a primitive precursor of NK, NKT, and CD4+ T cells. Specifically immature (CD127+) NK cells are closely related to LTi cells (Eberl et al. 2004). LTi cells promote the formation of lymphoid organs and sustain primed CD4+ T cell memory responses (Eberl et al. 2004). Thus, like IL-17 producing γδ T cells and NKT cells, LTi cells provide a rapidly available source of IL-17. Interestingly, it was recently recognized that innate lymphoid cells (ILCs) can be considered a family of non-T/non-B lymphocytes that includes not only NK and LTi cells, but also cells that produce IL-5, IL-13, IL-17 or IL-22. These ILC subsets are developmentally related and require cytokine signals through the common γ-chain of the IL-2 receptor. The distinct ILC subsets, which seem to have important roles in protective immunity analogous to helper T cell subsets, were recently reviewed by Spits and DiSanto (Spits and Di Santo 2011). Next to LTi and NK cells, other innate IL-17 producers have been postulated, including macrophages and neutrophils (reviewed by (Cua and Tato 2010; Song et al. 2008), however data is limited and further studies are needed to understand more of their role in mucosal tissue.

2.3 Interactions between Th17 and other cells of the immune system

Cells of the immune system modulate each other's function. Many cells may interact with Th17 cells including APCs, other T helper subsets, B cells and neutrophils (Figure 3). APCs play a central role in directing immune responses by secreting cytokines that polarize CD4+ T cells into distinct lineages. Several studies support the hypothesis that changes in APC function probably precede inappropriate development and expansion of Th17 cells. For example, monocytes from inflamed joints of rheumatoid arthritis patients promote the development to Th17 cells but not Th1 or Th2 cells via a cell-contact-dependent mechanism (Evans et al. 2009). Furthermore, it was found that monocyte-derived DCs from patients with multiple sclerosis secrete elevated levels of IL-23 when compared to healthy controls (Vaknin-Dembinsky, Balashov, and Weiner 2006). Additionally, in psoriasis DCs secrete IL-1β, IL-23 and CCL20, promoting both the development of Th17 cells and their migration to the skin (Kryczek et al. 2008). However, the initial stimuli that polarize APCs to produce cytokines that promote Th17 cells are still unclear.

It has long been known that Th1 and Th2 cells antagonize each other's differentiation and function. Not surprisingly, IFNγ produced by Th1 cells and IL-4 produced by Th2 cells inhibit Th17 development (Bettelli, Oukka, and Kuchroo 2007). For Treg cells and Th17 cells there appears to be an even closer developmental relationship because the differentiation of both of these cell types require transforming growth factor (TGF)β (Veldhoen et al. 2006). Additionally, Th17 differentiation is inhibited by Treg cells, via the production of IL-2. Th17 cells can also modulate B cell function as has been shown by their ability to promote antibody production (IgM, IgG and IgA but not IgE) (Acosta-Rodriguez, Napolitani et al. 2007).

There is growing evidence that T cells are involved in orchestrating sustained mobilization of neutrophils. In the lungs for instance, in a subpopulation of COPD patients there is an accumulation of CD4+ and CD8+ T cells, which is associated with the presence of neutrophils

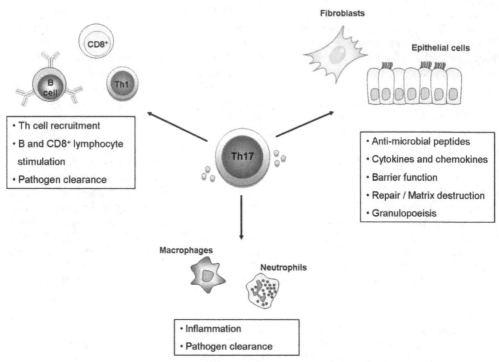

Fig. 3. Th17 cells act on other immune cells and on cells of non-hematopoietic origin. Cytokines produced by Th17 cells have the ability to act on other cells. This allows for a crosstalk between immune and non-immune cells to provide protection and promote inflammation.

(Turato et al. 2002). IL-17 seems to be an important mediator of linking activated T cells to accumulation of neutrophils, although solid data on T helper cells and neutrophils are lacking. In vitro work confirmed that IL-17 orchestrated neutrophilic influx by the production of CXCL8 (IL-8), CXCL1 (GRO-a), and granulocyte-macrophage colony stimulating factor (GM-CSF) in airway epithelial cells, smooth muscle cells, endothelial cells, and fibroblasts (Murphy et al. 2008). So, the importance of Th17 cells in neutrophilic inflammation lies in the ability of IL-17 to induce granulopoiesis, neutrophil chemotaxis, and the anti-apoptotic properties of G-CSF (Kolls and Linden 2004; Ouyang, Kolls, and Zheng 2008). Accordingly, administration of IL-17A to the lung induces robust neutrophil recruitment (Laan et al. 1999), although – by contrast - chronic IL-17A/F overexpression resulted in enhanced lymphocyte and macrophage but not neutrophil numbers (Park et al. 2005; Yang, Chang et al. 2008).

3. IL-17 in lung diseases

Although Th17 cells have only recently been recognized as a distinct lineage of CD4+ T cells, associations between IL-17 and human disease have been known for many years. Particularly disorders previously classified as typical Th1 disease, such as rheumatoid arthritis (Kotake et al. 1999), inflammatory bowel disease (Fujino et al. 2003), and psoriasis (Arican et al. 2005), are now considered to be primarily Th17-driven. For that reason (chronic) lung conditions previously believed to be Th1 cell disorders deserve special attention as Th17 cells might contribute to their pathogenesis. Moreover, immunity mediated by Th17 cells seems particularly important at epithelial and mucosal surfaces, as indicated by the distinct pattern of expression of Th17 subset-associated chemokine and cytokine receptors (Aujla et al. 2008; Ouyang, Kolls, and Zheng 2008).

Because Th17 cells and IL-17 play a role in regulating neutrophilic and macrophage inflammation in the lung, a potential role in many different lung diseases including asthma and chronic obstructive pulmonary disease (COPD), cystic fibrosis (CF), pulmonary infectious diseases, sarcoidosis and other interstitial lung diseases and rejection after lung transplantation, seems legitimate. Asthmatics were shown to have elevated levels of IL-17A mRNA and protein levels in induced sputum and these levels were positively correlated with disease severity (Bullens et al. 2006; Molet et al. 2001; Al-Ramli et al. 2009). In COPD, recent studies showed increased expression of Th17 cytokines in bronchial mucosa and sputum (Di Stefano et al. 2009; Doe et al. 2010). Airway neutrophilia is a major feature of CF exacerbations and it is shown that sputum IL-17 is upregulated and correlates with *Pseudomonas aeruginosa* colonization (Dubin and Kolls 2007). In infection models in mice, there is considerable evidence that IL-17 and/or IL-23 are important in host responses against *Klebsiella pneumoniae* (Tesmer et al. 2008). Furthermore, several studies have now linked IL-17 to fibrosis in the lung in mouse models of pulmonary fibrosis and idiopathic pulmonary fibrosis in humans (Braun et al. 2010; Kurasawa et al. 2000; Wilson et al. 2010). Similarly, Th17 cells and IL-17 may be important regulators of the airway fibrotic response driving the development of bronchiolitis obliterans syndrome (BOS) upon lung transplantation.

For functional analysis of IL-17 producing cells in relation to other immune cells or epithelial cells, it is important to consider their anatomical localization. Obviously, bronchoscopy-guided or surgically guided biopsies allow histopathologically examination in situ, but are not frequently performed because they are invasive techniques. Bronchoalveolar lavage (BAL) is again not commonly performed except in lung transplantation and interstitial lung disease. For this reason sputum and nasopharyngeal washes are often studied. Blood and serum might be ideal to study because they are easily accessible. However, it is not always clear to what extend these compartments reflect what is happening in the lung. The methodology to study IL-17+ T cells in biopsies or in serum and BAL represents only indirect evidence of Th17 cells. Flow cytometry does provide direct evidence as it can combine several parameters (Figure 2). In this way, identification of distinct IL17+ T cells and even separate subpopulations is relatively simple.

3.1 COPD and asthma

COPD and asthma represent two classes of chronic obstructive lung disorders that may share some similar immunological disease mechanisms. COPD is marked by a progressive and irreversible airway obstruction and emphysematic changes in the lung. In asthma the airway obstruction is reversible and there is a marked airway hyperresponsiveness and airway inflammation. Recent studies on the immunological mechanisms of COPD and asthma pathogenesis point towards a role for IL-17 and Th17 cells in both diseases.

3.1.1 COPD

In COPD, chronic inhalation of toxic particles and gases causes destruction of lung parenchyma, activates epithelial cells, increases mucus production and stimulates migration of many inflammatory cells (Hogg 2004; Hogg et al. 2004). This results in an abnormal inflammatory response in the small airways and alveoli. It is believed that both the innate and the adaptive immune system are involved in this inflammatory process (Barnes 2008; Hogg et al. 2004). Progression of the disease is associated with the presence of lymphoid follicles, a histological hallmark of an adaptive immune response and termed bronchus-associated lymphoid tissue (BALT) collections. The presence of neutrophils, BALT collections, autoantibodies in the lungs, and also autoreactive T cells in the periphery, indicate CD4+ T cell involvement in the pathogenesis of COPD (Curtis, Freeman, and Hogg 2007; Feghali-Bostwick et al. 2008; Hogg et al. 2004; Vanaudenaerde et al. 2011). A potential role for adaptive immune responses in COPD has also been suggested in studies that show expansion of lung T and B cells with oligoclonality in patients with COPD and in murine emphysema models (Motz et al. 2010; Sullivan et al. 2005). To date, there are only few studies examining the expression of IL-17A and IL-17F in COPD. However, since neutrophilic inflammation (including elevated CXCL8 levels) is a common feature of COPD (Barnes 2000), and infiltrating CD4+ T cells in COPD were previously considered to be Th1 cells, it is expected that Th17 cells play an important role in this disease.

Although direct evidence for the role of IL-17 and Th17 cells in COPD remains largely absent, the importance of IL-17 in stimulating chemokine production and the role of neutrophils and macrophages in promoting COPD pathogenesis have led to interest in a potential connection (Curtis, Freeman, and Hogg 2007). Another possible link derives from the ability of IL-17 to drive matrix metalloproteinases (MMP)9 production, a protein which is involved in the breakdown of extracellular matrix, as is observed in emphysema (Prause et al. 2004). It is also known that IL-17-mediated signalling induces target cells to produce various inflammatory mediators such as TNF-α, IL-6 and IL-1β. Interestingly, increased levels of IL-6 and TNFα are found in sputum and BAL fluid and have been associated with disease severity in patients with COPD (Hacievliyagil et al. 2006). TNFα promotes CXCL8 expression from airway epithelial cells. Elevated levels of serum TNFα have also been linked to exacerbations in COPD patients (Calikoglu et al. 2004). In addition TNFα production by mast cells is increased due to IL-17A, leading to neutrophil infiltration in the airways (Feldmann et al. 2001). Furthermore, IL-17 is capable of increasing mucin production from airway epithelial cells (Prause et al. 2004) and excessive mucus production is one of the characteristic of COPD. Recently it was shown that patients with stable COPD exhibited elevated numbers of IL-22- and IL-23-positive cells in the bronchial epithelium and IL-17-positive cells in the submucosa when compared to healthy controls (Di Stefano et al. 2009; Doe et al. 2010; Chang et al. 2011). Additionally, airway smooth muscle cells from COPD patients express IL-17RA and respond to IL-17 by inducing CXCL8 production (Rahman et al. 2005). In contrast to these findings, the levels of IL-17 in sputum from patients with COPD do not differ from control subjects (Barczyk, Pierzchala, and Sozanska 2003). In addition to human studies, mice exposed to cigarette smoke exhibit enhanced IL-17 production (Melgert et al. 2007; Harrison et al. 2008). Experiments on murine lung epithelial cells have also shown that overexpression of IL-17A induces a COPD-like lung inflammation (Park et al. 2005). Taken together, these findings indicate a role for Th17 cells in COPD, but it is still unclear whether and how these cells contribute to disease pathogenesis or progression. Moreover, to what extend Th1 and Th17-mediated immune responses affect airway obstruction, emphysematic changes, inflammation or COPD exacerbations are questions that need to be addressed.

3.1.2 Asthma

Asthma is usually characterized by concurrent airway inflammation, cytokine production, and airway hyperresponsiveness to relevant antigens and a specific trigger. The central role of the Th2 subset in the disease, inducing airway eosinophilia and bronchial hyperresponsiveness, is well accepted. Individually, the Th2 cytokines can explain many of the salient features of asthma, including IgE induction in B cells (IL-4), airway eosinophilia (IL-5) goblet cell hyperplasia (IL-4, IL-13) and bronchial hyperreactivity (IL-13 acting on bronchial smooth muscle cells) (Wills-Karp et al. 1998). However, some individuals with asthma display airway neutrophilia rather than eosinophilia (Anderson 2008). It appears that in those patients with asthma in which inflammation is nonatopic, non-IgE-dependent, and noneosinophilic, airway neutrophilia is correlated with asthma severity. This suggests a major role for neutrophils, at least in this subset of patients with asthma (Louis et al. 2000). Neutrophilic inflammation has also been described in sudden-onset fatal asthma and neutrophil numbers are highly elevated in status asthmaticus (Lamblin et al. 1998). These observations suggest a role for these cells in severe and fatal asthma (Cosmi et al. 2011). With the involvement of neutrophils, several studies tried to find an association between Th17 lymphocytes and asthma.

Asthmatics have elevated levels of IL-17A mRNA and protein in breath condensate, sputum, BAL, and airway biopsies (Bullens et al. 2006; Pene et al. 2008; Molet et al. 2001). Furthermore, increased IL-17A and IL-17F levels are positively correlated to disease severity, suggesting an important role for IL-17A and IL-17F in severe asthma (Al-Ramli et al. 2009). Indeed, elevated IL-17A levels also correlate to increased neutrophilic inflammation, a characteristic of severe and steroid-resistant asthma (Bullens et al. 2006). One could also hypothesize that IL-17 may have opposite pathophysiological roles in different disease stages, as would be supported by findings in an asthma mouse model, indicating that IL-17A is required for induction of disease but negatively regulates established asthma (Schnyder-Candrian et al. 2006). IL-17F may also play an important role in the development of asthma, as a polymorphism in IL-17F which results in a loss-of-function mutation, is inversely related to asthma risk (Hizawa et al. 2006). In these studies however, the cellular source of IL-17 remained unknown, but recent studies attributed the production of IL-17 primarily to CD4+ T cells (Pene et al. 2008; Tesmer et al. 2008). A novel subset of Th2 memory cells that co-express the key Th2 and Th17 transcription factors, GATA3 and RORCT, respectively, and coproduce Th2 and Th17 cytokines was recently described (Wang et al. 2010). Interestingly, the number of IL-17+ Th2 cells was significantly increased in peripheral blood of atopic asthma patients. Compared with classical Th17 or Th2 cells, these IL-17+ Th2 cells had an increased capacity to induce influx of inflammatory leukocytes, and therefore are thought to represent key pathogenic cells promoting exacerbation of allergic asthma.

3.2 Pulmonary infections

There is considerable evidence that IL-17 and other Th17 cytokines are important in pulmonary host responses to infection by a variety of different bacteria, fungi and protozoa, and viruses. Also in infection, the major function of IL-17 appears to be to promote chemokine and pro-inflammatory cytokine production and consequent recruitment and activation of neutrophils and macrophages. Additionally, Th17 cytokines can control the infection by induction of anti-microbial peptides during the early immune responses at mucosal sites. Upon stimulation with various microbial agents, activated DCs secrete cytokines which determine the type of adaptive immunity that develops, i.e., whether the immune response is skewed toward Th1 or Th17 cells. Nevertheless, Th17 responses do not always seem to have a protective effect in mucosal infections. Current studies suggest that limited and correctly timed Th17 responses are protective, when appropriately balanced with concurrent Th1 immunity, but that uncontrolled Th17 cell activity could lead to a counterproductive level of organ inflammation (Tesmer et al. 2008).

Human studies on the role of IL-17 and Th17 cells in pulmonary infections are limited. The best human "model" demonstrating the role of IL-17 and Th17 cells in clearing pulmonary infections is Job's syndrome or the hyper-IgE syndrome. This syndrome is caused by loss-of-function mutations in STAT3, resulting in the inability of naïve T cells to differentiate into Th17 cells. These patients manifest chronic, recurrent and severe bacterial and fungal infections (Milner et al. 2008). Although other factors such as disturbed neutrophil chemotaxis are also involved in hyper-IgE syndrome (Hill et al. 1974), the Th17 cell deficiency is prominent. This therefore suggests an essential role for Th17 cells in the host immune system.

3.2.1 Bacteria

The host response to bacteria is largely triggered by Toll like receptor (TLR) ligands stimulating the production of inflammatory mediators, such as the pro-inflammatory cytokines IL-1β, IL-6 and TNFα, and the recruitment of phagocytic cells to the lung (Akira, Uematsu, and Takeuchi 2006). Several components of the innate immune system have been identified as key mediators of bacterial clearance such as neutrophils and macrophages. The role of Th17 cells in bacterial pneumonia is less clear. However, HIV patients with depleted CD4+ T cells are more susceptible to bacterial infections in the lung (Wolff and O'Donnell 2003), indicating a role for T cells in bacterial pneumonia.

One of the best studied bacterial pathogens in pulmonary host defense is *Klebsiella pneumoniae*. *Klebsiella pneumoniae* is a virulent Gram-negative pathogen that can cause pneumonia. In mice infected with this organism, TLR4 activation in the lung leads to production of IL-23 by DCs, which then stimulates CD4+, CD8+ and even γδ T cells to release IL-17 (Happel et al. 2003). Interestingly, both IL17A and IL17F are induced in a dose-dependent fashion (Aujla et al. 2008; Happel et al. 2005). Accordingly, the protective effects of IL-17 in host defense against bacterial pathogens were shown in studies that compared the susceptibility of IL-17R-deficient and control mice to *K. pneumoniae* infection (Ye et al. 2001). After intranasal infection, IL-17R-deficient mice were more susceptible to lung infection with *K. pneumoniae* (Happel et al. 2005; Ye et al. 2001). The increased bacteraemia and mortality observed in these mice were associated with delayed neutrophil recruitment and reduced expression levels of CXCL1, CXCL2, and G-CSF in the lung 12–24 hrs after infection. Related experiments demonstrated the essential role of IL-23 in triggering IL-17 production during this infection. Also IL-23-deficient mice are highly susceptible to *K. pneumoniae* and do not upregulate IL-17 in response to infection, whereas IL-17 production readily occurs after infection in control mice (Happel et al. 2005). Furthermore, administration of recombinant IL-17 restores the early chemokine response, enhances local production of TNFα and IL-1β, and reduces the bacterial burden in IL-23-deficient mice after *K. pneumoniae* infection (Happel et al. 2005; Ye et al. 2001). Together, these findings demonstrate that IL-17 produced in an IL-23-dependent fashion is essential for early recruitment of neutrophils and other inflammatory cells to provide immunity to *K.*

pneumoniae infection. In these studies it was also shown that in addition to IL-17 also IL-22 is measurable during infection. In contrast to gene deletion of IL-17, which results in a substantial reduction of CXCL1 and G-CSF in response to bacterial challenge, antibody neutralization of IL-22 causes an even more profound defect in mucosal immunity that leads to rapid dissemination of bacteria from the lung to the spleen (Aujla et al. 2008). The loss of mucosal immunity was not associated with defects in G-CSF or CXCL1 but with loss of barrier function and anti-microbial protein expressed in lung epithelium. Thus while IL-17 production by Th17 cells is critically important in host defense against *K. pneumoniae* infection in the airway because of its role in neutrophil recruitment and activation, IL-22 acts by augmenting the barrier defense against pathogens by triggering the production of anti-microbial peptides and enhancing healing of the epithelium should it be breached (Aujla et al. 2008). Importantly, not only Th17 responses are necessary for optimal protective immunity to *K. pneumonia*. Also IL-12-driven Th1 responses, resulting in efficient IFNγ production, contribute to the optimal bacterial clearance in a mouse model of *K. pneumonia* (Happel et al. 2005).

Following these initial studies with *K. pneumoniae*, the importance of IL-23 and IL-17 in host defense has been further established for a growing list of pathogens. Similar to *K. pneumoniae*, in mice infected with *Mycoplasma pneumoniae*, infiltration of the lungs by neutrophils is dependent on IL-23–induced upregulation of IL-17 (Wu et al. 2007). Additionally, accumulating evidence suggests that another Gram-negative extracellular respiratory pathogen, *Bordetella pertussis* which causes the whooping cough, may bias the host response towards the production of Th17 cytokines by preferentially inhibiting IL-12 and inducing IL-23 (Fedele et al. 2008). The above-referenced studies clearly demonstrate a protective role for Th17 effector cytokines in host defense against primary challenges with specific extracellular Gram-negative pathogens. Th17 response may also play a role in controlling primary infection with intracellular pathogens such as *Mycobacterium tuberculosis*, although a much more limited one when compared with extracellular bacterial pathogens. It was shown that although Th17 cells are not critical to the primary response to *M. tuberculosis*, Th17 activation is clearly involved in response to vaccination against tuberculosis (Khader et al. 2007). In addition to this Th17-mediated vaccine-induced immunity to *M. tuberculosis*, Th17 cytokine responses have also been implicated in vaccine-induced immunity against *B. pertussis* (Higgins et al. 2006) and *Streptococcus pneumoniae* (Malley et al. 2006). This indicates that the host Th17 effector cytokines have evolved as protective immune mechanisms against extracellular bacteria but are dispensable for primary protection against most intracellular pathogens that require a Th1 pathway for protection, such as in tuberculosis infection.

Pseudomonas aeruginosa is another Gram-negative pathogen. Although not as virulent as *K. pneumoniae*, *P. aeruginosa* is a highly adaptable pathogen that causes both acute and chronic pulmonary infections. Chronic colonization and infection in the lung is associated with pre-existing airway disease such as CF. CF is a disease characterized by the excessive production of aberrantly hydrated mucus in the airways, resulting from mutations in the ion channel cystic fibrosis transmembrane conductance regulator (CFTR). This increased mucus production, blocks normal ciliary function and thereby enhances recurrent pulmonary infections. During pulmonary exacerbation, CF patients exhibit airway neutrophilia and elevated levels of IL-23 and both IL-17A and IL-17F in bronchoalveolar lavage fluid and sputum (McAllister et al. 2005). Recently it was shown that CD4+ Th17 cells are prominently featured in the airway walls of CF patients but that NKT cells and γδ T cells are also sources of IL-17 in patients with CF (Tan et al. 2011). In the latter study, IL-17+ cells were correlated with CF and non-CF bronchiectasis, but not with the presence of *P. aeruginosa*. It has been shown that clearance of *P. aeruginosa* is dependent on Th17 responses (Dubin and Kolls 2007).

3.2.2 Fungi, viruses and other opportunistic pathogens

Several reports from mouse and human studies have shown that Th17 cells are important for clearing opportunistic infections such as *Cryptococcus neoformans, Pneumocystis jirovecii* and *Candida albicans*. E.g. patients with Job's syndrome are extremely susceptible to mucocutaneous fungal infections caused by Candida species. It has been suggested that Th17 cytokines, particularly IL-17, contribute to tissue pathology in invasive *Aspergillus* infection in the lung particularly in the setting of NADPH oxidase deficiency (Romani et al. 2008). In respiratory tract models of fungal infections using *P. jirovecci*, induction of IL-23 and IL-17 following pathogen challenge is protective, since IL-23KO mice or neutralization of the IL-23/IL-17 axis resulted in impaired clearance of the pathogen (Rudner et al. 2007).

Human viruses can induce IL-17 responses, as shown for herpes simplex virus (Maertzdorf, Osterhaus, and Verjans 2002) and respiratory syncytial virus (Hashimoto et al. 2005). Human rhinovirus infections are associated with exacerbations of asthma and COPD and IL-17 was shown to function synergistically with human rhinovirus to induce IL-8 from epithelial cells. This may contribute to the recruitment of neutrophils, immature DCs and memory T cells to the lung contributing to severe inflammatory profiles seen during viral exacerbations of airway disease (Wiehler and Proud 2007).

Taken together, there is accumulating evidence for the involvement of IL-17 in bacterial, fungal and viral infection in the respiratory system in the mouse, whereas in human the role of IL-17 or Th17 cells is largely unexplored.

3.3 Sarcoidosis, pulmonary fibrosis and other interstitial lung diseases

Interstitial lung diseases (ILD) refer to a very heterogeneous group of lung diseases affecting the lung parenchyma. The exact nature of the initiating event and the subsequent cascade of mechanistic proceedings are most likely different in every single ILD. Multiple factors are likely to be involved but it is now clear that the immune system plays a major part in the pathogenesis of ILD. A similarity in every ILD is the interaction of growth factors, cytokines, and other mediators with cells that reside in the lung which seem to form part of the cascade of events that have been identified in the pathogenesis.

Recent data point to a potential role of IL-17 and Th17 cells in a number of ILD. E.g. Wegener granulomatosis (Abdulahad et al. 2008), Langerhans histiocytosis (Coury et al. 2008), and hypersensitivity pneumonitis (Joshi et al. 2009; Simonian et al. 2009) have been reported to be linked to IL-17. Pulmonary IL-17 producing γδ T cells have also been detected in response to bleomycin-induced tissue damage, a model for induced pulmonary fibrosis (Braun et al. 2010). Conversely, a particular subset of γδ T cells secreting IL-17 has been shown to contribute to hyperinflammatory granulomatous disease and fatal lung tissue damage during pulmonary aspergillosis (Romani et al. 2008). Recently, also sarcoidosis was suggested as a Th1/Th17 multisystem disorder (Facco et al. 2011), based on the presence of IL-17 positive CD4+ T cells in sarcoid lung tissue and their ability to respond to the chemotactic stimulus CCL20. Moreover IL-17A was expressed by macrophages infiltrating sarcoid tissue. Sarcoidosis is a systemic inflammatory disease characterized by non-caseating granulomas in various organs with pulmonary involvement in over 90% of patients (ATS 1999). These granulomas are compact, organized collections of macrophages and epithelioid cells, surrounded by and infiltrated with T lymphocytes, but the pathological processes that result in granulomatous inflammation are largely unknown. The accumulation in the lung of apparently oligoclonal IFNγ-producing T helper cells in sarcoidosis indicated an antigen-driven Th1 response (Rosen 2007; Zaba et al. 2010). Also because IL-17A has been implicated in the formation of a mycobacterial infection-induced granuloma in the lung (Curtis and Way 2009), we investigated Th17 cells by intracellular flow cytometry and immunohistochemistry in blood, BAL and bronchial mucosal biopsies from a cohort of newly diagnosed sarcoidosis patients and healthy controls. These studies provided evidence for the involvement of the Th17 lineage in sarcoidosis: IL-17A-expressing T cells were present in and around the granuloma and IL-22-expressing T cells were found in the subepithelial lamina propria in mucosal biopsies of sarcoidosis patients (Figure 4). This was accompanied by the presence of IL-17A⁺, IL-17A⁺IFNγ⁺ and IL-17A⁺IL-4⁺ memory T helper cells in BAL and by a significant increase in the proportions of these cells in the circulation (ten Berge et al. 2011).

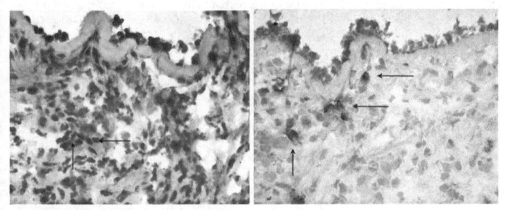

Fig. 4. IL-17A⁺ and IL-22⁺ cells in sarcoidosis lung biopsies containing granulomas. Hematoxylin nucleus staining and IL-17A (left) and IL-22 (right) staining of lung mucosal frozen sections from a granuloma-containing sarcoidosis biopsy (40 x magnifications). Arrows indicate IL-17A⁺ cells as well as diffuse IL-17A staining in red (left) and IL-22⁺ cells as well as diffuse IL-22 staining in the epithelium in red (right).

3.4 IL-17 in transplantation

Organ transplantation is currently a valid treatment option for selected patients with end-stage disease. Graft rejection is still the most severe complication following organ transplantation. In lung transplantation, episodes of acute rejection (AR) tend to lead to chronic rejection, which is the main cause of late graft loss and poor long-term survival (Lee, Christie, and Keshavjee 2010; Burton et al. 2007). The diagnosis of AR is based on clinical findings and/or histological confirmation in transbronchial biopsies (Vanaudenaerde et al. 2006). It has been shown that in addition to the frequency and severity of AR, also other risk factors such as ischemia-reperfusion injury (Lee, Christie, and Keshavjee 2010), gastro-oesophageal reflux (King et al. 2009), CMV pneumonitis and other infections (Valentine et al. 2009) are associated with an increased risk of chronic rejection. Chronic graft rejection, clinically known as BOS is defined as a progressive decline in lung function with other underlying conditions being absent (Estenne et al. 2002). More than 50% of the patients surviving five years after lung transplantation suffer from BOS (Christie et al. 2010).

Classically, graft rejection has been shown to be mediated by CD4+ and CD8+ T cells (Heeger 2003). Th1 cells were associated with graft rejection, whereas Th2 cells were considered to protect against rejection (Piccotti et al. 1997). Evidence is accumulating for an important role of IL-17 in allograft rejection, both in rodent models and humans. Prior to the first description of Th17 cells, IL-17 was implicated in the process of allograft rejection. Blocking IL-17 function in a rat cardiac allograft transplantation model increased graft survival significantly (Antonysamy et al. 1999). Around that same period, a number of reports highlighted the importance of IL-17 in the context of renal transplantation. Already in 1998 it was shown that IL-17 was detectable by immunofluorescent staining of acutely rejecting human renal transplant biopsies, but not in healthy kidneys or pre-transplant biopsies (Van Kooten et al. 1998). Moreover, elevated IL-17 mRNA and protein levels could be detected in renal biopsy specimens and urinary sediment from patients found to have subclinical rejection when compared with control samples without any evidence of rejections (Loong et al. 2002). Additionally, elevated IL-17 mRNA and protein levels were detectable as early as the second post-operative day in a rat renal allograft model and its appearance is followed by the local production of pro-inflammatory molecules known to be induced by IL-17 (Hsieh et al. 2001).

It is important to keep in mind that transplantation procedures themselves may have a direct effect on the cytokine profile within the graft. Following an organ harvest the ischemia-reperfusion injury results in the release of a number of inflammatory mediators. These mediators include some of the cytokines that are important in T cell differentiation such as TGFβ (Basile et al. 2001). A recent study demonstrated that factors released by human endothelial cells as a consequence of ischemia-reperfusion injury could enhance the production of both IL-17 and IFNγ by CD4+ T cells (Rao, Tracey, and Pober 2007). These findings indicate that perioperative factors might result in increased Th17 activity within the graft.

3.4.1 IL-17 in lung transplantation

In lung transplantation, IL-17 has been implicated in ischemia reperfusion injury, acute rejection, infection and BOS (Bobadilla et al. 2008; Vanaudenaerde, De Vleeschauwer et al. 2008; Yoshida et al. 2006). At day 28 after lung transplantation, IL-17 mRNA levels were found to be elevated in the bronchoalveolar lavage (BAL) fluid from patients with acute rejection when compared with those without rejection. This difference disappeared at longer follow up (Vanaudenaerde et al. 2006). These increased IL-17 levels were associated with increased numbers of both BAL lymphocytes and neutrophils and correlated with the severity of rejection (Vanaudenaerde et al. 2006). However, such a correlation with severity of rejection could not be confirmed in another study even though this study did show increased numbers of IL-17 positive cells in endobronchial biopsies early after lung transplantation (Snell et al. 2007). These apparently conflicting results may be explained by differences in the time of sampling, suggesting that early events after transplantation may be critical for inducing IL-17 production or that patient selection is crucial (Shilling and

Wilkes 2011). Additionally, patient heterogeneity may also cause conflicting results, e.g. by including both unilateral and bilateral transplant patients or by not discriminating between primary lung diseases.

Protein levels of IL-6 and IL-1β and mRNA levels for TGF-β, IL-17, IL-23 and IL-8 in BAL fluid were increased in lung transplant recipients with BOS when compared to controls (Vanaudenaerde, Wuyts et al. 2008). CXCL8, a potent chemoattractant for neutrophils, has previously been associated with BOS, but it was unclear whether the presence of neutrophils was just a marker of general inflammation or a key mediator of obliterative bronchiolitis (McDyer 2007). Since IL-17 promotes neutrophil chemotaxis, the presence of neutrophils has been suggested to be secondary to a Th17-mediated alloimmune or autoimmune response (Shilling and Wilkes 2011). In a mouse model increased levels of IL-6 and IL-17 also correlated with tracheal obliteration, and blockade of IL-6 decreased both allograft fibrosis and IL-17 transcripts (Nakagiri et al. 2010). Increased neutrophilic inflammation of the airways with upregulation of IL-8 is common in the BAL of BOS patients. However, there are also many of these patients without considerable BAL neutrophilia despite the fact that they seem to be in an identical clinical condition with progressive decline in lung function, compatible with BOS. This may indicate the existence of different phenotypes within BOS with possible different treatment strategies. BAL neutrophilia might therefore be an important tool to select patients who might benefit from azithromycin treatment, since it has been demonstrated that azithromycin significantly reduces airway neutrophilia and CXCL8 in patients with BOS (Gottlieb et al. 2008).

Th17 cell responses may also trigger BOS by facilitating autoimmune responses, because autoantibodies against collagen type V have been described to be involved in lung allograft rejection (Burlingham et al. 2007). Immunohistochemical analysis indicated that collagen V becomes exposed in the lung matrix after ischemia-reperfusion injury in rat lung isografts and allografts (Yoshida et al. 2006), and that collagen V peptides are released in the BAL (Haque et al. 2002). Additionally, in humans it has been shown that pre-transplant patients who exhibit collagen V reactivity have an increased incidence of early graft dysfunction following lung transplantation (Bobadilla et al. 2008).

Recent observations in our own group indicate that not only in BOS but also in stable lung transplantation patients IL-17 and other Th17 cytokines might play a role. We found enhanced Th17 differentiation of peripheral blood mononuclear cells (PBMC) in a group of stable lung transplantation patients, compared with both healthy individuals and patients on the waiting list for a lung transplantation. The increase in the proportions of circulating Th17 cells was not linked to donor-specific haploreactivity. Interestingly, increased proportions of circulating IL-17A+ CD4+ T cells co-expressing IFNγ were found, indicating that specific Th17 subpopulations may have a functional role in stable lung transplantation patients (Paats *et al.*, unpublished data).

4. Therapeutic potential

Accumulating evidence suggests that IL-17 and other cytokines involved in the Th17 pathway play an important role in the pathogenesis of various lung diseases. Interference with the activity of Th17 cells or the inflammatory mediators that either induce them (IL-1β, IL-6, and IL-23), act in concert with IL-17 (TNFα and IL-1β), or work downstream of IL-17 could be an effective treatment modality. One of these novel treatment modalities is cell blockade by monoclonal antibodies. Most antibody therapies have not yet been tested in lung pathology, which is remarkable because of the lung's continuous exposure to external triggers and pathogens. The risks of monoclonal antibody therapies must also be kept in mind. Adverse effects including infections, cancer and autoimmune disease are all issues that need consideration before antibody treatment can be introduced (Hansel et al. 2010).

The most direct way to control the biologic effects of Th17 cells would be to target production of their effector cytokines. Monoclonal antibodies against IL-17 or the IL-17R and a soluble IL-17R have been developed for clinical application. Administration of LY2439821, an anti-IL-17 monoclonal antibody, has been described in RA and improved signs and symptoms of the disease, without significant adverse events (Genovese et al. 2010). Additionally, it is promising that clinical trials with the fully human antibody, AIN457, in RA, psoriasis and noninfectious uveitis, show that targeting IL-17A interrupts inflammation and reduces disease activity (Hueber et al. 2010). Inhibitors of other products of Th17 cells such as IL-21 and IL-22 have not reached the clinical setting (Ma et al. 2008; Young et al. 2007). Another option might be to down-regulate IL-1β, IL-6 and IL-23, the cytokines that induce Th17 differentiation. Targeting the IL-6R with a monoclonal antibody (e.g., tocilizumab, a humanized monoclonal antibody against the receptor) and neutralizing the IL-1R with an antagonist (e.g., anakinra, a recombinant human IL-1R antagonist) are two effective approaches to the treatment of rheumatoid arthritis and other autoimmune inflammatory diseases (Dinarello 2005; Yokota et al. 2005). A monoclonal antibody (ustekinumab) targeting the shared IL-12/IL-23 p40 subunit, blocks both Th1 and Th17 cells and was shown to be efficient in the treatment of psoriasis and Crohn's disease (Griffiths et al. 2010). IL-17 induces the production of IL-1β and TNFα. Antibodies, antagonists or receptor antagonists to IL-1 and TNFα are already in use for a range of autoimmune and chronic inflammatory conditions (Sutton et al. 2009). Unfortunately, recurrence of immunoinflammatory disease when treatment with TNFα inhibitors is discontinued is common. A combination of IL-17 and TNFα inhibitors, administered either simultaneously or sequentially, might be a good alternative to better control inflammation (Nadkarni, Mauri, and Ehrenstein 2007; Miossec, Korn, and Kuchroo 2009). Targeting intracellular signaling molecules or transcriptional factors involved in the activation of IL-17 production e. g. by small molecule inhibitors is an alternative approach for the development of new drugs. However, it is complicated by the fact that many of the signaling pathways are not unique to the IL-23-IL-17 axis and may also inhibit responses of other cell types involved in protective immunity (Mills 2008).

Non-selective blockade of the adaptive immune system by the use of steroids or cyclosporine seem ineffective in patients with severe asthma, COPD and CF (Barnes 2008; Vanaudenaerde et al. 2011). This is probably due to the reported steroid resistance of the Th17 cell–neutrophil axis (McKinley et al. 2008). Other medication capable of dampening the innate immune system might be an alternative way to interfere with the Th17 pathway. The best documented therapy for reducing IL-17-T cell-mediated neutrophilia is macrolide therapy, which is being used effectively in clinical practice in patients with CF, asthma, COPD and BOS (Jaffe and Bush 2001; Seemungal et al. 2008). In addition, in vitro studies have shown that vitamin D inhibits Th17 cells (Mora, Iwata, and von Andrian 2008; Colin et al. 2010), hence vitamin D therapy might have potential in controlling Th17-mediated lung diseases. Clinical trials that could prove the importance of vitamin D in chronic lung diseases are currently in progress. Furthermore, other medication capable of interfering with the innate immune system, such as vitamin A or statins, merits attention (Vanaudenaerde et al. 2011).

5. Conclusions

We still have much to learn about the phenotype, function and regulation of human Th17 cells. It is however clear that IL-17 and other Th17 associated cytokines play a central role in regulating diverse immune responses. With their potential to induce a pronounced neutrophilic inflammation, which is a common feature of many pulmonary inflammatory conditions, Th17 cells are subject of great research interest. Important to realize is that besides Th17 cells there are also other sources of IL-17, including CD8+ T cells, γδ T cells, NK T cells, and LTi cells. Depending on the timing, the tissue, and the local microenvironment, IL-17 secreting cells appear to be able to play both beneficial and detrimental roles in lung immunity and disease. The exact balance of these roles during the processes of many autoimmune and infectious diseases is however not fully understood yet. Therefore, the challenge lies in uncovering strategies to maximize the protective effect of IL-17 producing cells while simultaneously preventing these cells from causing immune-mediated host damage. At present, therapies that modulate the Th17 cell pathway are being tested in the clinic with promising results.

6. Acknowledgement

We thank Bernt van den Blink, Alex Kleinjan and Ingrid Bergen (Erasmus MC Rotterdam) for their assistance and stimulating discussions.

7. References

Abdulahad, W. H., C. A. Stegeman, P. C. Limburg, and C. G. Kallenberg. 2008. Skewed distribution of Th17 lymphocytes in patients with Wegener's granulomatosis in remission. *Arthritis Rheum* 58 (7):2196-205.

Acosta-Rodriguez, E. V., G. Napolitani, A. Lanzavecchia, and F. Sallusto. 2007. Interleukins 1beta and 6 but not transforming growth factor-beta are essential for the differentiation of interleukin 17-producing human T helper cells. *Nat Immunol* 8 (9):942-9.

Acosta-Rodriguez, E. V., L. Rivino, J. Geginat, D. Jarrossay, M. Gattorno, A. Lanzavecchia, F. Sallusto, and G. Napolitani. 2007. Surface phenotype and antigenic specificity of human interleukin 17-producing T helper memory cells. *Nat Immunol* 8 (6):639-46.

Akira, S., S. Uematsu, and O. Takeuchi. 2006. Pathogen recognition and innate immunity. *Cell* 124 (4):783-801.

Al-Ramli, W., D. Prefontaine, F. Chouiali, J. G. Martin, R. Olivenstein, C. Lemiere, and Q. Hamid. 2009. T(H)17-associated cytokines (IL-17A and IL-17F) in severe asthma. *J Allergy Clin Immunol* 123 (5):1185-7.

Anderson, G. P. 2008. Endotyping asthma: new insights into key pathogenic mechanisms in a complex, heterogeneous disease. *Lancet* 372 (9643):1107-19.

Annunziato, F., L. Cosmi, V. Santarlasci, L. Maggi, F. Liotta, B. Mazzinghi, E. Parente, L. Fili, S. Ferri, F. Frosali, F. Giudici, P. Romagnani, P. Parronchi, F. Tonelli, E. Maggi, and S. Romagnani. 2007. Phenotypic and functional features of human Th17 cells. *J Exp Med* 204 (8):1849-61.

Antonysamy, M. A., W. C. Fanslow, F. Fu, W. Li, S. Qian, A. B. Troutt, and A. W. Thomson. 1999. Evidence for a role of IL-17 in alloimmunity: a novel IL-17 antagonist promotes heart graft survival. *Transplant Proc* 31 (1-2):93.

Arican, O., M. Aral, S. Sasmaz, and P. Ciragil. 2005. Serum levels of TNF-alpha, IFN-gamma, IL-6, IL-8, IL-12, IL-17, and IL-18 in patients with active psoriasis and correlation with disease severity. *Mediators Inflamm* 2005 (5):273-9.

ATS, ERS, WASOG. 1999. Statement on sarcoidosis. Joint Statement of the American Thoracic Society (ATS), the European Respiratory Society (ERS) and the World Association of Sarcoidosis and Other Granulomatous Disorders (WASOG) adopted by the ATS Board of Directors and by the ERS Executive Committee, February 1999. *Am J Respir Crit Care Med* 160 (2):736-55.

Aujla, S. J., Y. R. Chan, M. Zheng, M. Fei, D. J. Askew, D. A. Pociask, T. A. Reinhart, F. McAllister, J. Edeal, K. Gaus, S. Husain, J. L. Kreindler, P. J. Dubin, J. M. Pilewski, M. M. Myerburg, C. A. Mason, Y. Iwakura, and J. K. Kolls. 2008. IL-22 mediates mucosal host defense against Gram-negative bacterial pneumonia. *Nat Med* 14 (3):275-81.

Aujla, S. J., P. J. Dubin, and J. K. Kolls. 2007. Th17 cells and mucosal host defense. *Semin Immunol* 19 (6):377-82.

Barczyk, A., W. Pierzchala, and E. Sozanska. 2003. Interleukin-17 in sputum correlates with airway hyperresponsiveness to methacholine. *Respir Med* 97 (6):726-33.

Barnes, P. J. 2000. Chronic obstructive pulmonary disease. *N Engl J Med* 343 (4):269-80.

2008. Immunology of asthma and chronic obstructive pulmonary disease. *Nat Rev Immunol* 8 (3):183-92.

Basile, D. P., D. Donohoe, K. Roethe, and J. L. Osborn. 2001. Renal ischemic injury results in permanent damage to peritubular capillaries and influences long-term function. *Am J Physiol Renal Physiol* 281 (5):F887-99.

Bettelli, E., M. Oukka, and V. K. Kuchroo. 2007. T(H)-17 cells in the circle of immunity and autoimmunity. *Nat Immunol* 8 (4):345-50.

Bluestone, J. A., C. R. Mackay, J. J. O'Shea, and B. Stockinger. 2009. The functional plasticity of T cell subsets. *Nat Rev Immunol* 9 (11):811-6.

Bobadilla, J. L., R. B. Love, E. Jankowska-Gan, Q. Xu, L. D. Haynes, R. K. Braun, M. S. Hayney, A. Munoz del Rio, K. Meyer, D. S. Greenspan, J. Torrealba, K. M. Heidler, O. W. Cummings, T. Iwata, D. Brand, R. Presson, W. J. Burlingham, and D. S. Wilkes. 2008. Th-17, monokines, collagen type V, and primary graft dysfunction in lung transplantation. *Am J Respir Crit Care Med* 177 (6):660-8.

Boniface, K., K. S. Bak-Jensen, Y. Li, W. M. Blumenschein, M. J. McGeachy, T. K. McClanahan, B. S. McKenzie, R. A. Kastelein, D. J. Cua, and R. de Waal Malefyt. 2009. Prostaglandin E2 regulates Th17 cell differentiation and function through cyclic AMP and EP2/EP4 receptor signaling. *J Exp Med* 206 (3):535-48.

Braun, R. K., A. Martin, S. Shah, M. Iwashima, M. Medina, K. Byrne, P. Sethupathi, C. H. Wigfield, D. D. Brand, and R. B. Love. 2010. Inhibition of bleomycin-induced pulmonary fibrosis through pre-treatment with collagen type V. *J Heart Lung Transplant* 29 (8):873-80.

Bullens, D. M., E. Truyen, L. Coteur, E. Dilissen, P. W. Hellings, L. J. Dupont, and J. L. Ceuppens. 2006. IL-17 mRNA in sputum of asthmatic patients: linking T cell driven inflammation and granulocytic influx? *Respir Res* 7:135.

Burlingham, W. J., R. B. Love, E. Jankowska-Gan, L. D. Haynes, Q. Xu, J. L. Bobadilla, K. C. Meyer, M. S. Hayney, R. K. Braun, D. S. Greenspan, B. Gopalakrishnan, J. Cai, D. D. Brand, S. Yoshida, O. W. Cummings, and D. S. Wilkes. 2007. IL-17-dependent cellular immunity to collagen type V predisposes to obliterative bronchiolitis in human lung transplants. *J Clin Invest* 117 (11):3498-506.

Burton, C. M., J. Carlsen, J. Mortensen, C. B. Andersen, N. Milman, and M. Iversen. 2007. Long-term survival after lung transplantation depends on development and severity of bronchiolitis obliterans syndrome. *J Heart Lung Transplant* 26 (7):681-6.

Calikoglu, M., G. Sahin, A. Unlu, C. Ozturk, L. Tamer, B. Ercan, A. Kanik, and U. Atik. 2004. Leptin and TNF-alpha levels in patients with chronic obstructive pulmonary disease and their relationship to nutritional parameters. *Respiration* 71 (1):45-50.

Cella, M., A. Fuchs, W. Vermi, F. Facchetti, K. Otero, J. K. Lennerz, J. M. Doherty, J. C. Mills, and M. Colonna. 2009. A human natural killer cell subset provides an innate source of IL-22 for mucosal immunity. *Nature* 457 (7230):722-5.

Chang, Y., J. Nadigel, N. Boulais, J. Bourbeau, F. Maltais, D. H. Eidelman, and Q. Hamid. 2011. CD8 positive T cells express IL-17 in patients with chronic obstructive pulmonary disease. *Respir Res* 12:43.

Chen, Z., and J. J. O'Shea. 2008. Regulation of IL-17 production in human lymphocytes. *Cytokine* 41 (2):71-8.

Chen, Z., C. M. Tato, L. Muul, A. Laurence, and J. J. O'Shea. 2007. Distinct regulation of interleukin-17 in human T helper lymphocytes. *Arthritis Rheum* 56 (9):2936-46.

Christie, J. D., L. B. Edwards, A. Y. Kucheryavaya, P. Aurora, F. Dobbels, R. Kirk, A. O. Rahmel, J. Stehlik, and M. I. Hertz. 2010. The Registry of the International Society for Heart and Lung Transplantation: twenty-seventh official adult lung and heart-lung transplant report--2010. *J Heart Lung Transplant* 29 (10):1104-18.

Colin, E. M., P. S. Asmawidjaja, J. P. van Hamburg, A. M. Mus, M. van Driel, J. M. Hazes, J. P. van Leeuwen, and E. Lubberts. 2010. 1,25-dihydroxyvitamin D3 modulates Th17 polarization and interleukin-22 expression by memory T cells from patients with early rheumatoid arthritis. *Arthritis Rheum* 62 (1):132-42.

Cosmi, L., R. De Palma, V. Santarlasci, L. Maggi, M. Capone, F. Frosali, G. Rodolico, V. Querci, G. Abbate, R. Angeli, L. Berrino, M. Fambrini, M. Caproni, F. Tonelli, E. Lazzeri, P. Parronchi, F. Liotta, E. Maggi, S. Romagnani, and F. Annunziato. 2008. Human interleukin 17-producing cells originate from a CD161+CD4+ T cell precursor. *J Exp Med* 205 (8):1903-16.

Cosmi, L., F. Liotta, E. Maggi, S. Romagnani, and F. Annunziato. 2011. Th17 cells: new players in asthma pathogenesis. *Allergy* 66 (8):989-98.

Coury, F., N. Annels, A. Rivollier, S. Olsson, A. Santoro, C. Speziani, O. Azocar, M. Flacher, S. Djebali, J. Tebib, M. Brytting, R. M. Egeler, C. Rabourdin-Combe, J. I. Henter, M. Arico, and C. Delprat. 2008. Langerhans cell histiocytosis reveals a new IL-17A-dependent pathway of dendritic cell fusion. *Nat Med* 14 (1):81-7.

Crome, S. Q., A. Y. Wang, C. Y. Kang, and M. K. Levings. 2009. The role of retinoic acid-related orphan receptor variant 2 and IL-17 in the development and function of human CD4+ T cells. *Eur J Immunol* 39 (6):1480-93.

Crome, S. Q., A. Y. Wang, and M. K. Levings. 2010. Translational mini-review series on Th17 cells: function and regulation of human T helper 17 cells in health and disease. *Clin Exp Immunol* 159 (2):109-19.

Crotty, S. 2011. Follicular helper CD4 T cells (TFH). *Annu Rev Immunol* 29:621-63.

Cua, D. J., and C. M. Tato. 2010. Innate IL-17-producing cells: the sentinels of the immune system. *Nat Rev Immunol* 10 (7):479-89.

Curtis, J. L., C. M. Freeman, and J. C. Hogg. 2007. The immunopathogenesis of chronic obstructive pulmonary disease: insights from recent research. *Proc Am Thorac Soc* 4 (7):512-21.

Curtis, M. M., and S. S. Way. 2009. Interleukin-17 in host defence against bacterial, mycobacterial and fungal pathogens. *Immunology* 126 (2):177-85.

Di Stefano, A., G. Caramori, I. Gnemmi, M. Contoli, C. Vicari, A. Capelli, F. Magno, S. E. D'Anna, A. Zanini, P. Brun, P. Casolari, K. F. Chung, P. J. Barnes, A. Papi, I. Adcock, and B. Balbi. 2009. T helper type 17-related cytokine expression is increased in the bronchial mucosa of stable chronic obstructive pulmonary disease patients. *Clin Exp Immunol* 157 (2):316-24.

Dinarello, C. A. 2005. Blocking IL-1 in systemic inflammation. *J Exp Med* 201 (9):1355-9.

Doe, C., M. Bafadhel, S. Siddiqui, D. Desai, V. Mistry, P. Rugman, M. McCormick, J. Woods, R. May, M. A. Sleeman, I. K. Anderson, and C. E. Brightling. 2010. Expression of the T helper 17-associated cytokines IL-17A and IL-17F in asthma and COPD. *Chest* 138 (5):1140-7.

Dong, C. 2008. TH17 cells in development: an updated view of their molecular identity and genetic programming. *Nat Rev Immunol* 8 (5):337-48.

Dubin, P. J., and J. K. Kolls. 2007. IL-23 mediates inflammatory responses to mucoid Pseudomonas aeruginosa lung infection in mice. *Am J Physiol Lung Cell Mol Physiol* 292 (2):L519-28.

Duhen, T., R. Geiger, D. Jarrossay, A. Lanzavecchia, and F. Sallusto. 2009. Production of interleukin 22 but not interleukin 17 by a subset of human skin-homing memory T cells. *Nat Immunol* 10 (8):857-63.

Eberl, G., S. Marmon, M. J. Sunshine, P. D. Rennert, Y. Choi, and D. R. Littman. 2004. An essential function for the nuclear receptor RORgamma(t) in the generation of fetal lymphoid tissue inducer cells. *Nat Immunol* 5 (1):64-73.

Elias, K. M., A. Laurence, T. S. Davidson, G. Stephens, Y. Kanno, E. M. Shevach, and J. J. O'Shea. 2008. Retinoic acid inhibits Th17 polarization and enhances FoxP3 expression through a Stat-3/Stat-5 independent signaling pathway. *Blood* 111 (3):1013-20.

Estenne, M., J. R. Maurer, A. Boehler, J. J. Egan, A. Frost, M. Hertz, G. B. Mallory, G. I. Snell, and S. Yousem. 2002. Bronchiolitis obliterans syndrome 2001: an update of the diagnostic criteria. *J Heart Lung Transplant* 21 (3):297-310.

Evans, H. G., N. J. Gullick, S. Kelly, C. Pitzalis, G. M. Lord, B. W. Kirkham, and L. S. Taams. 2009. In vivo activated monocytes from the site of inflammation in humans specifically promote Th17 responses. *Proc Natl Acad Sci U S A* 106 (15):6232-7.

Facco, M., A. Cabrelle, A. Teramo, V. Olivieri, M. Gnoato, S. Teolato, E. Ave, C. Gattazzo, G. P. Fadini, F. Calabrese, G. Semenzato, and C. Agostini. 2011. Sarcoidosis is a Th1/Th17 multisystem disorder. *Thorax* 66 (2):144-50.

Fedele, G., M. Nasso, F. Spensieri, R. Palazzo, L. Frasca, M. Watanabe, and C. M. Ausiello. 2008. Lipopolysaccharides from Bordetella pertussis and Bordetella parapertussis differently modulate human dendritic cell functions resulting in divergent prevalence of Th17-polarized responses. *J Immunol* 181 (1):208-16.

Feghali-Bostwick, C. A., A. S. Gadgil, L. E. Otterbein, J. M. Pilewski, M. W. Stoner, E. Csizmadia, Y. Zhang, F. C. Sciurba, and S. R. Duncan. 2008. Autoantibodies in patients with chronic obstructive pulmonary disease. *Am J Respir Crit Care Med* 177 (2):156-63.

Feldmann, M., F. M. Brennan, B. M. Foxwell, and R. N. Maini. 2001. The role of TNF alpha and IL-1 in rheumatoid arthritis. *Curr Dir Autoimmun* 3:188-99.

Ferretti, S., O. Bonneau, G. R. Dubois, C. E. Jones, and A. Trifilieff. 2003. IL-17, produced by lymphocytes and neutrophils, is necessary for lipopolysaccharide-induced airway neutrophilia: IL-15 as a possible trigger. *J Immunol* 170 (4):2106-12.

Fossiez, F., O. Djossou, P. Chomarat, L. Flores-Romo, S. Ait-Yahia, C. Maat, J. J. Pin, P. Garrone, E. Garcia, S. Saeland, D. Blanchard, C. Gaillard, B. Das Mahapatra, E. Rouvier, P. Golstein, J. Banchereau, and S. Lebecque. 1996. T cell interleukin-17 induces stromal cells to produce proinflammatory and hematopoietic cytokines. *J Exp Med* 183 (6):2593-603.

Fujino, S., A. Andoh, S. Bamba, A. Ogawa, K. Hata, Y. Araki, T. Bamba, and Y. Fujiyama. 2003. Increased expression of interleukin 17 in inflammatory bowel disease. *Gut* 52 (1):65-70.

Genovese, M. C., F. Van den Bosch, S. A. Roberson, S. Bojin, I. M. Biagini, P. Ryan, and J. Sloan-Lancaster. 2010. LY2439821, a humanized anti-interleukin-17 monoclonal antibody, in the treatment of patients with rheumatoid arthritis: A phase I randomized, double-blind, placebo-controlled, proof-of-concept study. *Arthritis Rheum* 62 (4):929-39.

Godfrey, D. I., H. R. MacDonald, M. Kronenberg, M. J. Smyth, and L. Van Kaer. 2004. NKT cells: what's in a name? *Nat Rev Immunol* 4 (3):231-7.

Gottlieb, J., J. Szangolies, T. Koehnlein, H. Golpon, A. Simon, and T. Welte. 2008. Long-term azithromycin for bronchiolitis obliterans syndrome after lung transplantation. *Transplantation* 85 (1):36-41.

Griffiths, C. E., B. E. Strober, P. van de Kerkhof, V. Ho, R. Fidelus-Gort, N. Yeilding, C. Guzzo, Y. Xia, B. Zhou, S. Li, L. T. Dooley, N. H. Goldstein, A. Menter, and Accept Study Group. 2010. Comparison of ustekinumab and etanercept for moderate-to-severe psoriasis. *N Engl J Med* 362 (2):118-28.

Hacievliyagil, S. S., H. Gunen, L. C. Mutlu, A. B. Karabulut, and I. Temel. 2006. Association between cytokines in induced sputum and severity of chronic obstructive pulmonary disease. *Respir Med* 100 (5):846-54.

Hansel, T. T., H. Kropshofer, T. Singer, J. A. Mitchell, and A. J. George. 2010. The safety and side effects of monoclonal antibodies. *Nat Rev Drug Discov* 9 (4):325-38.

Happel, K. I., P. J. Dubin, M. Zheng, N. Ghilardi, C. Lockhart, L. J. Quinton, A. R. Odden, J. E. Shellito, G. J. Bagby, S. Nelson, and J. K. Kolls. 2005. Divergent roles of IL-23 and IL-12 in host defense against Klebsiella pneumoniae. *J Exp Med* 202 (6):761-9.

Happel, K. I., M. Zheng, E. Young, L. J. Quinton, E. Lockhart, A. J. Ramsay, J. E. Shellito, J. R. Schurr, G. J. Bagby, S. Nelson, and J. K. Kolls. 2003. Cutting edge: roles of Toll-like receptor 4 and IL-23 in IL-17 expression in response to Klebsiella pneumoniae infection. *J Immunol* 170 (9):4432-6.

Haque, M. A., T. Mizobuchi, K. Yasufuku, T. Fujisawa, R. R. Brutkiewicz, Y. Zheng, K. Woods, G. N. Smith, O. W. Cummings, K. M. Heidler, J. S. Blum, and D. S. Wilkes. 2002. Evidence for immune responses to a self-antigen in lung transplantation: role of type V collagen-specific T cells in the pathogenesis of lung allograft rejection. *J Immunol* 169 (3):1542-9.

Harrington, L. E., R. D. Hatton, P. R. Mangan, H. Turner, T. L. Murphy, K. M. Murphy, and C. T. Weaver. 2005. Interleukin 17-producing CD4+ effector T cells develop via a lineage distinct from the T helper type 1 and 2 lineages. *Nat Immunol* 6 (11):1123-32.

Harrison, O. J., J. Foley, B. J. Bolognese, E. Long, 3rd, P. L. Podolin, and P. T. Walsh. 2008. Airway infiltration of CD4+ CCR6+ Th17 type cells associated with chronic cigarette smoke induced airspace enlargement. *Immunol Lett* 121 (1):13-21.

Hashimoto, K., J. E. Durbin, W. Zhou, R. D. Collins, S. B. Ho, J. K. Kolls, P. J. Dubin, J. R. Sheller, K. Goleniewska, J. F. O'Neal, S. J. Olson, D. Mitchell, B. S. Graham, and R. S. Peebles, Jr. 2005. Respiratory syncytial virus infection in the absence of STAT 1 results in airway dysfunction, airway mucus, and augmented IL-17 levels. *J Allergy Clin Immunol* 116 (3):550-7.

Hayashi, N., T. Yoshimoto, K. Izuhara, K. Matsui, T. Tanaka, and K. Nakanishi. 2007. T helper 1 cells stimulated with ovalbumin and IL-18 induce airway hyperresponsiveness and lung fibrosis by IFN-gamma and IL-13 production. *Proc Natl Acad Sci U S A* 104 (37):14765-70.

Heeger, P. S. 2003. T-cell allorecognition and transplant rejection: a summary and update. *Am J Transplant* 3 (5):525-33.

Higgins, S. C., A. G. Jarnicki, E. C. Lavelle, and K. H. Mills. 2006. TLR4 mediates vaccine-induced protective cellular immunity to Bordetella pertussis: role of IL-17-producing T cells. *J Immunol* 177 (11):7980-9.

Hill, H. R., H. D. Ochs, P. G. Quie, R. A. Clark, H. F. Pabst, S. J. Klebanoff, and R. J. Wedgwood. 1974. Defect in neutrophil granulocyte chemotaxis in Job's syndrome of recurrent "cold" staphylococcal abscesses. *Lancet* 2 (7881):617-9.

Hizawa, N., M. Kawaguchi, S. K. Huang, and M. Nishimura. 2006. Role of interleukin-17F in chronic inflammatory and allergic lung disease. *Clin Exp Allergy* 36 (9):1109-14.

Hogg, J. C. 2004. Pathophysiology of airflow limitation in chronic obstructive pulmonary disease. *Lancet* 364 (9435):709-21.

Hogg, J. C., F. Chu, S. Utokaparch, R. Woods, W. M. Elliott, L. Buzatu, R. M. Cherniack, R. M. Rogers, F. C. Sciurba, H. O. Coxson, and P. D. Pare. 2004. The nature of small-airway obstruction in chronic obstructive pulmonary disease. *N Engl J Med* 350 (26):2645-53.

Hsieh, H. G., C. C. Loong, W. Y. Lui, A. Chen, and C. Y. Lin. 2001. IL-17 expression as a possible predictive parameter for subclinical renal allograft rejection. *Transpl Int* 14 (5):287-98.

Hueber, W., D. D. Patel, T. Dryja, A. M. Wright, I. Koroleva, G. Bruin, C. Antoni, Z. Draelos, M. H. Gold, Group Psoriasis Study, P. Durez, P. P. Tak, J. J. Gomez-Reino, Group Rheumatoid Arthritis Study, C. S. Foster, R. Y. Kim, C. M. Samson, N. S. Falk, D. S. Chu, D. Callanan, Q. D. Nguyen, Group Uveitis Study, K. Rose, A. Haider, and F. Di Padova. 2010. Effects of AIN457, a fully human antibody to interleukin-17A, on psoriasis, rheumatoid arthritis, and uveitis. *Sci Transl Med* 2 (52):52ra72.

Ito, Y., T. Usui, S. Kobayashi, M. Iguchi-Hashimoto, H. Ito, H. Yoshitomi, T. Nakamura, M. Shimizu, D. Kawabata, N. Yukawa, M. Hashimoto, N. Sakaguchi, S. Sakaguchi, H. Yoshifuji, T. Nojima, K. Ohmura, T. Fujii, and T. Mimori. 2009. Gamma/delta T cells are the predominant source of interleukin-17 in affected joints in collagen-induced arthritis, but not in rheumatoid arthritis. *Arthritis Rheum* 60 (8):2294-303.

Ivanov, II, B. S. McKenzie, L. Zhou, C. E. Tadokoro, A. Lepelley, J. J. Lafaille, D. J. Cua, and D. R. Littman. 2006. The orphan nuclear receptor RORgammat directs the differentiation program of proinflammatory IL-17+ T helper cells. *Cell* 126 (6):1121-33.

Jaffe, A., and A. Bush. 2001. Anti-inflammatory effects of macrolides in lung disease. *Pediatr Pulmonol* 31 (6):464-73.

Joshi, A. D., D. J. Fong, S. R. Oak, G. Trujillo, K. R. Flaherty, F. J. Martinez, and C. M. Hogaboam. 2009. Interleukin-17-mediated immunopathogenesis in experimental hypersensitivity pneumonitis. *Am J Respir Crit Care Med* 179 (8):705-16.

Khader, S. A., G. K. Bell, J. E. Pearl, J. J. Fountain, J. Rangel-Moreno, G. E. Cilley, F. Shen, S. M. Eaton, S. L. Gaffen, S. L. Swain, R. M. Locksley, L. Haynes, T. D. Randall, and A. M. Cooper. 2007. IL-23 and IL-17 in the establishment of protective pulmonary CD4+ T cell responses after vaccination and during Mycobacterium tuberculosis challenge. *Nat Immunol* 8 (4):369-77.

King, B. J., H. Iyer, A. A. Leidi, and M. R. Carby. 2009. Gastroesophageal reflux in bronchiolitis obliterans syndrome: a new perspective. *J Heart Lung Transplant* 28 (9):870-5.

Kolls, J. K., and A. Linden. 2004. Interleukin-17 family members and inflammation. *Immunity* 21 (4):467-76.

Kondo, T., H. Takata, F. Matsuki, and M. Takiguchi. 2009. Cutting edge: Phenotypic characterization and differentiation of human CD8+ T cells producing IL-17. *J Immunol* 182 (4):1794-8.

Kotake, S., N. Udagawa, N. Takahashi, K. Matsuzaki, K. Itoh, S. Ishiyama, S. Saito, K. Inoue, N. Kamatani, M. T. Gillespie, T. J. Martin, and T. Suda. 1999. IL-17 in synovial fluids from patients with rheumatoid arthritis is a potent stimulator of osteoclastogenesis. *J Clin Invest* 103 (9):1345-52.

Kryczek, I., A. T. Bruce, J. E. Gudjonsson, A. Johnston, A. Aphale, L. Vatan, W. Szeliga, Y. Wang, Y. Liu, T. H. Welling, J. T. Elder, and W. Zou. 2008. Induction of IL-17+ T cell trafficking and development by IFN-gamma: mechanism and pathological relevance in psoriasis. *J Immunol* 181 (7):4733-41.

Kurasawa, K., K. Hirose, H. Sano, H. Endo, H. Shinkai, Y. Nawata, K. Takabayashi, and I. Iwamoto. 2000. Increased interleukin-17 production in patients with systemic sclerosis. *Arthritis Rheum* 43 (11):2455-63.

Laan, M., Z. H. Cui, H. Hoshino, J. Lotvall, M. Sjostrand, D. C. Gruenert, B. E. Skoogh, and A. Linden. 1999. Neutrophil recruitment by human IL-17 via C-X-C chemokine release in the airways. *J Immunol* 162 (4):2347-52.

Lamblin, C., P. Gosset, I. Tillie-Leblond, F. Saulnier, C. H. Marquette, B. Wallaert, and A. B. Tonnel. 1998. Bronchial neutrophilia in patients with noninfectious status asthmaticus. *Am J Respir Crit Care Med* 157 (2):394-402.

Lee, J. C., J. D. Christie, and S. Keshavjee. 2010. Primary graft dysfunction: definition, risk factors, short- and long-term outcomes. *Semin Respir Crit Care Med* 31 (2):161-71.

Loong, C. C., H. G. Hsieh, W. Y. Lui, A. Chen, and C. Y. Lin. 2002. Evidence for the early involvement of interleukin 17 in human and experimental renal allograft rejection. *J Pathol* 197 (3):322-32.

Louis, R., L. C. Lau, A. O. Bron, A. C. Roldaan, M. Radermecker, and R. Djukanovic. 2000. The relationship between airways inflammation and asthma severity. *Am J Respir Crit Care Med* 161 (1):9-16.

Ma, C. S., S. Suryani, D. T. Avery, A. Chan, R. Nanan, B. Santner-Nanan, E. K. Deenick, and S. G. Tangye. 2009. Early commitment of naive human CD4(+) T cells to the T follicular helper (T(FH)) cell lineage is induced by IL-12. *Immunol Cell Biol* 87 (8):590-600.

Ma, H. L., S. Liang, J. Li, L. Napierata, T. Brown, S. Benoit, M. Senices, D. Gill, K. Dunussi-Joannopoulos, M. Collins, C. Nickerson-Nutter, L. A. Fouser, and D. A. Young. 2008. IL-22 is required for Th17 cell-mediated pathology in a mouse model of psoriasis-like skin inflammation. *J Clin Invest* 118 (2):597-607.

Maertzdorf, J., A. D. Osterhaus, and G. M. Verjans. 2002. IL-17 expression in human herpetic stromal keratitis: modulatory effects on chemokine production by corneal fibroblasts. *J Immunol* 169 (10):5897-903.

Malley, R., A. Srivastava, M. Lipsitch, C. M. Thompson, C. Watkins, A. Tzianabos, and P. W. Anderson. 2006. Antibody-independent, interleukin-17A-mediated, cross-serotype immunity to pneumococci in mice immunized intranasally with the cell wall polysaccharide. *Infect Immun* 74 (4):2187-95.

Manel, N., D. Unutmaz, and D. R. Littman. 2008. The differentiation of human T(H)-17 cells requires transforming growth factor-beta and induction of the nuclear receptor RORgammat. *Nat Immunol* 9 (6):641-9.

Mantel, P. Y., H. Kuipers, O. Boyman, C. Rhyner, N. Ouaked, B. Ruckert, C. Karagiannidis, B. N. Lambrecht, R. W. Hendriks, R. Crameri, C. A. Akdis, K. Blaser, and C. B. Schmidt-Weber. 2007. GATA3-driven Th2 responses inhibit TGF-beta1-induced FOXP3 expression and the formation of regulatory T cells. *PLoS Biol* 5 (12):e329.

McAllister, F., A. Henry, J. L. Kreindler, P. J. Dubin, L. Ulrich, C. Steele, J. D. Finder, J. M. Pilewski, B. M. Carreno, S. J. Goldman, J. Pirhonen, and J. K. Kolls. 2005. Role of IL-17A, IL-17F, and the IL-17 receptor in regulating growth-related oncogene-alpha and granulocyte colony-stimulating factor in bronchial epithelium: implications for airway inflammation in cystic fibrosis. *J Immunol* 175 (1):404-12.

McDyer, J. F. 2007. Human and murine obliterative bronchiolitis in transplant. *Proc Am Thorac Soc* 4 (1):37-43.

McGeachy, M. J., K. S. Bak-Jensen, Y. Chen, C. M. Tato, W. Blumenschein, T. McClanahan, and D. J. Cua. 2007. TGF-beta and IL-6 drive the production of IL-17 and IL-10 by T cells and restrain T(H)-17 cell-mediated pathology. *Nat Immunol* 8 (12):1390-7.

McKinley, L., J. F. Alcorn, A. Peterson, R. B. Dupont, S. Kapadia, A. Logar, A. Henry, C. G. Irvin, J. D. Piganelli, A. Ray, and J. K. Kolls. 2008. TH17 cells mediate steroid-resistant airway inflammation and airway hyperresponsiveness in mice. *J Immunol* 181 (6):4089-97.

Melgert, B. N., W. Timens, H. A. Kerstjens, M. Geerlings, M. A. Luinge, J. P. Schouten, D. S. Postma, and M. N. Hylkema. 2007. Effects of 4 months of smoking in mice with ovalbumin-induced airway inflammation. *Clin Exp Allergy* 37 (12):1798-808.

Michel, M. L., A. C. Keller, C. Paget, M. Fujio, F. Trottein, P. B. Savage, C. H. Wong, E. Schneider, M. Dy, and M. C. Leite-de-Moraes. 2007. Identification of an IL-17-producing NK1.1(neg) iNKT cell population involved in airway neutrophilia. *J Exp Med* 204 (5):995-1001.

Michel, M. L., D. Mendes-da-Cruz, A. C. Keller, M. Lochner, E. Schneider, M. Dy, G. Eberl, and M. C. Leite-de-Moraes. 2008. Critical role of ROR-gammat in a new thymic pathway leading to IL-17-producing invariant NKT cell differentiation. *Proc Natl Acad Sci U S A* 105 (50):19845-50.

Mills, K. H. 2008. Induction, function and regulation of IL-17-producing T cells. *Eur J Immunol* 38 (10):2636-49.

Milner, J. D., J. M. Brenchley, A. Laurence, A. F. Freeman, B. J. Hill, K. M. Elias, Y. Kanno, C. Spalding, H. Z. Elloumi, M. L. Paulson, J. Davis, A. Hsu, A. I. Asher, J. O'Shea, S. M. Holland, W. E. Paul, and D. C. Douek. 2008. Impaired T(H)17 cell differentiation in subjects with autosomal dominant hyper-IgE syndrome. *Nature* 452 (7188):773-6.

Miossec, P., T. Korn, and V. K. Kuchroo. 2009. Interleukin-17 and type 17 helper T cells. *N Engl J Med* 361 (9):888-98.

Molet, S., Q. Hamid, F. Davoine, E. Nutku, R. Taha, N. Page, R. Olivenstein, J. Elias, and J. Chakir. 2001. IL-17 is increased in asthmatic airways and induces human bronchial fibroblasts to produce cytokines. *J Allergy Clin Immunol* 108 (3):430-8.

Mora, J. R., M. Iwata, and U. H. von Andrian. 2008. Vitamin effects on the immune system: vitamins A and D take centre stage. *Nat Rev Immunol* 8 (9):685-98.

Mosmann, T. R., and R. L. Coffman. 1989. TH1 and TH2 cells: different patterns of lymphokine secretion lead to different functional properties. *Annu Rev Immunol* 7:145-73.

Motz, G. T., B. L. Eppert, S. C. Wesselkamper, J. L. Flury, and M. T. Borchers. 2010. Chronic cigarette smoke exposure generates pathogenic T cells capable of driving COPD-like disease in Rag2-/- mice. *Am J Respir Crit Care Med* 181 (11):1223-33.

Murphy, D. M., I. A. Forrest, P. A. Corris, G. E. Johnson, T. Small, D. Jones, A. J. Fisher, J. J. Egan, T. E. Cawston, C. Ward, and J. L. Lordan. 2008. Simvastatin attenuates release of neutrophilic and remodeling factors from primary bronchial epithelial cells derived from stable lung transplant recipients. *Am J Physiol Lung Cell Mol Physiol* 294 (3):L592-9.

Nadkarni, S., C. Mauri, and M. R. Ehrenstein. 2007. Anti-TNF-alpha therapy induces a distinct regulatory T cell population in patients with rheumatoid arthritis via TGF-beta. *J Exp Med* 204 (1):33-9.

Nakagiri, T., M. Inoue, E. Morii, M. Minami, N. Sawabata, T. Utsumi, Y. Kadota, K. Ideguchi, T. Tokunaga, and M. Okumura. 2010. Local IL-17 production and a decrease in peripheral blood regulatory T cells in an animal model of bronchiolitis obliterans. *Transplantation* 89 (11):1312-9.

Nurieva, R. I., Y. Chung, D. Hwang, X. O. Yang, H. S. Kang, L. Ma, Y. H. Wang, S. S. Watowich, A. M. Jetten, Q. Tian, and C. Dong. 2008. Generation of T follicular helper cells is mediated by interleukin-21 but independent of T helper 1, 2, or 17 cell lineages. *Immunity* 29 (1):138-49.

O'Shea, J. J., and W. E. Paul. 2010. Mechanisms underlying lineage commitment and plasticity of helper CD4+ T cells. *Science* 327 (5969):1098-102.

Ouyang, W., J. K. Kolls, and Y. Zheng. 2008. The biological functions of T helper 17 cell effector cytokines in inflammation. *Immunity* 28 (4):454-67.

Park, H., Z. Li, X. O. Yang, S. H. Chang, R. Nurieva, Y. H. Wang, Y. Wang, L. Hood, Z. Zhu, Q. Tian, and C. Dong. 2005. A distinct lineage of CD4 T cells regulates tissue inflammation by producing interleukin 17. *Nat Immunol* 6 (11):1133-41.

Pene, J., S. Chevalier, L. Preisser, E. Venereau, M. H. Guilleux, S. Ghannam, J. P. Moles, Y. Danger, E. Ravon, S. Lesaux, H. Yssel, and H. Gascan. 2008. Chronically inflamed human tissues are infiltrated by highly differentiated Th17 lymphocytes. *J Immunol* 180 (11):7423-30.

Piccotti, J. R., S. Y. Chan, A. M. VanBuskirk, E. J. Eichwald, and D. K. Bishop. 1997. Are Th2 helper T lymphocytes beneficial, deleterious, or irrelevant in promoting allograft survival? *Transplantation* 63 (5):619-24.

Prause, O., S. Bozinovski, G. P. Anderson, and A. Linden. 2004. Increased matrix metalloproteinase-9 concentration and activity after stimulation with interleukin-17 in mouse airways. *Thorax* 59 (4):313-7.

Rahman, M. S., J. Yang, L. Y. Shan, H. Unruh, X. Yang, A. J. Halayko, and A. S. Gounni. 2005. IL-17R activation of human airway smooth muscle cells induces CXCL-8 production via a transcriptional-dependent mechanism. *Clin Immunol* 115 (3):268-76.

Rao, D. A., K. J. Tracey, and J. S. Pober. 2007. IL-1alpha and IL-1beta are endogenous mediators linking cell injury to the adaptive alloimmune response. *J Immunol* 179 (10):6536-46.

Romani, L., F. Fallarino, A. De Luca, C. Montagnoli, C. D'Angelo, T. Zelante, C. Vacca, F. Bistoni, M. C. Fioretti, U. Grohmann, B. H. Segal, and P. Puccetti. 2008. Defective tryptophan catabolism underlies inflammation in mouse chronic granulomatous disease. *Nature* 451 (7175):211-5.

Rosen, Y. 2007. Pathology of sarcoidosis. *Semin Respir Crit Care Med* 28 (1):36-52.

Rouvier, E., M. F. Luciani, M. G. Mattei, F. Denizot, and P. Golstein. 1993. CTLA-8, cloned from an activated T cell, bearing AU-rich messenger RNA instability sequences, and homologous to a herpesvirus saimiri gene. *J Immunol* 150 (12):5445-56.

Rudner, X. L., K. I. Happel, E. A. Young, and J. E. Shellito. 2007. Interleukin-23 (IL-23)-IL-17 cytokine axis in murine Pneumocystis carinii infection. *Infect Immun* 75 (6):3055-61.

Sallusto, F., C. R. Mackay, and A. Lanzavecchia. 2000. The role of chemokine receptors in primary, effector, and memory immune responses. *Annu Rev Immunol* 18:593-620.

Santarlasci, V., L. Maggi, M. Capone, F. Frosali, V. Querci, R. De Palma, F. Liotta, L. Cosmi, E. Maggi, S. Romagnani, and F. Annunziato. 2009. TGF-beta indirectly favors the development of human Th17 cells by inhibiting Th1 cells. *Eur J Immunol* 39 (1):207-15.

Schnyder-Candrian, S., D. Togbe, I. Couillin, I. Mercier, F. Brombacher, V. Quesniaux, F. Fossiez, B. Ryffel, and B. Schnyder. 2006. Interleukin-17 is a negative regulator of established allergic asthma. *J Exp Med* 203 (12):2715-25.

Schwarzenberger, P., V. La Russa, A. Miller, P. Ye, W. Huang, A. Zieske, S. Nelson, G. J. Bagby, D. Stoltz, R. L. Mynatt, M. Spriggs, and J. K. Kolls. 1998. IL-17 stimulates granulopoiesis in mice: use of an alternate, novel gene therapy-derived method for in vivo evaluation of cytokines. *J Immunol* 161 (11):6383-9.

Seemungal, T. A., T. M. Wilkinson, J. R. Hurst, W. R. Perera, R. J. Sapsford, and J. A. Wedzicha. 2008. Long-term erythromycin therapy is associated with decreased chronic obstructive pulmonary disease exacerbations. *Am J Respir Crit Care Med* 178 (11):1139-47.

Shilling, R. A., and D. S. Wilkes. 2011. Role of Th17 cells and IL-17 in lung transplant rejection. *Semin Immunopathol.*

Simonian, P. L., C. L. Roark, F. Wehrmann, A. K. Lanham, F. Diaz del Valle, W. K. Born, R. L. O'Brien, and A. P. Fontenot. 2009. Th17-polarized immune response in a murine model of hypersensitivity pneumonitis and lung fibrosis. *J Immunol* 182 (1):657-65.

Snell, G. I., B. J. Levvey, L. Zheng, M. Bailey, B. Orsida, T. J. Williams, and T. C. Kotsimbos. 2007. Interleukin-17 and airway inflammation: a longitudinal airway biopsy study after lung transplantation. *J Heart Lung Transplant* 26 (7):669-74.

Song, C., L. Luo, Z. Lei, B. Li, Z. Liang, G. Liu, D. Li, G. Zhang, B. Huang, and Z. H. Feng. 2008. IL-17-producing alveolar macrophages mediate allergic lung inflammation related to asthma. *J Immunol* 181 (9):6117-24.

Spits, H., and J. P. Di Santo. 2011. The expanding family of innate lymphoid cells: regulators and effectors of immunity and tissue remodeling. *Nat Immunol* 12 (1):21-7.

Sullivan, A. K., P. L. Simonian, M. T. Falta, J. D. Mitchell, G. P. Cosgrove, K. K. Brown, B. L. Kotzin, N. F. Voelkel, and A. P. Fontenot. 2005. Oligoclonal CD4+ T cells in the lungs of patients with severe emphysema. *Am J Respir Crit Care Med* 172 (5):590-6.

Sutton, C. E., S. J. Lalor, C. M. Sweeney, C. F. Brereton, E. C. Lavelle, and K. H. Mills. 2009. Interleukin-1 and IL-23 induce innate IL-17 production from gammadelta T cells, amplifying Th17 responses and autoimmunity. *Immunity* 31 (2):331-41.

Szabo, S. J., S. T. Kim, G. L. Costa, X. Zhang, C. G. Fathman, and L. H. Glimcher. 2000. A novel transcription factor, T-bet, directs Th1 lineage commitment. *Cell* 100 (6):655-69.

Tan, H. L., N. Regamey, S. Brown, A. Bush, C. M. Lloyd, and J. C. Davies. 2011. The th17 pathway in cystic fibrosis lung disease. *Am J Respir Crit Care Med* 184 (2):252-8.

ten Berge, B., M.S. Paats, I. Bergen, B. van den Blink, H. C. Hoogsteden, B. N. Lambrecht, R. W. Hendriks, and A. KleinJan. 2011. Increased IL-17A expression in granulomas and in circulating memory T cells in sarcoidosis. *Rheumatology* in press.

Tesmer, L. A., S. K. Lundy, S. Sarkar, and D. A. Fox. 2008. Th17 cells in human disease. *Immunol Rev* 223:87-113.

Trifari, S., C. D. Kaplan, E. H. Tran, N. K. Crellin, and H. Spits. 2009. Identification of a human helper T cell population that has abundant production of interleukin 22 and is distinct from T(H)-17, T(H)1 and T(H)2 cells. *Nat Immunol* 10 (8):864-71.

Turato, G., R. Zuin, M. Miniati, S. Baraldo, F. Rea, B. Beghe, S. Monti, B. Formichi, P. Boschetto, S. Harari, A. Papi, P. Maestrelli, L. M. Fabbri, and M. Saetta. 2002. Airway inflammation in severe chronic obstructive pulmonary disease: relationship with lung function and radiologic emphysema. *Am J Respir Crit Care Med* 166 (1):105-10.

Vaknin-Dembinsky, A., K. Balashov, and H. L. Weiner. 2006. IL-23 is increased in dendritic cells in multiple sclerosis and down-regulation of IL-23 by antisense oligos increases dendritic cell IL-10 production. *J Immunol* 176 (12):7768-74.

Valentine, V. G., M. R. Gupta, J. E. Walker, Jr., L. Seoane, R. W. Bonvillain, G. A. Lombard, D. Weill, and G. S. Dhillon. 2009. Effect of etiology and timing of respiratory tract infections on development of bronchiolitis obliterans syndrome. *J Heart Lung Transplant* 28 (2):163-9.

Van Kooten, C., J. G. Boonstra, M. E. Paape, F. Fossiez, J. Banchereau, S. Lebecque, J. A. Bruijn, J. W. De Fijter, L. A. Van Es, and M. R. Daha. 1998. Interleukin-17 activates human renal epithelial cells in vitro and is expressed during renal allograft rejection. *J Am Soc Nephrol* 9 (8):1526-34.

Vanaudenaerde, B. M., S. I. De Vleeschauwer, R. Vos, I. Meyts, D. M. Bullens, V. Reynders, W. A. Wuyts, D. E. Van Raemdonck, L. J. Dupont, and G. M. Verleden. 2008. The role of the IL23/IL17 axis in bronchiolitis obliterans syndrome after lung transplantation. *Am J Transplant* 8 (9):1911-20.

Vanaudenaerde, B. M., L. J. Dupont, W. A. Wuyts, E. K. Verbeken, I. Meyts, D. M. Bullens, E. Dilissen, L. Luyts, D. E. Van Raemdonck, and G. M. Verleden. 2006. The role of interleukin-17 during acute rejection after lung transplantation. *Eur Respir J* 27 (4):779-87.

Vanaudenaerde, B. M., S. E. Verleden, R. Vos, S. I. Vleeschauwer, A. Willems-Widyastuti, R. Geenens, D. E. Raemdonck, L. J. Dupont, E. K. Verbeken, and I. Meyts. 2011. Innate and Adaptive Interleukin-17-producing Lymphocytes in Chronic Inflammatory Lung Disorders. *Am J Respir Crit Care Med* 183 (8):977-86.

Vanaudenaerde, B. M., W. A. Wuyts, N. Geudens, T. S. Nawrot, R. Vos, L. J. Dupont, D. E. Van Raemdonck, and G. M. Verleden. 2008. Broncho-alveolar lavage fluid recovery correlates with airway neutrophilia in lung transplant patients. *Respir Med* 102 (3):339-47.

Veldhoen, M., R. J. Hocking, C. J. Atkins, R. M. Locksley, and B. Stockinger. 2006. TGFbeta in the context of an inflammatory cytokine milieu supports de novo differentiation of IL-17-producing T cells. *Immunity* 24 (2):179-89.

Vogelzang, A., H. M. McGuire, D. Yu, J. Sprent, C. R. Mackay, and C. King. 2008. A fundamental role for interleukin-21 in the generation of T follicular helper cells. *Immunity* 29 (1):127-37.

Volpe, E., N. Servant, R. Zollinger, S. I. Bogiatzi, P. Hupe, E. Barillot, and V. Soumelis. 2008. A critical function for transforming growth factor-beta, interleukin 23 and proinflammatory cytokines in driving and modulating human T(H)-17 responses. *Nat Immunol* 9 (6):650-7.

Wang, Y. H., K. S. Voo, B. Liu, C. Y. Chen, B. Uygungil, W. Spoede, J. A. Bernstein, D. P. Huston, and Y. J. Liu. 2010. A novel subset of CD4(+) T(H)2 memory/effector cells that produce inflammatory IL-17 cytokine and promote the exacerbation of chronic allergic asthma. *J Exp Med* 207 (11):2479-91.

Weaver, C. T., and R. D. Hatton. 2009. Interplay between the TH17 and TReg cell lineages: a (co-)evolutionary perspective. *Nat Rev Immunol* 9 (12):883-9.

Weaver, C. T., R. D. Hatton, P. R. Mangan, and L. E. Harrington. 2007. IL-17 family cytokines and the expanding diversity of effector T cell lineages. *Annu Rev Immunol* 25:821-52.

Wiehler, S., and D. Proud. 2007. Interleukin-17A modulates human airway epithelial responses to human rhinovirus infection. *Am J Physiol Lung Cell Mol Physiol* 293 (2):L505-15.

Wills-Karp, M., J. Luyimbazi, X. Xu, B. Schofield, T. Y. Neben, C. L. Karp, and D. D. Donaldson. 1998. Interleukin-13: central mediator of allergic asthma. *Science* 282 (5397):2258-61.

Wilson, M. S., S. K. Madala, T. R. Ramalingam, B. R. Gochuico, I. O. Rosas, A. W. Cheever, and T. A. Wynn. 2010. Bleomycin and IL-1beta-mediated pulmonary fibrosis is IL-17A dependent. *J Exp Med* 207 (3):535-52.

Wilson, N. J., K. Boniface, J. R. Chan, B. S. McKenzie, W. M. Blumenschein, J. D. Mattson, B. Basham, K. Smith, T. Chen, F. Morel, J. C. Lecron, R. A. Kastelein, D. J. Cua, T. K.

McClanahan, E. P. Bowman, and R. de Waal Malefyt. 2007. Development, cytokine profile and function of human interleukin 17-producing helper T cells. *Nat Immunol* 8 (9):950-7.

Wolff, A. J., and A. E. O'Donnell. 2003. HIV-related pulmonary infections: a review of the recent literature. *Curr Opin Pulm Med* 9 (3):210-4.

Wu, Q., R. J. Martin, J. G. Rino, R. Breed, R. M. Torres, and H. W. Chu. 2007. IL-23-dependent IL-17 production is essential in neutrophil recruitment and activity in mouse lung defense against respiratory Mycoplasma pneumoniae infection. *Microbes Infect* 9 (1):78-86.

Yang, L., D. E. Anderson, C. Baecher-Allan, W. D. Hastings, E. Bettelli, M. Oukka, V. K. Kuchroo, and D. A. Hafler. 2008. IL-21 and TGF-beta are required for differentiation of human T(H)17 cells. *Nature* 454 (7202):350-2.

Yang, X. O., S. H. Chang, H. Park, R. Nurieva, B. Shah, L. Acero, Y. H. Wang, K. S. Schluns, R. R. Broaddus, Z. Zhu, and C. Dong. 2008. Regulation of inflammatory responses by IL-17F. *J Exp Med* 205 (5):1063-75.

Yao, C., D. Sakata, Y. Esaki, Y. Li, T. Matsuoka, K. Kuroiwa, Y. Sugimoto, and S. Narumiya. 2009. Prostaglandin E2-EP4 signaling promotes immune inflammation through Th1 cell differentiation and Th17 cell expansion. *Nat Med* 15 (6):633-40.

Yao, Z., W. C. Fanslow, M. F. Seldin, A. M. Rousseau, S. L. Painter, M. R. Comeau, J. I. Cohen, and M. K. Spriggs. 1995. Herpesvirus Saimiri encodes a new cytokine, IL-17, which binds to a novel cytokine receptor. *Immunity* 3 (6):811-21.

Ye, P., F. H. Rodriguez, S. Kanaly, K. L. Stocking, J. Schurr, P. Schwarzenberger, P. Oliver, W. Huang, P. Zhang, J. Zhang, J. E. Shellito, G. J. Bagby, S. Nelson, K. Charrier, J. J. Peschon, and J. K. Kolls. 2001. Requirement of interleukin 17 receptor signaling for lung CXC chemokine and granulocyte colony-stimulating factor expression, neutrophil recruitment, and host defense. *J Exp Med* 194 (4):519-27.

Yokota, S., T. Miyamae, T. Imagawa, N. Iwata, S. Katakura, M. Mori, P. Woo, N. Nishimoto, K. Yoshizaki, and T. Kishimoto. 2005. Therapeutic efficacy of humanized recombinant anti-interleukin-6 receptor antibody in children with systemic-onset juvenile idiopathic arthritis. *Arthritis Rheum* 52 (3):818-25.

Yoshida, S., A. Haque, T. Mizobuchi, T. Iwata, M. Chiyo, T. J. Webb, L. A. Baldridge, K. M. Heidler, O. W. Cummings, T. Fujisawa, J. S. Blum, D. D. Brand, and D. S. Wilkes. 2006. Anti-type V collagen lymphocytes that express IL-17 and IL-23 induce rejection pathology in fresh and well-healed lung transplants. *Am J Transplant* 6 (4):724-35.

Young, D. A., M. Hegen, H. L. Ma, M. J. Whitters, L. M. Albert, L. Lowe, M. Senices, P. W. Wu, B. Sibley, Y. Leathurby, T. P. Brown, C. Nickerson-Nutter, J. C. Keith, Jr., and M. Collins. 2007. Blockade of the interleukin-21/interleukin-21 receptor pathway ameliorates disease in animal models of rheumatoid arthritis. *Arthritis Rheum* 56 (4):1152-63.

Yusuf, I., R. Kageyama, L. Monticelli, R. J. Johnston, D. Ditoro, K. Hansen, B. Barnett, and S. Crotty. 2010. Germinal center T follicular helper cell IL-4 production is dependent on signaling lymphocytic activation molecule receptor (CD150). *J Immunol* 185 (1):190-202.

Zaba, L. C., G. P. Smith, M. Sanchez, and S. D. Prystowsky. 2010. Dendritic cells in the pathogenesis of sarcoidosis. *Am J Respir Cell Mol Biol* 42 (1):32-9.

Zheng, W., and R. A. Flavell. 1997. The transcription factor GATA-3 is necessary and sufficient for Th2 cytokine gene expression in CD4 T cells. *Cell* 89 (4):587-96.

Zheng, Y., P. A. Valdez, D. M. Danilenko, Y. Hu, S. M. Sa, Q. Gong, A. R. Abbas, Z. Modrusan, N. Ghilardi, F. J. de Sauvage, and W. Ouyang. 2008. Interleukin-22 mediates early host defense against attaching and effacing bacterial pathogens. *Nat Med* 14 (3):282-9.

3

Nocardia Infection in Lung Transplantation

Pilar Morales[1], Ana Gil-Brusola[2] and María Santos[2]
[1]LungTrasplant Unit, [2]Microbiology Department,
Hospital Universitario La Fe, Valencia
Spain

1. Introduction

Organ transplant recipients (OTR) in general and, in particular, lung transplant recipients (LTx) – due to their underlying disease, extensive surgery, and the continual and profound immunosuppression to which they are subjected – become perfect targets for the development of infections. These are more frequent and severe than in the non-transplanted population, and may be caused by either common or less frequent opportunistic pathogens such as the *Nocardia* species.

Nocardia are ubiquitous bacteria found mainly in soil, organic matter and water (Lerner, 1996). Based on the available literature and on our own experience, we know that they can cause infections in both immunocompetent (40%) and immunocompromised patients (B.L. Beaman & L. Beaman, 1994), with a low frequency in transplantations in general , which is somewhat higher in LTx. Onset of disease is generally insidious and it is difficult to diagnose and treat. It produces mainly respiratory symptoms, but complications can occur, spreading to other organs and causing high mortality. In this chapter, we intend to review various epidemiological, clinical, diagnostic, therapeutic and prophylactic aspects of *Nocardia* infections in adult LTx.

2. Epidemiology and pathogenesis

2.1 General aspects

The genus *Nocardia* includes aerobic, gram-positive, weakly acid-fast bacteria of the order Actinomycetales. Other microorganisms that belong to this order are *Corynebacterium*, *Rhodococcus*, *Gordonia*, *Tsukamurella*, *Actinomadura* and *Mycobacterium*, particularly rapidly growing nontuberculous mycobacteria (Sorrell et al., 2005), which can also cause infections in humans. More than 50 species of *Nocardia* have been defined either phenotypically or by molecular methods (Brown-Elliott et al., 2006). Originally, only 10-12 species were known to cause disease in humans, the most frequently described being *N. asteroides*, *N. nova*, *N. farcinica*, *N. transvalesis*, *N. brasiliensis*, *N. pseudobrasiliensis*, *N. otitidiscaviarum* and *N. brevicatena complex*, with variations according to different environments and authors. Nowadays, taxonomy of this genus has undergone considerable changes due to modern molecular techniques, such as identification by 16S ribosomal RNA gene sequencing. New species have been described, such as *N. cryacigeorgica* (Schlaberg et al., 2008), *N. veterana* (Pottumarthy et al., 2003), *N. abscessus* (Yassin et al., 2000), *N. paucivorans* (Eisenblatter et al.,

2002) and *N. kruczakiae* (Conville et al., 2004), which should be taken into account in case of isolation in LTx samples.

Immune response to *Nocardia* is T-cell mediated (Deem, 1983). Therefore, the reduced cellular immune response of solid OTR is one of the major factors predisposing a patient to infection; in fact, 60% of cases occurs in immunocompromised patients.

2.2 Frequency

Estimated frequency of *Nocardia* infection among solid OTR globally ranges from 0.1 to 3.5 (Peleg et al., 2007a). In the past, these cases were more frequent in kidney, heart and liver transplantations, and less in LTx (Husain et al., 2002), but recently infections in the latter have been described as the most frequent (3.5%, Peleg et al., 2007a; 1.8%, Santos et al., 2011; 1.9%, Ponyagariyagorn et al., 2008). This increased risk of *Nocardia* infection in LTx may be due to several factors: a) the graft may have anatomical deficiencies, including lung denervation, reduced cough reflex and poor mucociliary clearance (Kramer et al., 1993; Husain et al., 2002); b) the organ has been continuously exposed to the atmosphere, with constant stimulation of the lung by environmental antigens and an increased risk of rejection; and, therefore, c) a need for more intense immunosuppression than in other solid OTR. Moreover, high average levels of calcineurin inhibitors 30 days prior to infection have been independently associated with subsequent infection by *Nocardia* (Hewagama et al., 2011).

The most frequently reported species of *Nocardia* in LTx, with variations in percentage in different studies, are *N. nova*, *N. farcinica*, *N. asteroides* and *N. brasiliensis*.

2.3 Risk factors

There are two multivariate studies (Peleg et al., 2007a; Martinez-Tomás et al., 2007) which investigate the influence of several variables as risk factors for *Nocardia* infection in solid OTR. Among them, three have been described as independent: a) the doses of immunosuppressive therapy, as already mentioned; b) chronic use of corticosteroids; and c) cytomegalovirus disease in the previous 6 months (Paya, 1999).

The relationship between opportunistic infections, including nocardiosis, and alemtuzumab, a monoclonal antibody that targets the antigen D52 and is used to prevent graft rejection (Basu et al., 2005; Peleg et al., 2007 b) by causing profound lymphopaenia, has been also reported. Moreover, the use of rituximab (Kundranda et al., 2007), another immunomodulator that targets the CD20 protein found on B cells and used in solid OTR to prevent or treat antibody-mediated rejection, has also been described.

Finally, hypogammaglobulinaemia, combined with immunosuppression, may favour the development of *Nocardia* infections (Corales et al., 2000), as has been observed in heart transplantation.
Renal failure, prolonged respiratory support and early graft rejection may also be risk factors but have not yet been demonstrated in multivariate analysis.

2.4 Transmission

The main route for *Nocardia* infection is inhalation of aerosolised microorganisms. From the respiratory tract, bacteria can then move to other organs, the most commonly and seriously affected being the central nervous system (CNS). Involvement of skin and subcutaneous tissue, bones and joints, retina and, less frequently, other organs or structures (heart, kidney, peritoneum, endocardium, testicles, etc.) is also possible. Primary cutaneous infection can occur by direct inoculation in both immunocompetent and immunocompromised patients (Brown-Elliot et al., 2006). There is no evidence for human-to-human transmission and disease presents mainly as isolated cases, although an outbreak related to contamination by dust pollution (Sahathevan et al., 1991) in a liver transplantation unit and some spread by contamination of hands in a cardiovascular surgery unit (Wenger et al., 1998) have been documented based on molecular data.

3. Symptoms and radiology

Time of onset of infection after transplantation is variable, but tends to be late. It rarely occurs in the first month and may range from 1 to 28 years (Santos et al., 2011). The greatest risk is within the first year (Peleg et al., 2007a, Clark, 2009), but later cases have also been described (Peraira et al., 2003, Oszoyoglu et al., 2007). Pulmonary presentation is the most common, with subacute and insidious pneumonia. Less frequent is the cutaneous form, following a minor injury or by direct inoculation (Ambrosioni et al., 2010). Symptoms are usually non-specific and include fever, fatigue, dyspnoea, cough and pleuritic pain (Patel & Payá, 1997; Minero et al., 2009). Common radiographic abnormalities include irregular nodular lesions which may cavitate, diffuse interstitial infiltrates and lung consolidation with parapneumonic pleural effusion (Balikian et al., 1978; Morales et al., 2011) (Figure 1). Both lungs are usually affected, without significant anatomical or zonal distribution (Oszoyoglu et al., 2007). In the case of single-lung transplantation, *Nocardia* can infect both the native and the transplanted organ (Husain et al., 2002).

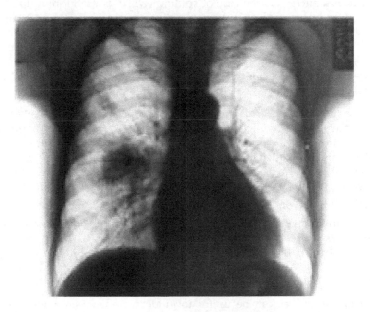

Fig. 1. Radiographic changes associated with Nocardia infection.

Haematogenous spread has been reported in up to 50% of cases (Clark, 2009), so it is important to exclude *Nocardia* clinically and/or radiologically in other organs, especially in the CNS (Singh & Husain, 2000). Moreover, and especially when the patient has a central venous catheter, blood should be cultured to rule out *Nocardia*. Cerebral involvement may be asymptomatic, therefore requiring neuroimaging with magnetic resonance or high resolution computed tomography (Ambrosini et al., 2010), or symptomatic, with headache, vomiting, altered level of consciousness, focal signs and seizures. Multiple radiographic cerebral lesions are observed in 40% (Singh & Husain, 2000). Meningitis is uncommon. Other forms of presentation of dissemination are cutaneous, ocular, intestinal, testicular and bone and joint disorders. Primary as well as disseminated cutaneous forms may present as subcutaneous nodules, cellulitis, abscess, mycetoma and sporotrichoid skin changes (Merigou et al., 1998). In this location, *N. brasiliensis* is the most common. The presence of the cutaneous form in organ transplant recipients should be followed by the exclusion of other forms of presentation of nocardiosis.

We must take into account the possible and frequent co-infections that occur with common and opportunistic bacteria, viruses, especially CMV, and fungi, mainly *Aspergillus* (Cabada et al., 2010) that make the patient's clinical and therapeutic management difficult (Santos et al., 2011). Differential diagnosis of pulmonary infection and brain nodule must include *Nocardia*, *Aspergillus* spp., *Cryptococcus neoformans*, *Mycobacteria*, *Rhodococcus equi*, post-transplant lymphoproliferative disease and primary lung cancer with metastasis.

4. Microbiological diagnosis

Definitive diagnosis of nocardiosis requires microscopic observation, isolation or nucleic acid detection of *Nocardia* in one or more samples from a suspected site. Specimen collection can be spontaneous, such as in the case of sputum (which is useful in up to 53% of cases), superficial such as in the case of a skin smear, or may require deeper samples such as bronchoaspirate, bronchoalveolar lavage or tissue biopsies. Smear staining with Gram stain, Ziehl-Neelsen (ZN) and modified ZN is the most useful and fastest diagnostic method. It can provide a diagnosis within the first few hours, showing abundant gram-positive or partially acid-fast branched bacilli (Figure 2), which are very characteristic of *Nocardia*, with moderate or abundant leukocytes resulting from the inflammatory response.

Differential diagnosis with *Rhodococcus*, *Gordonia* and rapidly growing mycobacteria must be considered, as discussed above. This information provides a reliable presumptive diagnosis and may guide empiric antibiotic therapy. Although *Nocardia* may grow in non-selective culture media, samples that can be contaminated with normal flora, such as those from the respiratory tract, should also be cultured in selective media such as Thayer-Martin agar with antibiotics (Shawar et al., 1990). Typical colonies appear chalky white (Figure 3) with aerial hyphae. Its growth is aerobic and may take from 2 to 5 days, sometimes even a week.

Species identification may by phenotypic, at least for the most common *Nocardia*, but genotypic methods such as polymerase chain reaction (PCR), restriction endonuclease analysis and sequencing of a portion of the 16S rRNA gene provide a safer and more accurate diagnosis. These techniques, however, are carried out by a limited number of laboratories (Brown-Elliot et al., 2006).

Identification of the species can be useful to guide treatment, since some have intrinsic resistance to several antibiotics, or to predict prognosis, since some species, such as *N.*

farcinica, are more virulent. In cases in which disseminated nocardiosis is suspected, *Nocardia* can also be isolated from a blood culture, although this is rare.

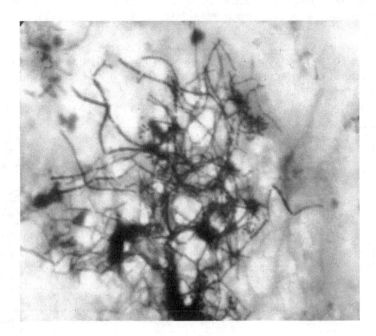

Fig. 2. Nocardia ZN stain.

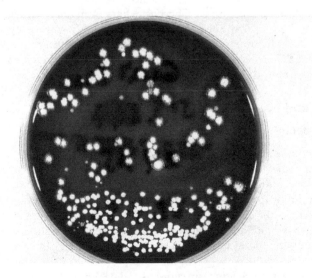

Fig. 3. Colonies of Nocardia.

Antimicrobial susceptibility testing of the *Nocardia* isolate is strongly recommended by the Clinical Laboratory Standard Institute (CLSI), which published the first approved methods in 2003 (Wayne, 2003). Primary susceptibility testing must include amikacin, amoxicillin/clavulanic acid, ceftriaxone, ciprofloxacin, clarithromycin, imipenem, linezolid, minocycline, trimethoprim-sulfamethoxazole (TMP/SMX) and tobramycin. Secondary recommendations include cefepime, cefotaxime, doxycycline, gentamicin and moxifloxacin. Some species of *Nocardia* have more predictable susceptibility patterns or, in other words, there are patterns of known resistance, such as *N. otitidiscaviarum* to imipenem, or the multi-resistance of *N. farcinica*, so it is sometimes necessary to perform *in vitro* synergy studies. The susceptibility patterns of the most common *Nocardia* can be seen in table 1.

	N. asteroides	*N. nova*	*N. farcinica*	*N. brasiliensis*
TMP/SMX	S (91-100)	S (89-100)	S (89-100)	S (100)
AMC	R (0-70)	R (3-50)	S (40-100)	S (65-100)
CEF	S (75-100)	S (70-100)	S (70-100)	V (50-100)
IMP	S (70-100)	S (100)	S (100)	V (0-100)
AMK	S (85-100)	S (100)	S (100)	S (100)
LZD	S (100)	S (100)	S (100)	S (100)
MIN	V (25-100)	V (29-100)	V (12-96)	S (0-100)
CIP	R(0-98)	R (0)	S (50-100)	R (0-30)
MXF	(50)	-	(88)	-

Table 1. Expected and reported antimicrobial susceptibility of selected *Nocardia* species (% of isolates susceptible in various series). Composite data from references (Clark, 2009; Hewagama et al., 2011; Brown-Elliott et al., 2001). TMP/SMX, trimethoprim-sulfamethoxazole; AMC, amoxicillin/clavulanic acid; CEF, ceftriaxone; IMP, imipenem; AMK, amikacin; LZD, linezolid; MIN, minocycline; CIP, ciprofloxacin; MXF, moxifloxacin; S, sensitive; R, resistant; V, variable.

5. Treatment and evolution

5.1 General aspects

Treatment of *Nocardia* infections in LTx is based primarily on antibiotics. In some cases, such as brain or cutaneous abscesses that do not respond to initial antibacterial therapy, surgical drainage is also required and, whenever possible, especially in more severe cases, a reduction of immunosuppressive therapy should be applied. The best treatment has not yet been determined. In the past, the antimicrobial of choice was TMP/SMX, but since the development of new antibiotics, *in vitro* synergy studies, the insidious nature of the disease and its high mortality, the recommendation is a combination of two or three drugs (Clark, 2009).

There are few studies correlating susceptibility data with clinical outcome (Sorrell et al., 2005), so the best combination is uncertain. Nevertheless, it is often chosen on the basis of: a) the species of *Nocardia* isolated; b) its sensitivity to antibiotics and possible interactions with the complex medication of transplanted patients; c) the location, extent and severity of the infection; and d) the experts' opinion and documented experience in the literature.

5.2 Empiric therapy

According to clinical experience, TMP/SMX remains the antimicrobial agent of choice for many *Nocardia* infections (Hewagama et al., 2011), supported by the *in vitro* synergy of its two components, the fact that it reaches high levels in lung, brain, skin and bone (Smego et al., 1983) and that it can be used as intravenous or oral maintenance therapy (Table 2). The main side effects include rash, nausea, vomiting, erythema multiforme, bone marrow suppression, hyperkalaemia and crystalluria, which may limit its use. Some species – *N. farcinica, N. otitidiscaviarum* and *N. nova* – may be resistant to sulphonamides, so it is important to determine the species and its *in vitro* susceptibility. These resistances and possible allergies to sulphonamides promoted the search for alternative antibiotics. Amikacin is universally active against most *Nocardia* species, except for *N. transvaliensis* and *N. brasiliensis*. The main limitations for its use are optical and renal toxicity. The combination of imipenem and amikacin is accepted as initial therapy in patients with severe nocardiosis (Minero et al., 2009) while the antibiogram is pending. This antibiotic combination is additive and synergic *in vitro* (Kanemitsu et al., 2003), maintains synergy when associated with sulphonamides (Gombert et al., 1986) and is effective in humans, so this triple combination has also been recommended as first-line treatment in patients with severe disease including dissemination to the CNS, where it is always better to use at least two drugs with good intracranial diffusion and, when severe, a triple combination (Ambrosioni et al., 2010). During the administration of amikacin and imipenem, doses should be adjusted according to renal function and auditory function should be monitored. In addition, in LTx, co-administration of cyclosporine or tacrolimus with amikacin may enhance the nephrotoxicity of aminoglycosides.

INFECTION	PRIMARY THERAPY	ALTERNATIVE THERAPY
Primary cutaneous	TMP/SMX*	TMP/SMX+ Fluoroquinolone
Pulmonary stable	TMP/SMX iv or po	Imipenem+amikacin or minocycline or linezolid
Pulmonary critical	Imipenem+amikacin or TMP/SMX	Linezolid
Cerebral	Imipenem+amikacin or TMP/SMX	Linezolid or ceftriaxone or cefotaxime or minocycline
Disseminated	Imipenem+amikacin or TMP/SMX	Ceftriaxone, cefotaxime, linezolid or minocycline

Table 2. Antibiotics suggested for Nocardia infections in organ recipients (Clark, 2009, Ambrosioni et al., 2010, modified). TMP/SMX, trimethoprim-sulfamethoxazole.

As regards the carbapenems, imipenem and meropenem have a similar spectrum of activity and effectiveness and, although the latter is somewhat less effective against *N. asteroides complex* (NAC) and more effective against *N. brasiliensis* and *N. otitidiscaviarum*, it is preferred in cases with CNS involvement, since imipenem has been associated with seizures. Ertapenem has slightly less activity against several species of *Nocardia* and doripenem, with a similar spectrum of antibiotic activity to meropenem (Lai et al., 2009) but without CNS penetration, has not been tested.

Other beta-lactam antibiotics such as the third-generation cephalosporins ceftriaxone or cefotaxime, due to their good CNS penetration, may be combined with other antimicrobials for treatment of intracranial infections with good results, depending on the species of *Nocardia*, since some may be intrinsically resistant (Garlando et al., 1992; Durmaz et al., 2001).

5.3 Other alternatives

The literature includes experiences of varying degrees of success with other antibiotic treatments, including minocycline and tigecycline, macrolides, ampicillin, piperacillin/ tazobactam, fluoroquinolones (ciprofloxacin, moxifloxacin and gatifloxacin), but experiences are limited and there is not enough scientific basis to include them in general recommendations. With moxifloxacin, which is active against *N. farcinica* (Hanse et al., 2008), good results have been obtained in some cases; however, in others there has been recurrence in the CNS, despite its activity and having achieved high levels of drug in the abscess material (Dahan et al., 2006).

In recent years, the oxazolidinone linezolid has been gathering attention due to its excellent activity against all species of *Nocardia*, including *N. farcinica* (Brown-Elliot et al., 2001). It has been used successfully, even in monotherapy, in six patients with disseminated nocardiosis (Moylett et al., 2003) and also in combination with other antimicrobials (Lewis et al., 2003; Rivero et al., 2008). It has extensive intravenous and oral bioavailability, crosses the blood-brain barrier, does not require renal or liver dose adjustments and has few interactions with immunosuppressive agents (Jodlowski et al., 2007), which makes it a very reasonable alternative as first- or second-line treatment of *Nocardia* infections in LTx (especially in cases of kidney involvement). Limitations on long-term use are conditioned by its high cost and possible toxicity, since, in addition to its minor adverse effects such as rash, nausea and vomiting, it may also induce, less frequently, thrombocytopaenia, aplastic anaemia, peripheral neuropathy, lactic acidosis and serotonin syndrome (Beekmann et al., 2008).

5.4 Duration of treatment

The optimal duration of treatment has not been standardised, but should be several months due to the difficulty of eradicating *Nocardia* and frequency of relapse (Sorrell et al., 2005). Most patients begin to improve in 1-2 weeks, but more severe cases must follow an additional 3 to 4 weeks of intravenous therapy before switching to oral treatment. Cerebral nocardiosis requires at least 9-12 months of treatment, whereas soft tissue and lung presentations require 6-12 months, depending on the clinical course and response to treatment (Clark, 2009). If the infection is associated with a central venous catheter, this must be removed and followed by administration of antibiotic treatment for several months.

5.5 Consolidation therapy

When the patient improves and intravenous treatment can be withdrawn, oral alternatives may include amoxicillin-clavulanate, TMP/SMX, linezolid, clarithromycin, ciprofloxacin and moxifloxacin as consolidation therapy. There are no trials comparing the effects of these antibiotics. Some studies recommend a dual oral combination after severe infections, such as those involving the CNS (Sullivan & Chapman, 2010).

After discontinuation of treatment, the patient should be monitored for a minimum of one year to detect possible relapses. In some hospitals, prophylaxis is maintained for as long as the patient remains immunosuppressed (King et al., 1993; Poonyagariyagorn et al., 2008).

5.6 Evolution

Despite combined treatment, the prognosis is variable and depends heavily on: the extent of infection, the underlying conditions of the organ recipients and co-infections that precede or coincide with *Nocardia* infection (Peleg et al., 2007b). Overall mortality is around 40% (Husain et al., 2002). In CNS infections it is 30-55% (Mamelak et al., 1994) and in the lung about 14-18% (Poonyagariyagorn et al., 2008; Morales et al., 2011). The prognosis is better in isolated skin lesions, in which some studies report up to 90% healing.

Delayed diagnosis and discontinuation of treatment has also been associated with poor prognosis. There is little information on the crude mortality rate, because in many cases the patient died due to multiple causes and it is difficult to determine the impact of *Nocardia* infection on the final outcome.

6. Prevention/Prophylaxis

Given the low incidence of *Nocardia* infection in LTx and that its onset tends to be late, primary chemoprophylaxis is not indicated. However, in patients with solid organ transplant in general, TMP/SMX is administered daily for at least six months post-transplant and then on alternate days indefinitely to prevent infection by *Pneumocystis jiroveci* (Hewayama et al., 2011). Some works suggest that this prophylaxis reduces infection by *Nocardia* and this benefit extends to other microorganisms. Nevertheless, there is an increasing number of reports of TMP/SMX susceptible *Nocardia* isolations in transplant recipients taking this antibiotic as prophylaxis (Roberts et al., 2000; Husain et al., 2002; Poonyagariyagorn et al., 2008; Khan et al., 2008; Minero et al., 2009). This fact raises doubts concerning the prophylactic role of TMP/SMX to prevent nocardiosis. The lack of efficacy may be due to different protocols in SOT recipients. Relapse has also been documented in LTx (Poonyagariyagorn, 2008; Roberts et al., 2000) after one cycle of antibiotic treatment, possibly due to short-term duration or interruption, but the data are controversial with regard to recommending secondary prophylaxis. Long-term prophylaxis to prevent these relapses is only suggested in a few hospitals.

Moreover, considering that *Nocardia* is a ubiquitous microorganism, it is important to teach LTx to alter their lifestyle and adopt a careful and alert attitude in order to reduce their high epidemiological risk of exposure, especially in the community. Recently, Avery and Michaels have published an excellent guide to strategies for avoiding infection following solid organ transplantation (Avery & Michaels, 2009).

7. Peri-Transplant considerations

7.1 Pre-Transplant

The future LTx may have had an infection that has already been treated or that is still active during the pre-transplant evaluation period. In fact, this happens with some frequency in patients with cystic fibrosis (CF). Neither situation, according to most experts and to our own experience, is an absolute contraindication for transplantation. Nevertheless, the patient must be monitored closely, being aware of possible relapses, complications or dissemination of infection, and ensuring full compliance with treatment.

7.2 Post-Transplant

Considerations are similar when nocardiosis occurs after transplantation, as we have previously discussed in the text, paying special attention to possible relapses.

7.3 Donor

Even though there is no documented case of *Nocardia* infection in the organ donor, nocardiosis would hypothetically be a relative contraindication for transplantation. In any case, treatment would be obligatory.

8. Final considerations

The practice of organ transplantation in general and lung transplantation in particular is a growing technique in the clinical setting and transplant recipients inevitably need immunosuppressive treatment. Therefore, the appearance of opportunistic infections, specifically nocardiosis, is expected. Given the nonspecific clinical and radiological signs, diagnosis of these infections is based on high clinical suspicion, proper sample collection and rapid microbiological diagnostic methods to confirm it and properly orient the antibiotic treatment as early as possible. The future challenge seems to be the application of molecular methods directly on the sample (Couble et al., 2005) and perhaps fewer but more effective and less toxic antibiotics, less aggressive immunosuppressive therapy and, overall, to try to avoid infection with a healthy lifestyle.

9. References

Avery, RK., Michaels, MG., & AST Infectious Diseases Community of Practice. 2009. Strategies for safe-living following solid organ transplantation. *Am J Transplant*, Vol 9, No 4 Suppl, (December 2009), pp. S252-S257.

Ambrosioni, J., Lew, D., Garbino, J. 2010. Nocardiosis: updated clinical review and experience at a tertiary center. *Infection*, Vol 38, No 2, (April 2010), pp. 89-97.

Balikian, JP., Herman, PG., & Kopit, S. 1978. Pulmonary nocardiosis. *Radiology*, Vol 126, No 3, (Mars 1978), pp. 569-573.

Basu, A., Ramkumar, M., Tan, HP., Marcos, A., Fung, JJ., Starzl, TE., Shapiro, TE., Khan A, & McCauley J. 2005. Reversal of acute cellar rejection after renal transplantation with Campath-1H. *Transplant Proc*, Vol 37, No 2, (Mars 2005), pp. 923-926.

Beaman, BL., & Beaman, L. 1994. Nocardia species: host-parasite relationships. *Clin Microbiol Rev*, Vol 7, No 2, (April 1994), pp. 213-264.

Beekmann, SE., Gilbert, DN., & Polgreen, PM. 2008. Toxicity of extended courses of linezolid: results of an Infectious Diseases Society of America Emerging Infections Network survey. *Diagn Microbiol Infect Dis*, Vol 62, No 4, (December 2008), pp. 407-410.

Brown-Elliott, BA., Ward, SC., Crist, CJ., Mann, LB., Wilson, RW., & Wallace, RJ, Jr. 2001. In vitro activities of linezolid against multiple Nocardia species. *Antimicrob Agents Chemother,* Vol 45, No 4, (April 2001), pp. 1295-1297.

Brown-Elliott, BA., Brown, JM., Conville, PS., & Wallace, RJ Jr. 2006. Clinical and laboratory features of the *Nocardia* spp. based on current molecular taxonomy. *Clin Microbiol Rev,* Vol 19, No 2, (April 2006), pp. 259-282.

Cabada, MM., Nishi, SP., Lea, AS., Schnadig, V., Lombrad, GA., Lick, SD., & Valentine, VG. 2010. Concomitant pulmonary infection with *Nocardia transvalensis* and *Aspergillus ustus* in lung transplantation. *J Heart Lung Transplant,* Vol 29, No 8,(August 2010), pp. 900-903.

Clark, NM., and the AST infectious diseases community of practice. 2009. *Nocardia* in solid organ transplant recipients. *Am J Transp,* Vol 9, No 4 Suppl, (December 2009), pp. S70-S77.

Conville, PS., Brown, JM., Steigertwalt, AG., Lee, JW., Anderson ,VL., Fishbain, JT., Holland, SM., & Witebsky, FG. 2004. *Nocardia kruczakiae* sp. nov., a pathogen in immunocompromised patients and a member of the "*N. nova complex*". *J Clin Microbiol,* Vol 42, No 11, (November 2004), pp. 5139-5145.

Corales, R., Chua, J., Mawhorter, S., Young, JB., Starling, R., Tomford, JW., McCarthy, P., Braun, WE., Smedira, N., Hobbs, R., Haas, G., Pelegrin, D., Majercik, M., Hoercher, K., Cook, D., & Avery, RK. 2002. Significant post-transplant hypogammaglobulinemia in six heart transplant recipients: An emerging clinical phenomenon? *Transpl Infect Dis,* Vol 2, No 3, (September 2002), pp. 133-139.

Couble, A., Rodriguez-Nava, V., de Montclos, MP., Boiron, P., & Laurent F. 2005. Direct detection of *Nocardia* spp. In clinical samples by a rapid molecular method. *J Clin Microbiol,* Vol 43, No 4, (April 2005), pp. 1921-1924.

Dahan, K., El Kabbaj, D., Venditto, M., Pastural, M., & Delahousse, M. 2006. Intracraneal Nocardia recurrence during fluorinated quinolones therapy. *Transpl Infect Dis,* Vol 8, No 3, (September 2006), pp. 161-165.

Deem, RL., Doughty, FA., & Beaman, BL. 1983. Immunologically specific direct T lymphocyte-mediated killing of *Nocardia asteroides*. *J Immunol,* Vol, 130, No 5, (May 1983), pp. 2401-2406.

Durmaz, R., Atasoy, MA., Durmaz, G., Adapinar, B., Arslantas, A., Aydinli, A., & Tel E. 2001. Multiple nocardial abscesses of cerebrum, cerebellum and spinal cord, causing quadriplegia. *Clin Neurol Neurosurg,* Vol 103, No 1, (April 2001), pp. 59-62.

Eisenblätter, M., Disko, U., Stoltenburg-Didinger, G., Scherübl, H., Schaal, KP., Roth, A., Ignatius, R., Keitz, M., Hahn, H., & Wagner, J. 2002. Isolation of Nocardia paucivorans from the cerebrospinal fluid of a patient with relapse of cerebral nocardiosis. *J Clin Microbiol,* Vol 40, No 9, (September 2002), pp. 3532-3534.

Garlando, F., Bodmer, T., Lee, C., Zimmerli, W., & Pirovino, M. 1992. Successful treatment of disseminated nocardiosis complicated by cerebral abscess with ceftriaxone and amikacin. Case Report. *Clin Infect Dis,* Vol 15, No 6, (December 1992), pp. 1039-1040.

Gombert, ME., Aulicino, TM., duBouchet, L., Silverman, GE., & Sheinbaum, WM. 1986. Therapy of experimental cerebral nocardiosis with imipenem, amikacin, trimethoprim sulfamethoxazole and minocycline antimicrob agents chemother. *Antimicrob Agents _Chemother,* Vol 30, No 2, (August 1986), pp. 270-273.

Hansen, G., Swanzy, S., Gupta, R., Cookson, B., & Limaye, AP. 2008. *In vitro* activity of fluoroquinolones against clinical isolates of *Nocardia* identified by partial 165 rRNAsequencing. *Eur J Clin Microbiol Infect Dis*, Vol 27, No 2, (February, 2008), pp. 115-120.

Hewagama, S., Langan, K., Nishi, SP., Valentine, VG., & Peleg AY. Chapter 17. Elsevier Inc.. ISHLT Monographseries. Diagnosis and management of infectious diseases in cardiothoracic transplantation and mechanical circulatory support. ed. Mooney ML, Hannan MM, Husain S, Kirklin JK. 2011, vol 5. pp 175-186. ISSN 1930-2134. Philadelphia.

Husain, S., McCurry, K., Dauber, J., Singh, N., & Kusne, S. 2002. *Nocardia* infection in lung transplant recipients. *J Heart Lung Transplant*, Vol 21, No 3, (Mars 2002), pp. 354-359.

Jodlowski, TZ., Melnychuk, I., & Conry, J. 2007. Linezolid for the treatment of *Nocardia* spp. infections. *Ann Pharmacother*, Vol 41, No 10, (October 2007), pp. 1694-1699.

Kanemitsu, K., Kunishima, H., Saga, T., Harigae, H., Ishikawa, S., Takemura, H., & Kaku, M. 2003. Efficacy of amikacin combinations for nocardiosis. *Tohoku J Exp Med*, Vol 201, No 3, (November, 2003), pp. 157-163.

Khan, BA., Duncam, M., Reynolds, J., & Wilkes, DS. 2008. *Nocardia* infection in lung transplant recipients. *Clin Transplant*, Vol 22, No 5, (September-October 2008), pp. 562-566.

King, CT., Chapman, SW., & Butkus, DE. 1993. Recurrent nocardiosis in a renal transplant recipient. *South Med J*, Vol 86, No 2, (February 1993), pp. 225-228.

Kramer, MR., Marshall, SE., Starnes, VA., Gamberg, P., Amitai, Z., & Theodore, J. 1993. Infectious complications in heart lung transplantation. Analysis of 200 episodes. *Arch Intern Med*, Vol 153, No 17, (September 1993), pp. 2010-2016.

Kundranda, MN., Spiro, TP., Muslimani, A., Gopalkrishna, KV., Melaragno, MJ., & Daw, HA. 2007. Cerebral nocardiosis in a patient with NHL treated with rituximab. *Am J Hematol*, Vol 82, No 11, (November, 2007), pp. 1033-1034.

Lai, CC., Tan, CK., Lin, SH., Liao, CH., Chou, CH., Hsu, HL., Huang, YT., & Hsueh, PR. 2009. Comparative in vitro activities of nemonxacin, doripenem, tigecycline, and 16 antimicrobials against *Nocardia brasiliensis*, *Nocardia asteroides* and unusual *Nocardia* species. *J Antimicrobial Chemother*, Vol 64, No 1, (July 2009), pp. 73-78.

Lerner, PI. 1996. Nocardiosis. *Clin Infect Dis*, Vol 22, No 6, (June 1996), pp. 891-903.

Lewis, KE., Ebden, P., Wooster, SL., Rees, J., & Harrison, GA. 2003. Multisystem infection with *Nocardia farcinica*-therapy with linezolid and minocycline. *J Infect*, Vol 46, No 3, (April 2003), pp. 199-202.

Mamelak, AN., Obana, WG., Flaherty, JF., & Rosenblum ML. 1994. Nocardial brain absceess: treatment strategies and factors influencing outcome. *Neurosurgery*, Vol 35, No 4, (October 1994), pp. 622-631.

Martinez-Tomás, R., Menéndez-Villanueva, R., Reyes-Calzada, S., Santos-Durantez, M., Vallés-Tarazona, JM., Modesto-Alapont, M., & Gobernado-Serrano, M. 2007. Pulmonary Nocardiosis: risk factors and outcomes. *Respirology*, Vol 12, No 3, (May 2007), pp. 394-400.

Merigou, D., Beylot-Barry, M., Ly, S., Doutre, MS., Texier-Maugein, J., Billes, P., & Beylot, C. 1998. Primary cutaneous *Nocardia asteroides* infection after heart transplantation. *Dermatology*, Vol 196, No,2, pp. 246-247.

Minero, MV., Marín, M., Cerenado, E., Rabadán, PM., Bouza, E., & Muñoz, P. 2009. Nocardiosis at the turn of the century. *Medicine (Baltimore)*, Vol 88, No 4, (July 2009), pp. 250-261.

Morales, P., Gil-Brusola, A., & Santos, M. 2011. *Nocardia* infection in lung transplant recipients: Twenty years review. *Am J Crit Care Med*, Vol 183, No 1, (May 2011), A4648.

Moylett, EH., Pacheco, SE., Brown-Elliott, BA., Perry, TR., Buescher, ES., Birmingham, MC., Schentag, JJ., Gimbel, JF., Apodaca, A., Schwartz, MA., Rakita, RM., & Wallace, RJ Jr. 2003. Clinical experience with linezolid for the treatment of *Nocardia* infection. *Clin Infect Dis,* Vol 36, No 3 (February 2003), pp. 313-318.

Oszoyoglu, AA., Kirsch, J., & Mohammed, TL. 2007. Pulmonary nocardiosis after lung transplantation: CT findings in 7 patients and review of literature. *J Thorac Imaging*, Vol 22, No 2, (May 2007), pp. 143-148.

Patel, R., & Payá, CV. 1997. Infections in solid-organ transplant recipients. *Clin Microbiol Rev*, Vol 10, No1, (January 1997), pp. 86-124.

Paya CV. 1999. Indirect effects of CMV in the solid organ transplant patient. *Transpl Infect Dis*, Vol 1, (suppl 1), pp. 8-12.

Peleg, AY., Husain, S., Qureshi, ZA., Silveira, FP., Sarumi, M., Shutt, KA., Kwak, EJ., & Paterson, DL. 2007. Risk factors, clinical characteristics, and outcome of *Nocardia* infection in organ transplant recipients: a matched case-control study. *Clin Infect Dis*, Vol 44, No 10, (May 2007), pp. 1307-1314.

Peleg, AY., Husain, S., Kwak, EJ., Silveira, FP., Ndirangu, M., Tran, J., Shutt, KA., Shapiro, R., Thai, N., Abu-Elmagd, K., McCurry, KR., Marcos, A., & Paterson, DL. 2007. Opportunistic infections in 547 organ transplant recipients receiving alemtuzumab, a humanized monoclonal CD-52 antibody. *Clin Infect Dis*, Vol 44, No 2, (January 2007), pp. 204-212.

Peraira, JR., Segovia, J., Fuentes, R., Jiménez-Mazuecos, J., Arroyo, R., Fuertes, B., Mendaza, P., & Pulpon, LA. 2003. Pulmonary nocardiosis in heart transplant recipients: treatment and outcome. *Transplant Proc*, Vol 35, No 5, (August 2003), pp. 2006-2008.

Poonyagariyagorn, HK., Gershman, A., Avery, R., Minai, O., Blazey, H., Asamoto, K., Alster, J., Murthy, S., Mehta, A., Petterson, G., Mason, DP., & Budev M. 2008. Challenges in the diagnosis and management of *Nocardia* infections in lung transplant recipients. *Transpl Infect Dis*, Vol 10, No 6, (December 2008), pp. 403-408.

Pottumarthy, S., Limaye, AP., Prentice, JL., Houze, YB., Swanzy, SR., & Cookson, BT. 2003. *Nocardia veterana*, a new emerging pathogen. *J Clin Microbiol*, Vol 41, No 4, (April 2003), pp. 1705-1709.

Roberts, SA., Franklin, JC., Mijch, A., & Spelman, D. 2000. Nocardia infection in heart-lung transplant at Alfred Hospital, Melbourne, Australia, 1989-1998. *Clin Infect Dis*, Vol 31, No 4, (October, 2000), pp. 968-972.

Rivero, A., García-Lázaro, M., Pérez-Camacho, I., Natera, C., del Carmen Almodovar, M., Camacho, A., & Torre-Cisneros J. 2008. Successful long-term treatment for dissemitad infection with multiresistant *Nocardia farcinica*. *Infection*, Vol 36, No 4, (August 2008), pp. 389-391.

Sahathevan, M., Harvey, FA., Forbes, G., O'Grady, J., Gimson, A., Bragman, S., Jensen, R., Philpott-Howard, J., Williams, R., & Casewell, MW. 1991. Epidemiology, bacteriology and control of an outbreak of *Nocardia asteroides* infection on a liver unit. *J Hosp Infect,* Vol 18, Suppl A, (June 1991), pp. 473-80.

Santos, M., Gil-Brusola, A., & Morales, P. 2011. Infection by *Nocardia* in solid organ transplantation: thirty years of experience. *Transplant Proc,* (in press).

Schlaberg, R., Huard, RC., & Della-Latta, P. 2008. *Nocardia cyriacigeorgica,* an emerging pathogen in the United States. *J Clin Microbiol,* Vol 46, No 1, (January 2008), pp. 265-273.

Shawar, RM., Moore, DG., & LaRocco, MT. 1990. Cultivation of *Nocardia* spp on chemically defined media for selective recovery of isolates from clinical specimens. *J Clin Microbiol,* Vol 28, No 3, (Mars 1990), pp. 508-512.

Singh, N., Husain, S. 2000. Infections of the central nervous system in transplant recipients. *Transpl Infect Dis,* Vol 2, No 3, (September 2000), pp. 101-11.

Smego, RA Jr., Moeller, MB., & Gallis, HA. 1983. Trimetoprim-sulfamethoxazole therapy for *Nocardia* infections. *Arch Intern Med,* Vol 143, No 4, (April, 1983), pp. 711-718.

Sorrell, TC., Mitchell, DH., & Iredell, JR. In: Mandel GL, Bennett JE, Dolin R, eds. Principles and Practice of Infectious Diseases. 6th Ed. Philadelphia, PA: Churchill Livingstone 2005, pp. 2916-2914.

Sullivan, DC., & Chapman, SW. 2010. Bacteria that masquerade as fungi: actinomycosis/nocardia. *Proc Am Thorac Soc,* Vol 7, No 3, (May 2010), pp. 216-221.

Wayne, PA. 2003. Susceptibility testing of mycobacteria, nocardiae and other aerobic actinomycetes. M24-A. Clinical and Laboratory Standards Institute (CLSI/NCCLS).

Wenger, PN., Brown, JM., McNeil, MM., & Jarvis, WR. 1998. *Nocardia farcinica* sternotomy site infections in patients following open heart surgery. *J Infect Dis,* Vol, 178, No 5, (November, 1998), pp. 1539-1543.

Yassin, AF., Rainey, FA., Mendrock, U., Brzezinka, H., & Schaal, KP. 2000. *Nocardia abscessus* sp. nov. *Int J Syst Evol Microbiol,* Vol 50, No 4, (July, 2000), pp. 1487-1493.

4

In Vivo Models of Lung Disease

Tracey L. Bonfield

Inflammatory Mediator and Cystic Fibrosis Lung Disease Modeling CORE Center
Department of Pediatric Pulmonology
Case Western Reserve University
Cleveland, Ohio
USA

1. Introduction

Development of new therapeutics for lung diseases requires good modeling systems in which to test hypotheses. Often, how lung diseases are modeled *in vivo*, are not at all initiated by the same events that cause the disease in humans. The models for interstitial pulmonary fibrosis or chronic obstructive lung disease for example, require the use of toxic reagents and models for asthma do not use the same antigenic stimuli. What this means is what is used to initiate disease *in vivo* using animal models is not necessarily totally responsible for the same disease in humans. Even in situations of generating genetic models focusing on identified genes associated with specific disease entities modeled *in vivo*, the disease in the animal model is still not the same as the disease in humans even if the gene is most certainly involved. The focus of this chapter is to describe a variety of the animal models that have been developed to study specific lung disease entities including understanding the strength and the weaknesses of the *in vivo* modeling systems. The main goal of animal modeling is to provide an *in vivo* complex scenario which allows for the pursuit of defining the underlying mechanisms of diseases or importantly to provide a format for studying new interventional therapeutics. The focus of the chapter will start with basic anatomy, physiological differences and immunological responses which either enhance the selection of the model or are used to study specific components of the disease process.

Anatomy and Lung Models: For an *in vivo* model to provide the appropriate conditions, modeling the anatomy and the physiology of the lung model must first be considered. Whether dealing with small rodents such as mice, rats, and ferrets or larger animal such as pigs, sheep or monkeys, a detailed understanding of the model's anatomy and physiology must be considered for the correlation to human diseases (1,2). The issues to consider include the anatomical patterns of the alveolar spaces, the bronchial tree, milieu differences including the changes in the surfactant proteins, phospholipids, and physiological differences including the respiratory rate and airway clearance mechanisms (3,4). Some of the issues of correlating with human disease have to do with how the lung structure is different with the human lung and how this relates to differences in lung structure and function. This also relates to size, oxygenation and gaseous exchange. Another important issue is how the lung structure relates to the physiology and whether the mechanisms for homeostasis maintenance the same? This complicates things further since in most instances a direct cross-over between animal models and human disease is not complete. The relevant comparative anatomy of the lung would include all of the variables outlined in Figure 1.

Comparative Lung Anatomy, Structure and Function

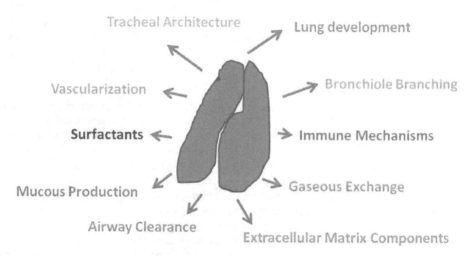

Fig. 1. Contributions to *In vivo* Lung Models. Here we show the lung and the variables associated with model selection regardless of the lung disease to be studied.

Function and Lung Model: The selection of an *in vivo* model must take into consideration not just the similarities and differences between the model and the human disease but also the question being asked in the disease application. The more common comparisons are listed in Table 1, when evaluating murine and rat models. Certainly, some animal models provide good *in vivo* correlates to the clinical situation; other are not so realistic. Choosing the model has to do with the question being answered and the reasoning behind selecting the model. For examples, cats and horses have been shown to develop spontaneous airway hyper-responsiveness, which would be consistent with human asthma (5,6). However, given the size of the animals, the inability to generate congenic species makes these models economically unrealistic. The opposite perspective is the ability to use mice for diseases such as asthma and cystic fibrosis (CF). Although the specific disease can be mimicked, the spectrum of the pathophysiology is different. For example, the mouse model for CF does not develop spontaneous lung disease (4,7). The model does provide an invaluable tool to study infection induced inflammation and in some case cell specific contribution of disease (8). In the murine asthma model, a variety of antigens can be used to induce disease, but it has been shown that many of the pathways associated with disease in humans are not played out in the murine model of the disease (9,10). It is a balance between the clinical or mechanistic question and the goal of the study for the selection of the appropriate model. Animal models afford the opportunity for investigators to experimentally manipulate a number of controlled variables such as strain of animal, and environment to investigate the molecular interactions involved in the pathogenesis of many lung diseases. The selection is based upon the basic pathophysiology, anatomy and the ability to induce the disease in a time sensitive fashion for comparative and economic consistency.

Mechanism of Study	Mouse	Rat
Lung Remodeling and Repair	Offers the ability to study specific genes associated with repair and remodeling. Depends on species susceptibility to either the Th_1 or Th_2 process.	Enhanced susceptibility to develop Th_2 driven cellular immune responses. Larger airways, easier to measure breathing dynamics.
Inflammation	Mechanisms involve similar but often different proteins. Careful experimental design for a focused approach on the similarities but remembering the differences.	Functionally similar but several components and events which are different. Understanding the similarities and differences are important in the context of disease.
Response to Infection	Similar processes and players with proteins being both the same and different. This all depends on protein homology or even presence.	Similar processes with players of proteins being often times similar. The issue is the availability of reagents for studying the mechanisms of interests.
Response to Injury	Injury response is relative to the total surface area at the air-liquid interface. Mouse models use chemicals, which are not the initiators in human disease.	Injury associated with chemicals of mechanical contributions can be used due to the size difference from the murine counterparts. Chemicals used are always associated with real human disease.

Table 1. In Vivo Models and Studies of Lung Disease Pathophysiology

Acute Lung Injury: Acute lung injury (ALI) and acute respiratory distress syndrome (ARDS) results from severe injury to the lung parenchyma (11). Animal modeling experiments of ALI and ARDS have been very useful in providing some directions into the mechanisms related to disease pathogenesis and providing opportunities to explore new and innovative therapeutic targets. As with most lung disease modeling systems, the design of the model and its manipulation is predominately dictated by the hypothesis and the focal point of pathology. The pathology associated with ALI and ARDS includes inflammatory cell recruitment, exudation with edema in the small airways potentially resulting in alveolar collapse (12). The recruitment of inflammatory cells, the changes in tonicity at the tissue interface are all pathologies which contribute to the injurious process. This occurs through enhancing the production of inflammatory proteins, proteases and reactive oxygen radicals at the tissue interface. This gets to the mechanisms associated with the development of ALI and ARDS including the processes involving the injury and down-stream response to the injury which also contributes to tissue damage (13,14). There are three different models that are used for inducing different aspects of ALI and ARDS. These include the surfactant washout (LAV) model, oleic acid intravenous injection (OAI) model and the lipopolysaccharide (LPS) model (15). The LAV model utilizes a series of broncholaveolar lavages which requires larger animals like rats and ferrets. In the surfactant washout models, the focus is removing the protective anti-inflammatory molecules such as surfactant protein A (SP-A) potentially altering the air-liquid interface surface tension, resulting in changes in oxygenation efficiency. The change in surface milieu signals the production of pro-inflammatory cytokines with results in recruitment of inflammatory cells which ultimately ctonritbutes to interstitial tissue damage (15). The OAI model uses an infusion of oleic acid into the central vein or the right atrium (16,17), necessitating the requirement of larger animals. There is considerable diversity in terms of the dosing and the timing of the administration of OAI, making the model highly variable and not well accepted. The precise mechanisms by which the oleic acid induces lung edema, and the mechanisms associated with the recruitment of inflammatory cells and injury are not completely understood. The response of the animal to the oleic acid, results in a series of inflammatory events that create ALI/ARDS which has been theroretically associated with anhanced pro-inflammatory cytokine production.

The production of the pro-inflammatory cytokines in the LPS model is the common process involved with ALI development, as discussed in reference to the OAI and LAV models. The LPS model uses the product of gram negative bacteria (LPS) to induce cytokines and the down-stream events which result in inefficiency in the ability to resolve infection (15,18). In a sense it is a process that confuses the immune system so that it is unable to perform efficiently. The LPS is usually extracted from *Escherichia coli*, but could be from other gram negatives such as *Pseudomonas aeruginosa*, a common pathogen associated with community acquired pneumonia and ventilator associated pneumonia (19,20). The development of stable lung injury is dependent on dosage, time, route of administration and size of the model selected. In the murine models of the ALI/ARDS the LPS is administered intra-tracheally. The process of infection induced ALI and/or ARDS may include sepsis in the animal model but also in human disease. In fact, about 50% of sepsis cases ultimately account for ALI and ARDS ventilator support (21). The development of sepsis, results from a sustained and uncontrolled inflammatory response to the infectious insult contributing to dysfunction of at least one organ system. The sequences of events which lead to sepsis are unknown as well as the events that result in pulmonary failure (22,23). In the models of sepsis induced ALI/ARDS, LPS is administered intra-tracheally or induced by surgically clipping the gastrointestinal tract (11,15).

In Vivo Models, Clinical Relevance and Limitations. Histologically, human ALI/ARDS can be sub-divided into an exudative and fibroproliferative phase (24). The exudative phase is characterized by the accumulation of inflammatory proteins containing neutrophils (25), followed by the accumulation of macrophages initiating the fibroproliferative phase of the disease (26,27). In some patients the process and side-effects of the acute inflammatory response completely resolves whereas others progress with chronic inflammation, fibrosis and neovascularization (28). Each of the different models used to develop ALI/ARDS have both valid and controversial contributions to studying these diseases *in vivo*. How these models compare and provide insight into ALI/ARDS is outlined in Figure 2. In the surfactant washout model, it is a useful tool in studying the importance of surfactant maintenance in airway-interface surface tension and pathophysiology of ALI. The issue is that most clinical conditions do not result in clinically significant surfactant abnormalities in the adult population (29). In the OAI model, the ability to induce the pathophysiology of ALI/ARDS is dependent on using injectable oleic acid, which is obviously not similar to the *in vivo* clinical development of the disease. However, it is still a useful model for studying the pathology of ARDS especially with a focus on membrane injury (16,17). Since infection has been closely associated with the development of ALI/ARDS, the LPS model seems to be the most translatable. However the other two models probably represent up-stream events in the exposure, specificity and sensitivity of the development of infection based ALI/ARDS (30-32). As with most *in vivo* animal models it does not appear that the model is consistent with all of the components of the human disease. The LPS model does not appear to develop the fibroproliferative phase of ALI/ARDS; which limits the use of these models for studying the secondary issues associated with ALI/ARDS chronic inflammation and fibrosis (15,30).

Acute Lung Injury In vivo Models
Strengths and Weaknesses

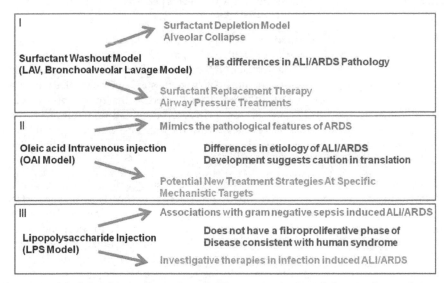

Fig. 2. In Vivo Models of Acute Lung Injury. Three principal models exist for studying ALI/ARDS. In each case the model has important contribution to the pathophysiology shown in blue, and potential therapies shown in green. The important caveats and limitations are shown in red.

Chronic Obstructive Pulmonary Disease (COPD) and Emphysema: COPD is the fifth leading cause of death worldwide and is associated with pollution and smoking history (33). COPD is a very complex disease with four described traits: emphysema, small airway remodeling, chronic bronchitis and pulmonary hypertension (34). The underlying pathophysiology of COPD is dependent on the structure and function of the lung along with the immunological processes that occur post-insult. Although patients present with variations and combinations of these pathologies, all patients progress into severe pulmonary failure. The kinetics of disease progression is dependent on the patient, patient compliance to therapeutic intervention and the ability to respond to current therapeutics. In this case the animal model of choice should require a close attention to lung anatomy and physiology since these play very important roles in the overall development of COPD and emphysema (35), especially as it relates to the overall development of new therapeutics. Besides the basics of understanding the similarities and differences between lung anatomy of the animal model and that of the human disease some consideration must also be given to the overall lung mechanics.

The *in vivo* model most commonly used to study COPD includes cigarette smoke (36). The issue lies with the ability to deliver a homogenous dosing of cigarette smoke over a defined time range, and that these models do not completely recapitulate the human disease. Further, since there are genomic differences which increase susceptibility to COPD, the translatable ability is always in the background. Additionally, the pulmonary pathology produced in the context of the cigarette model produces subtle pathologies which may also introduce subjective interpretation in quantifying the histopathology (37). Better computerized-microscopic programs need to be developed that can better quantify and minimize subjective interpretation of the studies (26,38).

Non-specific inflammation is another indicator of COPD, with a predominance of neutrophils and the inflammation approach to studying COPD focuses on apoptosis and elastase (39,40). The apoptosis model focuses on the failure of the COPD lung to repair itself post-injury focusing on dysregulated normal lung tissue turnover. The mechanism associated with apoptosis induced COPD has been linked to the production of vascular endothelial growth factor (VEGF) and/or the VEGF receptor (40). It is not clear whether this VEGF/VEGF receptor dysfunction is by itself critical for inducing endothelial cell apoptosis and the processes that result in decreased vascularization in the lung or whether it is in the context of a variety of other factors which ultimately contribute to COPD.

The elastase model uses a product of the inflammatory response to initiate and perpetuate the inflammatory response seen in COPD. The original hypothesis for the importance of elastase came patients α_1-anti-trypsin deficiency (41,42). Individuals with this disease develop emphysema and COPD. These patients are treated with exogenous α_1-anti-trypsin, the endogenous inhibitor of elastase. In COPD/emphysema, the recruitment of inflammatory cells and the disproportionate production of proteases without the appropriate anti-protease counter-part ultimately results in extracellular matrix degradation, inflammatory cell recruitment, matrix metalloprotease activity, cellular activation which all contribute to the lung damage similar to the mechanisms in α_1-anti-trypsin deficiency (43,44). The disadvantage of the elastase model, is that the function of elastase and cigarette smoke in COPD emphysema are potentially mediated through very different pathophysiological mechanisms which again brings up the issue of clinical translation. It is efficient to have a very specific inducer of emphysema for investigating specific mechanisms and therapeutic development. However, results obtained from specific products need to be taken into consideration as compared to the complex *in vivo* environment post complex insult (45,46). Some investigators have used LPS to induce airway and parenchymal changes, although the pathophysiology is more reminiscent of ALI/ARDS than COPD (33,47). Table 2 lists the pros and cons of each of the COPD models.

Model	Pathology	Positives of Model	Negatives of Model
Cigarette Induced COPD	Dilated alveolar ducts, abnormal parenchyma and increased numbers of goblet cells. Pulmonary function tests show decrease in effectiveness.	The most similar to the human disease in terms of inducing agent that produces emphysema.	It is not debilitating in animals. Lesions do not progress beyond a certain point to mimic the human disease.
Apoptosis Induced COPD	Induction of air space enlargement. Matrix breakdown.	Induces enlarged airspaces in short period of time.	Pathophysiological mechanisms are not permanent.
Elastase Induced COPD	Increased numbers of neutrophils, elevated elastase.	Rapid and easy onset, easy to measure functional changes and possibly relevant to the repair and remodeling issues in COPD.	Mechanism of disease induction is secondary to the initiators of clinical COPD.
Starvation-Induced COPD	Decreased lung volume, changes in lung structure and function.	Limited variability and short term impact on disease development.	Compassionate care of animals. The pathology may be due to decreased repair mechanisms.
LPS Induced COPD	Produces enlarged airways in chronic scenarios. Matrix metalloproteinase production	Short-term model with parenchymal changes.	Inflammatory differential is not the same as pollutant induced insult which may reflect different mechanisms of pathophysiology.

Table 2. Models of COPD

Bronchopulmonary Dysplasia: Bronchopulmonary dysplasia (BPD) remains the leading cause of respiratory morbidity and mortality in severely pre-term infants (48,49). The treatment of prematurity itself induces BPD, which complicates matters including ventilator induced surfactant deficiency and inflammation (44,50). Intrinsic BPD is characterized by immaturity, decreased growth, and immature vascularization (51). The main model for BPD is hyperoxic exposure in animal models such as rats and mice (49). Hyperoxia inhibits the normal budding and branching of the bronchi (52) leading to arrest in lung development resembling pre-term infant BPD (53). In these studies, it appears that both the airways and capillary vessels are affected requiring ventilation which can also contribute to inflammation and dysplasia (48,49,51). To understand the mechanisms and outcomes in BPD, animal models must contain elements of the normal fetal lung and the mechanisms associated with development and function. For the pulmonary mechanics studies, the *in vivo* models consist of larger animal models including lamb, rabbits and guinea pigs (49). The change in lung mechanics and the accumulation of fluid, changes the airway surface tension contributing to robust inflammatory cytokine production contributing further to the histopathology. Using these models, studies have provided avenues for understanding the role of surfactant therapy, decreased tidal volumes, improved control of oxygenation on BPD development and translation clinically (49,54).

Alveolar Proteinosis: The lung faces physical and environmental challenges, due to changing in lung volumes as well as exposure to foreign pathogens. The pulmonary surfactant system is integral in protecting the lung from these challenges via two different and distinct groups of surfactant proteins (55). Surfactant protein (SP)-B and SP-C are small molecular weight hydrophobic surfactant proteins that regulate air liquid interface surface tension. SP-A and SP-D are the larger hydrophilic surfactant proteins which aide in surface tension but which also have microbicidal function. Additionally, there are other non-surfactant proteins called defensins which also aid in inflammation and host defense (56). Pulmonary alveolar proteinosis (PAP) is a process by which there is a surfactant accumulation in the lungs potentially due to the inability to catabolize surfactant (57). There are three forms of the disease: genetic, exposure induced and idiopathic (58). The genetic disease specifically impacts children, and is associated with mutations in some of the surfactant protein genes (59-61). Exposure induced PAP is found in scenarios of particulate inhalation including silica and titanium (62-65). The idiopathic form is associated with circulating auto-antibodies against the macrophage growth and differentiation factor granulocyte-macrophage colony stimulating factor (GM-CSF) (66,67). Clinical studies have correlated the presence of the neutralizing antibody to PAP (66,68,69). Clinical trials of GM-CSF, plasmapheresis and whole lung lavage have shown limited successes with some sustainable relief, but none of the treatments are curative (70). In terms of animal models, most have been done with mice since the defects are most often associated with the absence of surfactant or GM-CSF proteins and murine GM-CSF knockout development of alveolar proteinosis (71-73). The surfactant protein knockouts develop diseases very reminiscent of pediatric interstitial proteinosis (50). The GM-CSF knockout mouse has many pathophysiological outcomes which are reminiscent of the human PAP adult disease (74). The nice part of these models is that they do not have to be induced, so there is relatively little variability between animal to animal. There have been some attempts to develop an autoimmune model of idiopathic PAP using monkeys and mice (75,76). These efforts have provided important insight into the potential mechanisms of development in early and late stages of PAP due to autoimmunity against GM-CSF.

Agent utilized	Pathology	Advantages	Disadvantages
Bleomycin	Induced lung damage and repair.	Ease of administration.	Requires specific dosing regimen. Toxic to investigators.
Silica	Chronic inflammatory response and repair mechanisms associated with fibrosis.	Sustained inflammation since silica is not resolved by macrophages.	Not a natural inducer of fibrosis. The mechanisms may not be translatable.
FITC	Inflammatory response and repair mechanisms. Natural hapten induced inflammatory mechanisms.	Visualize areas of repair and fibrosis.	Some characteristics of the lung disease are absent. There is significant variability depending on the FITC batch.
Irradiation	Induces direct cell death via DNA damage with a subsequent influx of inflammatory cells. The radiation may also directly induce the fibrotic processes.	Ease of study, no chemical requirement. Mimics human process in terms of initiation and progress.	Long time for the fibrosis to develop, limited to modeling radiation induced pneumonitis.
Viral Induced Transgenes	Viruses used to up-regulate mediators of fibrosis.	Specific *in vivo* molecules associated with IPF formation such as TNF or TGFB.	Deal with potential mechanisms but is not realistic to defining disease process.

Table 2. In vivo Models for Interstitial Pulmonary Fibrosis

Interstitial Pulmonary Fibrosis: Fibrosis is an important cause of morbidity and mortality in a variety of lung diseases, but it has a very prominent role in idiopathic pulmonary fibrosis (IPF)—(77). IPF presents with a homogenous phenotype with both definable physiologic and radiographic presentation but without identifiable etiology (78) although, the literature suggests that alveolar type II cell injury is an important early feature in the pathogenesis of pulmonary fibrosis (79). The source of injury is unknown. Different approaches to modeling pulmonary fibrosis have been used by investigating exposure to bleomycin, silica, fluorescein isothiocyannate (FITC) and irradiation (77). At the genetic level, some models of IPF have included over-expression of 'hypothesized" genes in the pathogenesis of IPF or utilization of transgenics for cell specific contribution to IPF. Bleomycin is the most frequently used agent in modeling IPF (80,81). The advantage of bleomycin is the ease with which it can be administered and the consistency of the IPF pathophysiology. Bleomycin is a chemotherapeutic agent which induces lung damage through direct DNA strand breakage and the generation of free radicals. The response to the injury is healing and fibrosis. Silica aerosolized into the lung induces pulmonary fibrosis through inducing chronic inflammation and frustrated phagocytosis by macrophages (77,82). Post-ingestion, the macrophages constitutively produce pro-fibrotic cytokines (83). The greatest advantage of the silica based system is that the silica particles are not easily cleared from the lungs creating a persistent stimulus and a non-reversible fibrotic process. Regardless of the model fibrosis is dependent on the strain of animals, suggesting immune dependent contribution to the overall susceptibility of IPF development. FITC is another chemical used to induce pulmonary fibrosis (77,84). Fluorescein, delivered directly into the airway acts as a hapten attaching to lung proteins providing a depot for continuous lung exposure to antigen. The advantage of the FITC model is the ability to actually image the processes as they occur in the lung.

Asthma: Asthma is a very complex and heterogeneous disease affecting 300 million people worldwide especially in Westernized countries (85). Why developing countries seem to be somewhat protective has been the foundation for the hygiene hypothesis (86). Asthma is a complex trait caused by multiple environmental factors with the main characteristics being airway inflammation and airway hyper-reactivity (AHR) (87). The pathogenesis of asthma is associated with many environmental factors, many cell types and several molecular and cellular pathways. Some specific presentations of asthma are outlined in Figure 3 (88,89). The majority of the induced asthmas are due to exposure to an irritant such as air pollution, allergen or viral exposure. Even aspirin and drug induced asthma can be associated with changes in the pulmonary milieu upon dosing. Interestingly, some asthma phenotypes are not associated with identifiable exposures, such as exercise induced and metabolic syndrome associated asthma.

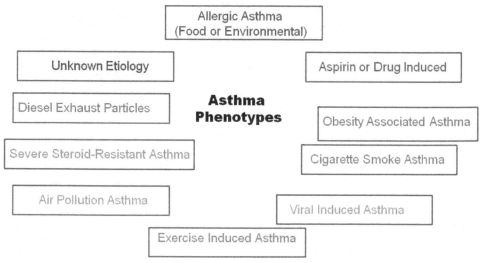

Fig. 3. Asthma Phenotypes. Asthma is a heterogeneous disease with multiple factors associated with the development and response to therapy. Given these issues, designing experiments and translating into clinical significance become a challenge.

These different pathways and phenotypes probably suggest mechanisms that are co-existent but also synergistic depending on the patient, environment, compliance and documentation.

Animal models of asthma have helped to clarify some of the underlying pathophysiological mechanisms contributing to the development of asthma (5,9,10). Much of the focus of these models is on T cell driven allergic responses contributing to understanding of the heterogeneity of asthma (90). The murine model of asthma using Balb/C mice has defined the important role of allergen-specific Th_2 cells in recruiting eosinophils into the airway, their activation and the release of histamine associated with atopic airway reactive disease. The major caveat in the murine asthma studies is that the allergen sensitization process does not completely recapitulate the allergic response in humans complicating the ability to utilize these models for therapeutic development (91). This has been quite frustrating in asthma therapy development, even though certain biomarkers have been identified in the *in vivo* models they have ultimately not translated into efficient therapeutic care for patients with asthma (10). The inability to translate the observations from the animal models to patient care were very disappointing and increased the lack of the appreciation of the animal models toward mechanisms and pathogenesis of asthma. The fortunate component of the murine asthma model is the ability to sensitize the animals to a variety of foreign proteins and to use transgenic animals for studying mechanisms and response to different exposures. In most scenarios, the challenge results in a Th_2 polarization and enhanced allergen-specific IgE production (92). Pathologically the lungs have eosinophilia, mucus secretion and goblet cell hyperplasia, airway hyper-responsiveness and remodeling with fibrosis (5,88). These asthmatic phenomena have suggested that cytokines and cells other than T-cells, such as $IFN\gamma$, IL-17 and/or neutrophils, may also play a significant role in the lung pathology (93,94). Further, Th_2 targeted therapies have not been as effective as hoped in many clinical trials of asthma, suggesting alternative pathways to the lung inflammation and remodeling. These have resulted in several distinct alternatives to the traditional allergen challenge model. Table 3 outlines the different animal models currently available to study various aspects of the pathophysiology associated with asthma.

Lung Cancer: Several *in vivo* models exist which provide the opportunity to study cancer (95). The complications in these models are their inability to completely correlate with histologic patterns of the malignancies, natural strain susceptibility and time frames for cancer induction in humans. One important difference between the animal models and the human disease is that these animals have higher basal metabolic rates changing metastatic potential (33). Failure to develop specific tumor types is probably due to the variability of the transgene expression early in lung development. The most common compound utilized for the development of tumors in animal models is urethane (96). Mouse models have been used to study the roll of mutant oncogenes in the genesis of lung adenocarcinomas (97-99). These models have also proven useful for studying potential therapeutics. The development of a tyrosine kinase inhibitor which blocks epidermal growth factor receptor (EGFR) was found to benefit some patients after testing in mouse models. The deletion of other genes associated with human small-cell lung cancers could also be mimicked in a murine lung model aiding in therapeutic development of inhibitors (33,95).

Malignant mesothelioma is a cancer associated with environmental exposure to asbestos (95). The disease has a poor prognosis, with little to offer patients in terms of therapy. Mouse models of pleural mesothelioma have been produced by exposing mice to asbestos

Model	Advantage	Disadvantage	Pathology Association	Translation into the Clinic
Allergen Challenge	Similar to atopic induced asthmatic disease. Can be defined by the route, dosage and duration of the sensitization and challenge regime.	The model does not recapitulate all of the components of the allergic disease.	Airway hyper-reactivity, systemic IgE, mucous production, goblet cell hyperplasia.	Variability in species, sensitization/challenge regimes, and duration of studies. Has introduced some clinical failures.
Viral Respiratory Infection	Independent of Th_2 mechanism, Induced using sendai virus (parainfluenza) or respiratory syncitial virus (RSV).	Maybe considered a contributor to the human disease but may precede the start of asthma symptoms in humans.	Airway hyper-reactivity, alternatively activated macrophages and natural killer cells.	Evidence for viruses has been found in patients with severe asthma and in children with asthma with pre-exposure to RSV.
Air Pollution	Ozone is a common inducer. This appears to be concentration, route and dosage dependent.	Difficult to obtain consistency due to inhalation variability.	Severe airway hyper-reactivity associated with neutrophils. Also requires the presence of IL-17.	May lead to some understanding of the down-stream event in severe chronic asthma.
Intrinsic AHR	Requires strain specific manipulation and is associated with specific proteases.	Is strain specific and appears to associate with the asthma susceptibility gene.	Appears to regulate the control of airway hyper-reactivity through smooth muscle cell activation and bronchospasm.	The association of the proteases to human asthma.

Table 3. In Vivo Models for the Versatility of the Asthma Phenotypes

fibers. A wide range of natural and synthetic fibers, chemicals and metals have also been shown to induce pleural and peritoneal mesotheliomas (100,101). Recently the technology of xenographic transplantation of human malignant mesotheliomas into rats or mice has been used to study new chemotherapeutic agents including immunotherapy, gene therapy and multimodality therapy (95). Asbestos-induced malignant mesotheliomas produced in rodents resemble the human disease with respect to latency and growth of the tumor cells. Even with these similarities, mice are not perfect models for humans.

Cystic Fibrosis: Cystic fibrosis (CF) is the result of defects in the gene encoding the cystic fibrosis transmembrane regulator (CFTR) and is the most common genetic disease among Caucasians (102).. Even though new therapeutics including correctors and activators like VX-770 has shown great promise in new phases of CF therapy, the cure has been elusive (103). The development of the *in vivo* models has focused on four major points of pathophysiology: anatomy, physiology, airway clearance and intrinsic and/or induced inflammation. The mouse model been the main model in CF research for several years, however, the model does not develop spontaneous lung disease requiring the introduction of bacteria to initiate the pathophysiological events associated with CF infection and inflammation (104). There are several different models of CFTR deficiency ranging from the complete absence of CFTR (null) to the partial expression and/or function (4). There have also been murine models developed in which the lung mutation remains but the gastrointestinal phenotype is corrected or it is cell specific (105). The reason for these later series of animals is that the murine CFTR null mutant consistently has gastrointestinal blockage once the mice have been weaned, increasing mortality and expense of the animals. To prevent obstruction, the animals are put on a laxative. Investigators have a choice whether to use laxative treated animals or gut corrected animals. In either case, it is likely that gastrointestinal obstruction is important in the overall immunity and host response to infection in CF. Therefore, observations in the gut corrected mouse may ultimately have to be verified in the null mouse depending on the focus of the studies. Even with the differences in the gastrointestinal constitution, the severity of the different murine models is defined by CFTR protein function related to the mRNA expressed, protein synthesis or folding of the complete CFTR protein (4). In addition to the gastrointestinal obstruction, most of the models display inflammation (106), failure to thrive (107), decreased survival (108,109) and hyper-responsiveness to stimulation (110). To improve the ability to look at CF globally, larger models of CFTR deficiency have been developed to better investigate the airway pathogenesis and progression of lung disease. Further, unique models have been developed using transgenic technology to induce CFTR deficiency in specific cell types, allowing for the sequential investigation of all of the contributing cellular abnormalities and how they contribute to the CF pathophysiology (105,107,111).

The pig has become an exciting new direction for CF model development. The pig lungs and human lungs have similar comparative anatomy (112,113) and have been used to study a variety of aspects of lung pathophysiology including surfactant homeostasis, airway hyper-responsiveness and lung injury (114). The first studies have shown that there were no differences in the newborn pig birth weight or appearance (4). Deficient CFTR in the pigs did not appear to alter normal birth weight, appearance and/or lung anatomy or function. The absence of CFTR however, did result in defective nasal transepithelial cell potential and all piglets developed severe gastrointestinal obstruction. Further, with piglet aging there appears to changes in lung physiology and function resembling that of infant with CF. However, the development of lung disease is still being investigated as to whether it is an intrinsic phenomena due to the absence of CFTR, or the result of environmental exposure (112). The pig is a great model for studies in CF lung pathophysiology, however husbandry and cost and reproductive cycle play a major part in being able to conduct several studies with reasonable numbers of animals.

The ferret has been shown to also be a good animal model for studying CFTR lung biology (7,115). The ferret lung shows CFTR expression in the airway epithelium and submucosal glands, identical to that in humans (4,7). Like the pig model, the majority of the CFTR deficient ferrets also developed gastrointestinal obstruction with "failure to thrive" (115,116).

To study CF, the availability of three established *in vivo* model systems provides ample ability to study various components of CF pathophysiology. Besides CFTR deficient mice, pigs and ferrets, other models have also been developed or observed (117) including the sheep (118) and monkey models (119). These have been less studied for a variety of reasons. Although these models have provided invaluable insight into the development of new CF therapeutics, new model systems should be considered to get even closer to the overall mechanisms associated with CF.

Summary: Human lung disease is a major cause of morbidity and mortality in the world. The pulmonary dysfunction may be primary or secondary to a variety of events. The pathophysiological mechanisms associated with the disease processes are different depending upon whether the insult is external as in the case of infection or injury or internal as in the case of genetic anomalies associated with important pulmonary or secretion functions. Studying lung disease requires models that attempt to recapitulate the human phenomena. There are no perfect models, and the selection for studies must be based upon the criteria of study and the ability of the model to meet the needs of the study. In this chapter we have highlighted a variety of pulmonary diseases and syndromes with a focus on the models used to study the various pathophysiological mechanisms associated with that specific disease entity. In the end, model development and usage will continue as a conduit with which to test mechanisms and to explore the development of new and innovative therapeutics.

2. References

[1] Hoymann, H. G. 2006. New developments in lung function measurements in rodents. *Exp. Toxicol. Pathol.* 57 Suppl 2: 5-11.

[2] Sadikot, R. T., J. W. Christman, and T. S. Blackwell. 2004. Molecular targets for modulating lung inflammation and injury. *Curr. Drug Targets.* 5: 581-588.

[3] Fisher, J. H., V. Sheftelyevich, Y. S. Ho, S. Fligiel, F. X. McCormack, T. R. Korfhagen, J. A. Whitsett, and M. Ikegami. 2000. Pulmonary-specific expression of SP-D corrects pulmonary lipid accumulation in SP-D gene-targeted mice. *Am. J. Physiol Lung Cell Mol. Physiol* 278: L365-L373.

[4] Fisher, J. T., Y. Zhang, and J. F. Engelhardt. 2011. Comparative biology of cystic fibrosis animal models. *Methods Mol. Biol.* 742: 311-334.

[5] Braun, A., and T. Tschernig. 2006. Animal models of asthma: innovative methods of lung research and new pharmacological targets. *Exp. Toxicol. Pathol.* 57 Suppl 2: 3-4.

[6] Herszberg, B., D. Ramos-Barbon, M. Tamaoka, J. G. Martin, and J. P. Lavoie. 2006. Heaves, an asthma-like equine disease, involves airway smooth muscle remodeling. *J. Allergy Clin. Immunol.* 118: 382-388.

[7] Li, Z., and J. F. Engelhardt. 2003. Progress toward generating a ferret model of cystic fibrosis by somatic cell nuclear transfer. *Reprod. Biol. Endocrinol.* 1: 83.

[8] Mueller, C., S. A. Braag, A. Keeler, C. Hodges, M. Drumm, and T. R. Flotte. 2011. Lack of cystic fibrosis transmembrane conductance regulator in CD3+ lymphocytes leads to aberrant cytokine secretion and hyperinflammatory adaptive immune responses. *Am. J. Respir. Cell Mol. Biol.* 44: 922-929.

[9] Braun, A., T. Tschernig, and D. A. Groneberg. 2008. Editorial: Experimental models of asthma. *J. Occup. Med. Toxicol.* 3 Suppl 1: S1.

[10] Kumar, R. K., and P. S. Foster. 2002. Modeling allergic asthma in mice: pitfalls and opportunities. *Am. J. Respir. Cell Mol. Biol.* 27: 267-272.

[11] Jugg, B. J., A. J. Smith, S. J. Rudall, and P. Rice. 2011. The injured lung: clinical issues and experimental models. *Philos. Trans. R. Soc. Lond B Biol. Sci.* 366: 306-309.

[12] Matthay, M. A. 2008. Treatment of acute lung injury: clinical and experimental studies. *Proc. Am. Thorac. Soc.* 5: 297-299.

[13] Rubenfeld, G. D., E. Caldwell, E. Peabody, J. Weaver, D. P. Martin, M. Neff, E. J. Stern, and L. D. Hudson. 2005. Incidence and outcomes of acute lung injury. *N. Engl. J. Med.* 353: 1685-1693.

[14] Matthay, M. A. 1999. Conference summary: acute lung injury. *Chest* 116: 119S-126S.

[15] Wang, H. M., M. Bodenstein, and K. Markstaller. 2008. Overview of the pathology of three widely used animal models of acute lung injury. *Eur. Surg. Res.* 40: 305-316.

[16] Wang, H. M., M. Bodenstein, B. Duenges, S. Ganatti, S. Boehme, Y. Ning, B. Roehrig, and K. Markstaller. 2010. Ventilator-associated lung injury superposed to oleic acid infusion or surfactant depletion: histopathological characteristics of two porcine models of acute lung injury. *Eur. Surg. Res.* 45: 121-133.

[17] Davidson, K. G., A. D. Bersten, H. A. Barr, K. D. Dowling, T. E. Nicholas, and I. R. Doyle. 2000. Lung function, permeability, and surfactant composition in oleic acid-induced acute lung injury in rats. *Am. J. Physiol Lung Cell Mol. Physiol* 279: L1091-L1102.

[18] Liu, D. D., Y. H. Hsu, and H. I. Chen. 2007. Endotoxin-induced acute lung injury is enhanced in rats with spontaneous hypertension. *Clin. Exp. Pharmacol. Physiol* 34: 61-69.

[19] Cash, H. A., D. E. Woods, B. McCullough, W. G. Johanson, Jr., and J. A. Bass. 1979. A rat model of chronic respiratory infection with Pseudomonas aeruginosa. *Am. Rev. Respir Dis.* 119: 453-459.

[20] Carrillo-Marquez, M. A., K. G. Hulten, W. Hammerman, L. Lamberth, E. O. Mason, and S. L. Kaplan. 2011. Staphylococcus aureus pneumonia in children in the era of community-acquired methicillin-resistance at Texas Children's Hospital. *Pediatr. Infect. Dis. J.* 30: 545-550.

[21] Lever, A., and I. Mackenzie. 2007. Sepsis: definition, epidemiology, and diagnosis. *BMJ* 335: 879-883.

[22] Fisher, C. J., and S. B. Yan. 2000. Protein C levels as a prognostic indicator of outcome in sepsis and related diseases. *Crit. Care Med.* 28: S49-S56.

[23] Lyn-Kew, K., and T. J. Standiford. 2008. Immunosuppression in sepsis. *Curr. Pharm. Des* 14: 1870-1881.

[24] Morrison, R. J., and A. Bidani. 2002. Acute respiratory distress syndrome epidemiology and pathophysiology. *Chest Surg. Clin. N. Am.* 12: 301-323.

[25] Chollet-Martin, S., C. Gatecel, N. Kermarrec, M. Gougerot-Pocidalo, and D. M. Payen. 1996. Alveolar neutrophil functions and cytokine levels in patients with the adult respiratory distress syndrome during nitric oxide inhalation. *Am. J. Respir. Crit. Care Med.* 153: 985-990.

[26] Desai, S. R. 2002. Acute respiratory distress syndrome: imaging of the injured lung. *Clin. Radiol.* 57: 8-17.

[27] Matute-Bello, G., W. C. Liles, F. Radella, K. P. Steinberg, J. T. Ruzinski, L. D. Hudson, and T. R. Martin. 2000. Modulation of neutrophil apoptosis by granulocyte colony-stimulating factor and granulocyte/macrophage colony-stimulating factor during the course of acute respiratory distress syndrome. *Crit. Care Med.* 28: 1-7.

[28] Mosser, D. M., and J. P. Edwards. 2008. Exploring the full spectrum of macrophage activation. *Nat. Rev. Immunol.* 8: 958-969.

[29] Anzueto, A., R. Baughman, K. Guntupalli, J. Weg, H. Wiedemann, A. Raventos, F. Lemaire, W. Long, D. Zaccardelli, and E. Pattishall. 1996. Aerosolized surfactant in adults with sepsis-induced acute respiratory distress syndrome. *N. Engl. J. Med.* 334: 1417-1421.

[30] Cockcroft, D. W. 2001. Defining the lung's response to endotoxin. *Am. J. Respir. Crit. Care Med.* 163: 1520-1523.

[31] Andersson, U., and K. J. Tracey. 2003. HMGB1 in sepsis. *Scand. J. Infect. Dis.* 35: 577-584.

[32] O'Grady, N. P., H. L. Preas, J. Pugin, C. Fuiza, M. M. Tropea, D. Reda, S. M. Banks, and A. F. Suffredini. 2001. Local inflammatory responses following bronchial endotoxin instillation in humans. *Am. J. Respir. Crit. Care Med.* 163: 1591-1598.

[33] Green, F. H., V. Vallyathan, and F. F. Hahn. 2007. Comparative pathology of environmental lung disease: an overview. *Toxicol. Pathol.* 35: 136-147.

[34] Hansel, N. N., L. Gao, N. M. Rafaels, R. A. Mathias, E. R. Neptune, C. Tankersley, A. V. Grant, J. Connett, T. H. Beaty, R. A. Wise, and K. C. Barnes. 2009. Leptin receptor polymorphisms and lung function decline in COPD. *Eur. Respir. J.* 34: 103-110.

[35] Winkler, A. R., K. H. Nocka, T. H. Sulahian, L. Kobzik, and C. M. Williams. 2008. In vitro modeling of human alveolar macrophage smoke exposure: enhanced inflammation and impaired function. *Exp. Lung Res.* 34: 599-629.

[36] Martin, J. G., and M. Tamaoka. 2006. Rat models of asthma and chronic obstructive lung disease. *Pulm. Pharmacol. Ther.* 19: 377-385.

[37] Tuder, R. M., T. Yoshida, I. Fijalkowka, S. Biswal, and I. Petrache. 2006. Role of lung maintenance program in the heterogeneity of lung destruction in emphysema. *Proc. Am. Thorac. Soc.* 3: 673-679.

[38] McCullough, B., X. Ying, T. Monticello, and M. Bonnefoi. 2004. Digital microscopy imaging and new approaches in toxicologic pathology. *Toxicol. Pathol.* 32 Suppl 2: 49-58.

[39] Taraseviciene-Stewart, L., I. S. Douglas, P. S. Nana-Sinkam, J. D. Lee, R. M. Tuder, M. R. Nicolls, and N. F. Voelkel. 2006. Is alveolar destruction and emphysema in chronic obstructive pulmonary disease an immune disease? *Proc. Am. Thorac. Soc.* 3: 687-690.

[40] Marwick, J. A., C. S. Stevenson, J. Giddings, W. MacNee, K. Butler, I. Rahman, and P. A. Kirkham. 2006. Cigarette smoke disrupts VEGF165-VEGFR-2 receptor signaling complex in rat lungs and patients with COPD: morphological impact of VEGFR-2 inhibition. *Am. J. Physiol Lung Cell Mol. Physiol* 290: L897-L908.

[41] Petrache, I., I. Fijalkowska, T. R. Medler, J. Skirball, P. Cruz, L. Zhen, H. I. Petrache, T. R. Flotte, and R. M. Tuder. 2006. alpha-1 antitrypsin inhibits caspase-3 activity, preventing lung endothelial cell apoptosis. *Am. J. Pathol.* 169: 1155-1166.

[42] Karaaslan, C., H. Hirakawa, R. Yasumatsu, L. Y. Chang, R. A. Pierce, J. D. Crapo, and S. Cataltepe. 2011. Elastase Inhibitory Activity of Airway alpha1-Antitrypsin Is Protected by Treatment With a Catalytic Antioxidant in a Baboon Model of Severe Bronchopulmonary Dysplasia. *Pediatr. Res.* 70: 363-367.

[43] Stolk, J., B. Veldhuisen, L. Annovazzi, C. Zanone, E. M. Versteeg, T. H. van Kuppevelt, W. Nieuwenhuizen, P. Iadarola, J. H. Berden, and M. Luisetti. 2006. Correction: Short-term variability of biomarkers of proteinase activity in patients with emphysema associated with type Z alpha-1-antitrypsin deficiency. *Respir. Res.* 7: 20.

[44] Podowski, M., C. L. Calvi, C. Cheadle, R. M. Tuder, S. Biswals, and E. R. Neptune. 2009. Complex integration of matrix, oxidative stress, and apoptosis in genetic emphysema. *Am. J. Pathol.* 175: 84-96.

[45] Rohrer, J., B. R. Wuertz, and F. Ondrey. 2010. Cigarette smoke condensate induces nuclear factor kappa-b activity and proangiogenic growth factors in aerodigestive cells. *Laryngoscope* 120: 1609-1613.

[46] Rose, J. E., F. M. Behm, T. Murugesan, and F. J. McClernon. 2010. Silver acetate interactions with nicotine and non-nicotine smoke components. *Exp. Clin. Psychopharmacol.* 18: 462-469.

[47] Barnes, P. J. 2004. Alveolar Macrohages as Orchestrators of COPD., 1 ed. 59-70.

[48] Cerny, L., J. S. Torday, and V. K. Rehan. 2008. Prevention and treatment of bronchopulmonary dysplasia: contemporary status and future outlook. *Lung* 186: 75-89.

[49] Bourbon, J. R., O. Boucherat, J. Boczkowski, B. Crestani, and C. Delacourt. 2009. Bronchopulmonary dysplasia and emphysema: in search of common therapeutic targets. *Trends Mol. Med.* 15: 169-179.

[50] Kishore, U., A. L. Bernal, M. F. Kamran, S. Saxena, M. Singh, P. U. Sarma, T. Madan, and T. Chakraborty. 2005. Surfactant proteins SP-A and SP-D in human health and disease. *Arch. Immunol. Ther. Exp. (Warsz.)* 53: 399-417.

[51] Abman, S. H. 2008. The dysmorphic pulmonary circulation in bronchopulmonary dysplasia: a growing story. *Am. J. Respir. Crit Care Med.* 178: 114-115.

[52] Baleeiro, C. E. O., S. E. Wilcoxen, S. B. Morris, T. J. Standiford, and R. Paine. 2003. Sublethal hyperoxia impairs pulmonary innate immunity. *J. Immunol.* 171: 955-963.

[53] Paine, R., III, S. E. Wilcoxen, S. B. Morris, C. Sartori, C. E. Baleeiro, M. A. Matthay, and P. J. Christensen. 2003. Transgenic overexpression of granulocyte macrophage-colony stimulating factor in the lung prevents hyperoxic lung injury. *Am. J. Pathol.* 163: 2397-2406.

[54] Soll, R. F., and F. Blanco. 2003. Natural surfactant extract versus synthetic surfactant for neonatal respiratory distress syndrome. *The Cochrane Library* 1: 1-35.

[55] Clark, H. W., K. B. M. Reid, and R. B. Sim. 2000. Collectins and innate immunity in the lung. *Microbes and Infection* 2: 273-278.

[56] Krasnodembskaya, A., Y. Song, X. Fang, N. Gupta, V. Serikov, J. W. Lee, and M. A. Matthay. 2010. Antibacterial effect of human mesenchymal stem cells is mediated in part from secretion of the antimicrobial peptide LL-37. *Stem Cells* 28: 2229-2238.

[57] DeMello, D. E., and Z. Lin. 2001. Pulmonary alveolar proteinosis: a review. *Pediatr. Pathol. Mol. Med.* 20: 413-432.

[58] Presneill, J. J., K. Nakata, Y. Inoue, and J. F. Seymour. 2004. Pulmonary alveolar proteinosis. *Clin. Chest Med.* 25: 593-613, viii.

[59] Mahut, B., C. Delacourt, P. Scheinmann, J. de Blic, T. M. Mani, J. C. Fournet, and G. Bellon. 1996. Pulmonary alveolar proteinosis: experience with eight pediatric cases and a review. *Pediatrics* 97: 117-122.

[60] Nogee, L. M., D. E. de Mello, L. P. Dehner, and H. R. Colten. 1993. Brief report: deficiency of pulmonary surfactant protein B in congenital alveolar proteinosis. *N. Engl. J. Med.* 328: 406-410.

[61] Nogee, L. M. 2004. Alterations in SP-B and SP-C expression in neonatal lung disease. *Annu. Rev. Physiol* 66: 601-623.

[62] Carnovale, R., J. Zornoza, A. M. Goldman, and M. Luna. 1977. Pulmonary alveolar proteinosis: its association with hematologic malignancy and lymphoma. *Radiology* 122: 303-306.

[63] Cordonnier, C., J. Fleury-Feith, E. Escudier, K. Atassi, and J. F. Bernaudin. 1994. Secondary alveolar proteinosis is a reversible cause of respiratory failure in leukemic patients. *Am. J. Respir. Crit Care Med.* 149: 788-794.

[64] Keller, C. A., A. Frost, P. T. Cagle, and J. L. Abraham. 1995. Pulmonary alveolar proteinosis in a painter with elevated pulmonary concentrations of titanium. *Chest* 108: 277-280.

[65] McCunney, R. J., and R. Godefroi. 1989. Pulmonary alveolar proteinosis and cement dust: a case report. *J. Occup. Med.* 31: 233-237.

[66] Kitamura, T., N. Tanaka, J. Watanabe, K. Uchida, S. Kanegasaki, Y. Yamada, and K. Nakata. 1999. Idiopathic pulmonary alveolar proteinosis as an autoimmune disease with neutralizing antibody against granulocyte/macrophage colony-stimulating factor. *J. Exp. Med.* 190: 875-880.

[67] Bonfield, T. L., D. Russell, S. Burgess, A. Malur, M. S. Kavuru, and M. J. Thomassen. 2002. Autoantibodies against granulocyte macrophage colony-stimulating factor are diagnostic for pulmonary alveolar proteinosis. *Am. J. Respir. Cell Mol. Biol.* 27: 481-486.

[68] Seymour, J. F., I. R. Doyle, K. Nakata, J. J. Presneill, O. D. Schoch, E. Hamano, K. Uchida, R. Fisher, and A. R. Dunn. 2003. Relationship of anti-GM-CSF antibody concentration, surfactant protein A and B levels, and serum LDH to pulmonary parameters and response to GM-CSF therapy in patients with idiopathic alveolar proteinosis. *Thorax* 58: 252-257.

[69] Bonfield, T. L., M. S. Kavuru, and M. J. Thomassen. 2002. Anti-GM-CSF titer predicts response to GM-CSF therapy in pulmonary alveolar proteinosis. *Clin. Immunol.* 105: 342-350.

[70] Kavuru, M. S., T. L. Bonfield, and M. J. Thomassen. 2003. Plasmapheresis, GM-CSF, and alveolar proteinosis. *Am. J. Respir. Crit. Care Med.* 167: 1036.

[71] Trapnell, B. C., and J. A. Whitsett. 2002. GM-CSF regulates pulmonary surfactant homeostasis and alveolar macrophage-mediated innate host defense. *Annu. Rev. Physiol.* 64: 775-802.

[72] Trapnell, B. C., J. A. Whitsett, and K. Nakata. 2003. Pulmonary alveolar proteinosis. *N. Engl. J. Med.* 349: 2527-2539.

[73] Shibata, Y., Y. P. Berclaz, Z. C. Chroneos, M. Yoshida, J. A. Whitsett, and B. C. Trapnell. 2001. GM-CSF regulates alveolar macrophage differentiation and innate immunity in the lung through PU.1. *Immunity* 15: 557-567.

[74] Reed, J. A., M. Ikegami, L. Robb, C. G. Begley, G. Ross, and J. A. Whitsett. 2000. Distinct changes in pulmonary surfactant homeostasis in common beta-chain- and GM-CSF-deficient mice. *Am. J. Physiol Lung Cell Mol. Physiol* 278: L1164-L1171.

[75] Sakagami, T., D. Beck, K. Uchida, T. Suzuki, B. C. Carey, K. Nakata, G. Keller, R. E. Wood, S. E. Wert, M. Ikegami, J. A. Whitsett, M. Luisetti, S. Davies, J. P. Krischer, A. Brody, F. Ryckman, and B. C. Trapnell. 2010. Patient-derived granulocyte/macrophage colony-stimulating factor autoantibodies reproduce pulmonary alveolar proteinosis in nonhuman primates. *Am. J. Respir. Crit Care Med.* 182: 49-61.

[76] Uchida, K., K. Nakata, B. C. Trapnell, T. Terakawa, E. Hamano, Y. Inoue, A. Mikami, I. Matsushita, J. F. Seymour, M. Oh-eda, I. Ishige, Y. Eishi, T. Kitamura, Y. Yamada, K. Hanaoka, and N. Keicho. 2004. High affinity autoantibodies specifically eliminate granulocyte-macrophage colony stimulating factor activity in the lung of patients with idopathic pulmonary alveolar proteinosis. *Blood* 103: 1089-1098.

[77] Degryse, A. L., and W. E. Lawson. 2011. Progress toward improving animal models for idiopathic pulmonary fibrosis. *Am. J. Med. Sci.* 341: 444-449.

[78] Cook, D. N., D. M. Brass, and D. A. Schwartz. 2002. A matrix for new ideas in pulmonary fibrosis. *Am. J. Respir. Cell Mol. Biol.* 27: 122-124.

[79] Lawson, W. E., J. E. Loyd, and A. L. Degryse. 2011. Genetics in pulmonary fibrosis--familial cases provide clues to the pathogenesis of idiopathic pulmonary fibrosis. *Am. J. Med. Sci.* 341: 439-443.

[80] Hattori, N., J. L. Degen, T. H. Sisson, H. Liu, B. B. Moore, R. G. Pandrangi, R. H. Simon, and A. F. Drew. 2000. Bleomycin-induced pulmonary fibrosis in fibrinogen-null mice. *J. Clin. Invest.* 106: 1341-1350.

[81] Swaisgood, C. M., E. L. French, C. Noga, R. H. Simon, and V. A. Ploplis. 2000. The development of bleomycin-induced pulmonary fibrosis in mice deficient for components of the fibrinolytic system. *Am. J. Pathol.* 157: 177-187.

[82] Barbarin, V., Z. Xing, M. Delos, D. Lison, and F. Huaux. 2005. Pulmonary overexpression of IL-10 augments lung fibrosis and Th2 responses induced by silica particles. *Am. J. Physiol Lung Cell Mol. Physiol* 288: L841-L848.

[83] Kang, J. L., K. Lee, and V. Castranova. 2000. Nitric oxide up-regulates DNA-binding activity of nuclear factor-κB in macrophages stimulated with silica and inflammatory stimulants. *Mol. Cell. Biol.* 215: 1-9.

[84] Cochand, L., P. Isler, F. Songeon, and L. P. Nicod. 1999. Human lung dendritic cells have an immature phenotype with efficient mannose receptors. *Am J Respir Cell Mol. Biol.* 21: 547-554.

[85] Belvisi, M. G., D. J. Hele, and M. A. Birrell. 2004. New advances and potential therapies for the treatment of asthma. *BioDrugs.* 18: 211-223.

[86] Elias, J. A., C. G. Lee, T. Zheng, B. Ma, R. J. Homer, and Z. Zhu. 2003. New insights into the pathogenesis of asthma. *J Clin. Invest* 111: 291-297.

[87] Brutsche, M. H., L. Joos, I. E. A. Carlen Brutsche, R. Bissinger, M. Tamm, A. Custovic, and A. Woodcock. 2002. Array-based diagnostic gene-expression score for atopy and asthma. *J. Allergy Clin. Immunol.* 109: 271-273.

[88] Ballow, M. 2006. Biologic immune modifiers: Trials and tribulations--are we there yet? *J. Allergy Clin. Immunol.* 118: 1209-1215.

[89] Boyton, R. J., and D. M. Altmann. 2004. Asthma: new developments in cytokine regulation. *Clin. Exp. Immunol.* 136: 13-14.

[90] Shapiro, S. D. 2006. Animal models of asthma: Pro: Allergic avoidance of animal (model[s]) is not an option. *Am. J. Respir. Crit Care Med.* 174: 1171-1173.

[91] Finotto, S., M. F. Neurath, J. N. Glickman, S. Qin, H. A. Lehr, F. H. Green, K. Ackerman, K. Haley, P. R. Galle, S. J. Szabo, J. M. Drazen, G. T. De Sanctis, and L. H. Glimcher. 2002. Development of spontaneous airway changes consistent with human asthma in mice lacking T-bet. *Science* 295: 336-338.

[92] Shaver, J. R., J. G. Zangrilli, S. Cho, R. A. Cirelli, M. Pollice, A. T. Hastie, J. E. Fish, and S. P. Peters. 1997. Kinetics of the development and recovery of the lung from IgE-mediated inflammation. *Am. J. Respir. Crit. Care Med.* 155: 442-448.

[93] Elias, J. A., R. J. Homer, Q. Hamid, and C. G. Lee. 2005. Chitinases and chitinase-like proteins in TH2 inflammation and asthma. *J. Allergy Clin. Immunol.* 116: 497-500.

[94] D'Ambrosio, D., P. Panina-Bordignon, and F. Sinigaglia. 2003. Chemokine receptors in inflammation: an overview. *J Immunol. Methods* 273: 3-13.

[95] Hoenerhoff, M. J., H. H. Hong, T. V. Ton, S. A. Lahousse, and R. C. Sills. 2009. A review of the molecular mechanisms of chemically induced neoplasia in rat and mouse models in National Toxicology Program bioassays and their relevance to human cancer. *Toxicol. Pathol.* 37: 835-848.

[96] Taguchi, A., K. Politi, S. J. Pitteri, W. W. Lockwood, V. M. Faca, K. Kelly-Spratt, C. H. Wong, Q. Zhang, A. Chin, K. S. Park, G. Goodman, A. F. Gazdar, J. Sage, D. M. Dinulescu, R. Kucherlapati, R. A. Depinho, C. J. Kemp, H. E. Varmus, and S. M. Hanash. 2011. Lung cancer signatures in plasma based on proteome profiling of mouse tumor models. *Cancer Cell* 20: 289-299.

[97] Naltner, A., S. Wert, J. A. Whitsett, and C. Yan. 2000. Temporal/spatial expression of nuclear receptor coactivators in the mouse lung. *Am. J. Physiol Lung Cell Mol. Physiol* 279: L1066-L1074.

[98] Heissig, B., S. Rafii, H. Akiyama, Y. Ohki, Y. Sato, T. Rafael, Z. Zhu, D. J. Hicklin, K. Okumura, H. Ogawa, Z. Werb, and K. Hattori. 2005. Low-dose irradiation promotes tissue revascularization through VEGF release from mast cells and MMP-9-mediated progenitor cell mobilization. *J. Exp. Med.* 202: 739-750.

[99] Rozakis-Adcock, M., R. Fernley, J. Wade, T. Pawson, and D. Bowtell. 1993. The SH2 and SH3 domains of mammalian Grb2 couple the EGF receptor to the Ras activator mSos1. *Nature* 363: 83-85.

[100] Kane, A. B. 2006. Animal models of malignant mesothelioma. *Inhal. Toxicol.* 18: 1001-1004.

[101] Altomare, D. A., C. A. Vaslet, K. L. Skele, R. A. De, K. Devarajan, S. C. Jhanwar, A. I. McClatchey, A. B. Kane, and J. R. Testa. 2005. A mouse model recapitulating molecular features of human mesothelioma. *Cancer Res.* 65: 8090-8095.

[102] Konstan, M. W., D. R. VanDevanter, L. Rasouliyan, D. J. Pasta, A. Yegin, W. J. Morgan, and J. S. Wagener. 2010. Trends in the use of routine therapies in cystic fibrosis: 1995-2005. *Pediatr. Pulmonol.* 45: 1167-1172.

[103] Shah, S. 2011. VX-770, a CFTR potentiator, may have a potential clinical benefit in a subgroup of people with cystic fibrosis. *Thorax.*

[104] Chroneos, Z. C., S. E. Wert, J. L. Livingston, D. J. Hassett, and J. A. Whitsett. 2000. Role of cystic fibrosis transmembrane conductance regulator in pulmonary clearance of Pseudomonas aeruginosa in vivo. *J. Immunol.* 165: 3941-3950.

[105] Hodges, C. A., C. U. Cotton, M. R. Palmert, and M. L. Drumm. 2008. Generation of a conditional null allele for Cftr in mice. *Genesis.* 46: 546-552.

[106] Bruscia, E. M., P. X. Zhang, E. Ferreira, C. Caputo, J. W. Emerson, D. Tuck, D. S. Krause, and M. E. Egan. 2009. Macrophages directly contribute to the exaggerated inflammatory response in cystic fibrosis transmembrane conductance regulator-/- mice. *Am. J. Respir. Cell Mol. Biol.* 40: 295-304.

[107] Hodges, C. A., B. R. Grady, K. Mishra, C. U. Cotton, and M. L. Drumm. 2011. Cystic Fibrosis growth retardation is not correlated with loss of Cftr in the intestinal epithelium. *Am. J. Physiol Gastrointest. Liver Physiol.*

[108] van Heeckeren, A. M., M. D. Schluchter, W. Xue, and P. B. Davis. 2006. Response to acute lung infection with mucoid Pseudomonas aeruginosa in cystic fibrosis mice. *Am. J. Respir. Crit Care Med.* 173: 288-296.

[109] van Heeckeren, A. M., J. Tscheikuna, R. W. Walenga, M. W. Konstan, P. B. Davis, B. Erokwu, M. A. Haxhiu, and T. W. Ferkol. 2000. Effect of Pseudomonas infection on weight loss, lung mechanics, and cytokines in mice. *Am. J. Respir. Crit Care Med.* 161: 271-279.

[110] van Heeckeren, A. M., and M. D. Schluchter. 2002. Murine models of chronic Pseudomonas aeruginosa lung infection. *Lab Anim* 36: 291-312.

[111] Hodges, C. A., M. R. Palmert, and M. L. Drumm. 2008. Infertility in females with cystic fibrosis is multifactorial: evidence from mouse models. *Endocrinology* 149: 2790-2797.

[112] Wine, J. J. 2010. The development of lung disease in cystic fibrosis pigs. *Sci. Transl. Med.* 2: 29ps20.

[113] Rogers, C. S., D. A. Stoltz, D. K. Meyerholz, L. S. Ostedgaard, T. Rokhlina, P. J. Taft, M. P. Rogan, A. A. Pezzulo, P. H. Karp, O. A. Itani, A. C. Kabel, C. L. Wohlford-Lenane, G. J. Davis, R. A. Hanfland, T. L. Smith, M. Samuel, D. Wax, C. N. Murphy, A. Rieke, K. Whitworth, A. Uc, T. D. Starner, K. A. Brogden, J. Shilyansky, P. B. McCray, Jr., J. Zabner, R. S. Prather, and M. J. Welsh. 2008. Disruption of the CFTR gene produces a model of cystic fibrosis in newborn pigs. *Science* 321: 1837-1841.

[114] Meyerholz, D. K., D. A. Stoltz, E. Namati, S. Ramachandran, A. A. Pezzulo, A. R. Smith, M. V. Rector, M. J. Suter, S. Kao, G. McLennan, G. J. Tearney, J. Zabner, P. B. McCray, Jr., and M. J. Welsh. 2010. Loss of cystic fibrosis transmembrane conductance regulator function produces abnormalities in tracheal development in neonatal pigs and young children. *Am. J. Respir. Crit Care Med.* 182: 1251-1261.

[115] Sun, X., H. Sui, J. T. Fisher, Z. Yan, X. Liu, H. J. Cho, N. S. Joo, Y. Zhang, W. Zhou, Y. Yi, J. M. Kinyon, D. C. Lei-Butters, M. A. Griffin, P. Naumann, M. Luo, J. Ascher, K. Wang, T. Frana, J. J. Wine, D. K. Meyerholz, and J. F. Engelhardt. 2010. Disease phenotype of a ferret CFTR-knockout model of cystic fibrosis. *J. Clin. Invest* 120: 3149-3160.

[116] Rogers, C. S., W. M. Abraham, K. A. Brogden, J. F. Engelhardt, J. T. Fisher, P. B. McCray, Jr., G. McLennan, D. K. Meyerholz, E. Namati, L. S. Ostedgaard, R. S. Prather, J. R. Sabater, D. A. Stoltz, J. Zabner, and M. J. Welsh. 2008. The porcine

lung as a potential model for cystic fibrosis. *Am. J. Physiol Lung Cell Mol. Physiol* 295: L240-L263.

[117] Spadafora, D., E. C. Hawkins, K. E. Murphy, L. A. Clark, and S. T. Ballard. 2010. Naturally occurring mutations in the canine CFTR gene. *Physiol Genomics* 42: 480-485.

[118] Williams, S. H., V. Sahota, T. Palmai-Pallag, S. J. Tebbutt, J. Walker, and A. Harris. 2003. Evaluation of gene targeting by homologous recombination in ovine somatic cells. *Mol. Reprod. Dev.* 66: 115-125.

[119] Wine, J. J., D. Glavac, G. Hurlock, C. Robinson, M. Lee, U. Potocnik, M. Ravnik-Glavac, and M. Dean. 1998. Genomic DNA sequence of Rhesus (M. mulatta) cystic fibrosis (CFTR) gene. *Mamm. Genome* 9: 301-305.

5

Pulmonary Paracoccidioidomycosis: Clinical, Immunological and Histopathological Aspects

Luz E. Cano[1,2,*], Ángel González[1,2], Damaris Lopera[1],
Tonny W. Naranjo[1,3] and Ángela Restrepo[1]
[1]*Corporación para Investigaciones Biológicas (CIB)*,
[2]*Escuela de Microbiología, Universidad de Antioquia (UdeA)*,
[3]*Escuela Ciencias de la Salud, Universidad Pontificia Bolivariana (UPB)*,
Medellín,
Colombia

This chapter is dedicated to the memory of a great scientist, a man of vision, a true mentor,
Professor Henrique Leonel Lenzi, Emeritus Professor, Laboratory of Pathology,
Instituto Oswaldo Cruz (Fiocruz), Rio de Janeiro,
Brazil

1. Introduction

The systemic endemic mycoses are a group of microbial pathologies affecting primarily the lower respiratory tract, often overlooked in the evaluation of community-acquired pneumonia. They form a heterogeneous group caused by dimorphic fungi that share similar characteristics. All of them have the respiratory tract as the portal of entry and from the lungs they may disseminate to the mucous membranes, the skin, and many other organs. Nonetheless, each fungal disease has specific characteristics concerning its clinical course, diagnosis, and management. Interestingly, specific geographical areas of the world have been associated with acquisition of these mycoses. The diagnosis may be difficult and delayed owing to the varied manifestations and the multitude of differential diagnoses (Bonifaz et al., 2011; Hsu et al., 2010).

The major endemic systemic mycoses include histoplasmosis, coccidioidomycosis, blastomycosis, paracoccidioidomycosis (PCM), and penicilliosis. All of them can cause disease in both immunocompetent and immunocompromised hosts, in particular, AIDS and organ transplantation patients, and more recently recipients of biological therapies, such as TNF inhibitors or antagonists. These mycoses have similar clinical and radiologic presentations but require different treatments. Furthermore, when they have spread to the lymph nodes or skin, they may mimic other pathologies such as leishmaniasis, lymphoma, and syphilis, among others (Bonifaz et al., 2011).

---

* Corresponding Author

In addition, some of them have been reported outside of the endemic areas (Europe, Japan, USA), all cases occurring in immigrants, tourists, or workers returning from endemic countries (Buitrago et al., 2011; Poisson et al., 2007).

For these reasons, it is essential that physicians around the world be informed of the clinical characteristics of these fungal diseases in order to include them in their differential diagnosis of patients coming from or visiting the recognized endemic areas.

2. Defining paracoccidioidomycosis (PCM)

Paracoccidioidomycosis (PCM) is an endemic systemic mycosis caused by the thermally dimorphic fungus, *Paracoccidioides brasiliensis*. The infection is acquired after inhalation of the infectious particles (conidia) produced by the fungus's mycelia form present in its as yet unknown natural habitat (Restrepo & Tobón, 2009; Restrepo et al., 2011). This fungal pathogen has two morphotypes, a mold at temperatures under 28°C that frequently reveals chlamydoconidia and more rarely conidia (size <5 µm): the latter can transform into yeast cells under the influence of body temperature. In tissues and cultures at 35°C-37°C, this fungus grows as a yeast resembling a pilot's wheel due to its multiple buds (Figure 1). Yeast cells are round to oval but quite variable in size (4–40 µm).

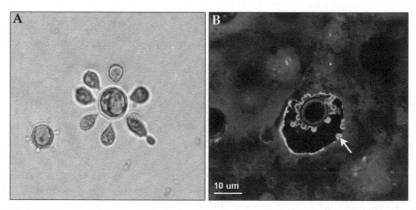

Fig. 1. *P. brasiliensis* budding yeast cells. (A) Pilot's wheel-like appearance of yeasts observed in a lactophenol cotton blue preparation from a colony grown at 36°C. (B) Multiple budding yeast cells observed in lung tissue with small spheric buds (arrow), attached to or released (arrow) from a large mother cell. Confocal indirect immunofluuorescence for fibronectin-covered *P.brasiliensis* yeast cells.

P.brasiliensis is only known in its asexual (anamorph) stage, but through molecular techniques it has been classified in the phylum Ascomycota, order Onygenales, family Onygenacea, close to *Histoplasma capsulatum*, *Blastomyces dermatitidis*, and *Emmonsia parva* phylogenetic tree, all of which have a teleomorphic, sexual stage in the genus *Ajellomyces* (Bialek et al., 2000b; Brummer et al., 1993).

More recently, the presence and expression of the mating type locus in several isolates of this fungus have been reported (Torres et al., 2010). Other studies have revealed that there are at least three distinct phylogenetic species, or clades, which are recognized within the genus (PS2, PS3, and S1) (Matute et al., 2006). In addition and based on high polygenetic diversity and exclusive morphogenetic characteristics, a different species, designated as *P.lutzi*, has been proposed (Teixeira et al., 2009).

2.1 General concepts on ecology

Geography sets PCM apart from other endemic mycoses of the Americas, such as histoplasmosis and coccidioidomycosis, as it is strictly confined to Latin America from Mexico at 23° North to Argentina at 34° South (Colombo et al., 2011; Nucci et al., 2009; Restrepo et al., 2011). The endemic areas are thus contained within the Tropics of Cancer and Capricorn (Bonifaz, 2010). PCM, however, is much more frequently reported in South-than in Central-American countries respecting Chile, Surinam, the Guyana, Nicaragua and Belize and with rare exceptions (one case each in Trinidad, Grenada and Guadeloupe), also the Caribbean Islands (Lacaz et al., 2002; Restrepo et al., 2011). Brazil accounts for over 80% of all reported cases with Venezuela, Colombia, Ecuador, Bolivia and Argentina informing lesser proportion of cases (Colombo et al., 2011; Restrepo et al., 2011).

Additionally, this mycosis is not distributed homogeneously within a particular endemic territory but is concentrated in tropical and subtropical regions with abundant forests and waterways, high annual rainfall indices (1400–2999 mm), and mild temperatures (17°C–24°C) predominating throughout the year (Borelli, 1972; Calle et al., 2001; Restrepo et al., 2001). Soil texture and moisture availability are also important (Conti-Díaz, 2007; Restrepo et al., 2001), as found in Brazil by spatial and ecologic correlate analyses (Simões et al., 2004). Studies on this aspect discovered a cluster of juvenile patients with the acute or subacute form who were potentially connected to the 1982–83 El Niño Southern Oscillation (ENSO) climatic anomalies (Barrozo et al., 2010).

P. brasiliensis's microniche has not been pinpointed precisely because the few isolations from natural sources have been sporadic, with soil being the substrate most frequently mentioned (Franco et al., 2000). Presently, there are indications that the habitat is to be found near waterways or in humid areas also propitious to agricultural crops such as coffee, tobacco and sugar cane (Calle et al., 2001; Restrepo et al., 2001). One hypothesis postulated that fish and aquatic birds would be required around the microniche to allow survival and dispersion of the fungus in nature (Conti-Díaz, 2007). Of ecological importance is the regular isolation of the fungus from armadillos (*Dassypus novemcinctus, Cabassous centralis*) captured in the endemic areas, some of which revealed internal lesions (Bagaggli et al., 2003). Dogs and other domesticated and feral animals have also been implicated (Ricci et al., 2004; Richini-Pereira et al., 2008). Nonetheless, *P. brasiliensis*'s microniche remains unknown despite many attempts to isolate it from suspected sites such as the permanent areas of residence of patients, in and around armadillos' burrows and their foraging areas (Restrepo et al., 2001).

Another circumstance that has hindered tracing the habitat has been the lack of information on outbreaks, which could have facilitated detection of the common source of infection (Lacaz et al., 2002; Restrepo et al., 2001). An increased number of childhood cases in areas where this disorder had previously been considered rare was noted by Coimbra et al. (1994) and Gonçalves et al. (1998), who suggested that colonization, gradual felling of the original native forests or changes in agricultural practices had probably exposed children to aerosolized fungal propagules, leading to increased disease rates. By the same token, in their study of 1,000 patients, Bellissimo-Rodrigues et al. (2011) pinpointed an area with the highest number of juvenile PCM cases, all of whom had resided close to coffee plantations, thereby raising the possibility of aerosol infection through agriculture-related work. None of the above reports, however, mentioned attempts at isolating the fungus from the environment.

Another important blocking factor in the search for the fungus's habitat is its capacity to enter prolonged quiescent stages, which has been demonstrated by the approximately 90 imported cases reported from nonendemic countries, as exemplified by the patients recently diagnosed in Europe (Buitrago et al., 2011; Mayayo et al., 2007; Poisson et al., 2007). All patients corresponded to emigrants living in Japan, the USA, Canada or several of the European countries where they had lived for a mean of 14 years after abandoning their native PCM-endemic homelands (Lacaz et al., 2002; Nucci et al., 2009; Shankar et al., 2011). These data clearly reveal *P. brasiliensis*'s ability to enter prolonged latency, to revive without notice and cause clinically manifested disease. This latency period prompted Borelli to create the term *reservarea* to indicate the site where the primary infection is thought to have occurred and distinguishing it from the site, the *endemic* area, where the infection was diagnosed (Borelli 1972).

2.2 General concepts on epidemiology
2.2.1 Distribution by age
The disease is relatively uncommon in children and adolescents with approximately 2% of all patients less than 10 years of age and 8% less than 20 years old. (Bellissimo-Rodrigues et al., 2011; Paniago et al., 2003; Shankar et al., 2011). Clinically manifested PCM occurs, consequently, more often (>80%) in adult patients 30–60 years old with the fourth decade of life presenting the largest number of cases (Colombo et al., 2011; Nucci et al., 2009; Paniago et al., 2003). The predominance of adult patients is reflected in higher mortality rates for those within this age group (Bittencourt et al., 2005; Coutinho et al., 2002; Prado et al., 2009; Santo, 2008). Although co-existence of the mycosis with HIV infection is relatively uncommon, 4%–5% according to data in the two largest series of cases published in Brazil (Belissimo-Rodrigues et al., 2011; Morejon et al., 2009), this dual infection has introduced a significant change in age distribution as these patients are younger (mean, 34 years of age) than the PCM non-AIDS cases (mean, 45 years of age).

2.2.2 Distribution by gender
Gender differences are also important markers of this fungal disorder, with adult males exhibiting overt disease much more often than females (Bellisimo-Rodrigues et al., 2011; Lacaz et al., 2002; Restrepo et al., 2011). Data taken from different series encompassing 5,500 patients revealed that 5,045 were males and 455 females for a male-to-female ratio of 11.1 to 1 (Shankar et al., 2011). In the largest Brazilian series totaling 1,000 patients, the male-to-female ratio was lower: 6 to 1. It should be noted that important variations have become apparent when comparing the series with the lowest ratio of 5.3 to 1 reported in Brazil by Blotta et al. (1999) and the highest 70.6 to 1 reported by Shankar et al. (2011) for Colombia. These findings indicate that present knowledge is insufficient to explain the male-to-female differences according to country of residence and indicate that inter-country variability needs further study.

The difference in the incidence of overt PCM between adult men and women has also been explained on hormonal grounds. In 27 women with the mycosis, 70% had menopausal signs and in 11% hysterectomy had been performed (Severo et al., 1998). Interestingly, in a series of 95 children with PCM collected from various Brazilian reports, there were 51 boys and 44 girls for a 1.16 to 1 ratio (Shankar et al., 2011). Such results contrast sharply with the 11.1 to 1 ratio recorded for overt PCM in adults. Since in children hormonal expression has not yet been fully developed, the finding of an almost equal gender distribution in prepubertal patients strengthens the protective role of hormones in this fungal disorder.

Additionally, in the experimental mouse model of PCM infection, differences in male and female animals have been noted. The fungus secretes a 17 beta estradiol-binding protein that attaches to the female hormone, regulating protein expression and hindering the mycelia to yeast transition so that in females fungal development is halted and the infection is controlled. On the other hand, in males conidia transform promptly into yeast cells and these multiply actively, resulting in progressive infection (Shankar et al., 2011). Additionally and as will be explained below, females exhibit a more active cellular immune response capable of halting the progress of the infection.

2.2.3 Distribution by occupation

Approximately 60% of the patients with active PCM work or have worked in agriculture-related jobs, notably in tobacco, coffee and sugarcane fields (Calle et al., 2001; Colombo et al., 2011; Nucci et al., 2009; Paniago et al., 2003). Other occupations mentioned in large series are masonry, bricklaying and mining, as well as lumberjacking in indigenous forests. These occupations are, ultimately, associated with inhalation of dust (Conti-Diaz & Calegari, 1979; Lacaz et al., 2002; Paniago et al., 2003; Restrepo et al., 2011). Even though residence in rural areas is a common trait among PCM patients, migration to urban settlements would be accompanied by a change in jobs so that when the diagnosis is established in these secondary localities, the medical history may record a different, non-PCM-related occupation. Additionally, recent land exploitation methods rely on insecticide application and soil burning, as done in sugarcane plantations, which should kill the fungus if present in the soil (Nucci et al., 2009; Restrepo et al., 2011). As a consequence, human exposure would no longer be as common; however, further observations are required to fully understand this point.

2.2.4 Incidence and prevalence

Despite the measures being implemented in Brazil, PCM is not yet a reportable disease, with the exception of the States of Mato Grosso do Sul, Minas Gerais and São Paulo (Bellissimo-Rodrigues et al., 2011). Consequently, prevalence and incidence rates are not fully dependable. Coutinho et al. (2002) reported an annual incidence rate of 1–3 per 100,000 inhabitants, and, based on 3,181 deaths known to have occurred as a result of PCM, a mean annual mortality rate of 1.45 per million inhabitants was estimated with a nonhomogenous spatial distribution among Brazil's regions and states. The authors concluded that PCM was important because it was the eighth cause of death from predominantly chronic or recurrent types of infections and parasitic diseases. It also had the highest mortality rate among the systemic mycoses but had low visibility. The great majority of deaths occurred in males (84.75%) and in the older age groups.

Bittencourt et al. (2005) analyzed 551 deaths of the mycosis in Parana State, Brazil, with an average annual mortality rate of 3.48 per million inhabitants, accounting not only for the fifth cause of death among the predominantly chronic infectious diseases, but also the highest mortality rate among the systemic mycoses. Santo (2008) reviewed 1,950 PCM death certificates finding that the largest number of deaths had occurred in men in the older age groups and among rural workers. The largest series of cases ever published (Bellissimo-Rodrigues et al., 2011) analyzed 1,000 Brazilian PCM patients and indicated that in the 1980–1999 period, the incidence rates for the Riberão Preto district in São Paulo State were equivalent to a mean of 2.70 cases per 100,000 inhabitants. Colombian estimates show a much lower incidence rate, with the highest being 0.24 per 100,000 inhabitants. Since these were annual mean mortality rates calculated on the basis of 7,482 deaths reported to be caused by PCM, the figures varied from 1.45 to 3.48 per one million inhabitants (Bellissimo-Rodrigues et al., 2011).

The importance of this mycosis can be inferred by the high burden of deaths occurring among the working population in individuals aged 30–60 years, mostly men engaged in agriculture (Bellissimo-Rodrigues et al., 2011).

2.3 Clinical presentations

PCM presents a gamut of clinical manifestations grouped according to the organs involved and the duration of the disease (Franco et al., 1987; Restrepo et al., 2008). Depending on the age and immune status of the host and on the size of the inhaled fungal inoculum, infection could be asymptomatic or may give rise to several different forms of disease. In immunocompetent individuals, they usually overcome fungal invasion; nonetheless, the fungus could remain quiescent, and a latent infection may be established. Four different clinical presentations are recognized, as follows.

2.3.1 Subclinical infection

After inhalation of the fungal particles, individuals may develop minor pulmonary symptoms that cannot be differentiated from those produced by other agents of pneumonia. The clinical manifestations often resolve spontaneously without medical intervention; however, the fungus could persist in a latent form and may later give rise to disease through endogenous reactivation, an event that may coincide with an alteration of the host's immune response (Benard et al., 2005). In some cases, the initial infection may leave a residual lung lesion. The latter situation presents the so-called regressive form of PCM. The latency process is known to exist and is frequently prolonged (mean, 14 years), as revealed by the cases reported outside the endemic areas (Buitrago et al., 2011; Walker et al., 2008; Shankar et al., 2011).

2.3.2 Acute/subacute or juvenile-type disease

This form of the mycosis is the result of the progression of a unresolved initial infection. The *acute/subacute progressive form* is seen mainly in undernourished children and adults less than 30 years of age and is the form observed in immunosuppressed individuals, such as those with HIV infection. The *juvenile form* is characterized by predominant involvement of the reticuloendothelial system. The mean duration of symptoms at consultation is 60 days and the most frequently involved organs are lymph nodes, skin, liver and spleen; less frequently bone marrow, stomach, small bowel, bones and joints are also invaded (Benard et al., 1994; Londero et al., 1996; Mendes, 1994; Morejon et al., 2009; Pereira et al., 2004).

2.3.3 Chronic or adult-type disease

This is the most frequently reported form of PCM, it has a prolonged course (months to years) and is diagnosed mainly in patients ranging from 30 to 50 years of age. This clinical form is characterized by significant lung damage as well as extrapulmonary manifestations. The respiratory symptoms become apparent only after several years with productive cough seen in 50% of the patients. Physical examination reveals few abnormalities even if extensive radiographic alterations are noted. The scarcity of respiratory symptoms explains why patients seek medical consultation based mainly on extrapulmonary manifestations, such as the presence of mucosal and skin lesions (Gomes et al., 2008; Marchiori et al., 2011; Mendes, 1994; Tuder et al., 1985). Besides the lungs, the most frequently compromised organs are the oral mucosa (involving oropharynx and larynx), skin and adrenal glands. Less frequently, the nasal and anal mucosa, genital organs and central nervous system may also be attacked. Mucosal lesions may be single or multiple, are progressive and destructive, giving rise to bleeding and pain, and are accompanied by dysphonia, dysphagia and sialorrhea.

2.3.4 Residual form

This form manifests the sequelae of prior disease at a moment when fungal growth has been arrested and the patient has overexpressed his immune responses to the point of developing fibrosis. This is exemplified by the *chronic form* of the mycosis where the lungs support the most prominent fibrotic changes, a complication recorded in approximately 60% of the patients (Funari et al., 1999; Naranjo et al., 1990; Tobón et al., 1995, 2003; Tuder et al., 1985).

The chronic progressive adult form often precedes the establishment of the *residual form*. In most cases, when the patient is finally diagnosed, this sequela is already present, reflecting the corresponding structural and functional alterations (Benard et al., 2005; Bethlem et al., 1999; Lacaz et al., 2002; Restrepo et al., 2008). It is noteworthy that residual lesions do not respond to antifungal treatment. Pulmonary fibrosis is an incapacitating disorder that may lead to core pulmonale and, finally, to death (Tobón et al., 2003; Tuder et al., 1985).

In the differential diagnosis of PCM, various diseases including tuberculosis, histoplasmosis, leishmaniasis, malignancies, lymphomatous disorders and certain abdominal syndromes should be considered (Campos et al., 2008; Nogueira et al., 2006; Ramos & Saraiva, 2008). It is important to note that PCM may coexist with tuberculosis in approximately 10% of the cases (Gomes et al., 2008; Quagliato et al., 2007).

2.4 Establishing the diagnosis

Diagnosis of PCM is based on the identification and isolation of the fungus. The microscopic visualization in representative clinical samples (including respiratory specimens or biopsies) of multiple budding yeast cells with a pilot's wheel-like appearance by direct KOH preparations or special stains, establishes the diagnosis (Lacaz et al., 2002; Nucci et al., 2009; Restrepo et al., 2009, 2011). Isolation of the fungus in culture is considered the gold standard and is successful in 60-85% of the cases. Additionally, serologic and immune-based tests [including agar gel immunodiffusion, complement fixation, enzyme-linked immunosorbent assays (ELISA) and antigen detection] are also frequently employed. These laboratory tests have great value and can also be employed in follow-up studies (Gómez et al., 1997, 1998; Lacaz et al., 2002; Nucci et al., 2009; Restrepo et al., 2009, 2011). In addition, in the last decade, molecular tests to diagnose PCM have been implemented; these tests require further research (Buitrago et al., 2011; Gomes et al., 2000; Bialek et al., 2000a; Koishi et al., 2010).

2.5 Therapeutic options

Treatment of PCM should be implemented according to the disease form; in addition, adequate nutrition, control of associated diseases, and measures to stop smoking must be implemented. Treatment of this mycosis includes sulfonamides, amphotericin B and azoles (Quagliato et al., 2007). Thus, in the case of minor and moderate forms of PCM, the combination of trimethoprim-sulfamethoxazole can be used (Shikanai-Yasuda et al., 2008). In cases of severe illness, treatment must be implemented using amphotericin B and continued with an oral antifungal, preferably itraconazole (Quagliato et al., 2007). Among the azoles, the latter is the drug of choice as it is effective in 98% of cases, irrespective of the clinical form, and has a low relapse rate (3%) (Naranjo et al., 1990; Shikanai-Yasuda et al., 2002). Nonetheless, it may not be possible to eradicate the etiologic agent completely, and the risk of endogenous reactivation may persist. Treatment of PCM is prolonged, usually taking 6 months to 1 or maximum 2 years, but in general it should continue until clinical manifestations are resolved, except for those due to residual fibrotic sequelae (Hahn et al., 2000; Shikanai-Yasuda et al., 2002).

3. Pathogenesis of experimental PCM in mice

Animal models are excellent tools to study the pathogenesis of the different infectious diseases. In order to understand the pathogenesis of PCM, different animal models of this mycosis have been established, using different hosts such as mice (Calich et al., 1985; Cano et al., 2000; Defaveri et al., 1982; McEwen et al., 1987; Moscardi & Franco, 1980), hamsters (Essayag et al., 2002; Iabuki & Montenegro, 1979; Peraçoli et al., 1982), guinea pigs (Fava-Netto et al., 1961) and rats (Iovannitti et al., 1999). All of these are powerful tools to explore the molecular and cellular aspects of PCM pathogenesis. The ability to control multiple variables in the establishment of the experimental models allows simulation of the human disease states and monitoring their course quantitatively. Therefore, animal models are a useful alternative to study the kinetics of the mechanisms involved in the pathogenesis of PCM.

3.1 Establishment of a pulmonary PCM model induced by *Pb*-conidia

Problems determining the initial stages of the host–*P. brasiliensis* interaction in humans when the fungal habitat is unknown indicate that an animal model of pulmonary PCM that would mimic, as closely as possible, human disease is needed. Such a model was established by the intranasal administration of *Pb*-conidia to male BALB/c mice to be studied sequentially during the course of infection (McEwen et al., 1987; Restrepo et al., 1992). In this model, we have determined certain immune, histological and radiological aspects of pulmonary lesions by histopathology (early and chronic periods) (González et al., 2008a, b, c; Lopera et al., 2010, 2011) as well as by high-resolution computed tomography-HRCT (chronic periods) (Lopera et al., 2010). The local immune response has been measured by determining different cytokines in supernatants of pulmonary homogenates (González et al., 2003, 2005b, 2008d; Naranjo et al., 2010).

3.2 Early immunological and histopathological findings in the model

It has been hypothesized that once *P. brasiliensis* conidia reach the lung, they interact initially with the extracellular matrix (ECM) proteins (expressed predominantly in lung tissue), lung epithelial cells (which also express these ECM proteins on their own surface), alveolar macrophages (Mɸs) and pulmonary dendritic cells. In addition, it has been reported that the different fungal morphotypes of *P. brasiliensis* (conidia, yeast cells and mycelia) exhibit on their surface adhesin-type molecules that allow both binding to several ECM proteins –

mainly fibronectin, fibrinogen and laminin – and adherence to epithelial cells (Caro et al., 2008; González et al., 2005a, 2008a, b; Hernández et al., 2010). Activation of pulmonary cells, mainly Mφs, took place after fungal interaction, thus initiating the inflammatory process through production of pro-inflammatory cytokines and chemokines, which in turn induced the expression of adhesion molecules on the leukocytes' surface (González et al., 2003, 2005b).

3.2.1 Early pulmonary inflammatory process

During the first 4 days post-infection, an acute inflammatory process, composed mainly of polymorphonuclear neutrophils (PMNs) and Mφs, was observed in the lungs (Cock et al., 2000; González et al., 2003, 2005b; Restrepo et al., 1992). At the histopathological level, this inflammatory event concurred with a bronchopneumonic process in which PMNs and Mφs accumulated and fused with each other to constitute extensive, ill-defined masses, located inside the alveolar and the surrounding peribronchiolar spaces, resulting in involvement of approximately 40% of the lung's area (Cock et al., 2000; González et al., 2005b; Restrepo et al., 1992). It should be noted that during the first 3 days post-challenge, eosinophils and lymphocytes were also observed at the perivascular level (González et al., 2005b). After the 4th day post-challenge, the cellular infiltrate was replaced by mononuclear cells, mainly Mφs. The results of additional studies conducted in bronchoalveolar lavage fluids (BALs) coincided with the *in situ* description, with predominance of PMNs and Mφs during the period indicated (González et al., 2003). Interestingly, at the end of the 2nd week post-infection, the inflammatory process decreased, indicating transient control of fungal invasion (González et al., 2005b).

Similarly, high levels of pro-inflammatory cytokines [interleukin (IL)-1β, IL-6, tumor necrosis factor-alpha (TNF-α) and chemokine, macrophage inflammatory protein (MIP)-2)] were recorded, especially in the pulmonary compartments and during the first 4 days post-challenge, (González et al., 2003). The production of these molecules by both inflammatory and endothelial cells accounted for the recruitment of certain inflammatory cells indirectly through induction of adhesion molecule expression, which in turn mediated migration of the inflammatory cells into the injured tissue (Tracey & Cerami, 1994). In accordance with the above results, a significant decrease in the mouse pulmonary fungal burden occurred after the first 2 days post-challenge (Cock et al., 2000; González et al, 2005b).

3.2.2 Expression of adhesion molecules and extracellular matrix proteins in the lungs

Adhesion molecules expressed on the cell's surface of both leukocytes and endothelial cells are important mediators in the recruitment of leukocytes to sites of inflammation including the lungs (Albeda et al., 1994; Pilewski & Albelda, 1993). Expression of these adhesion molecules is induced by the production of pro-inflammatory cytokines such as TNF-α and IL-1 (Osborn et al., 1989; Masinovsky et al., 1990), which have been reported as important inflammatory components in a variety of lung diseases including those caused by fungi (Hamacher & Schaberg, 1994; Izzo et al., 1998; Yokomura et al., 2001; Yu & Limper, 1997). In our PCM mouse model, we have observed that lungs of mice infected intranasally with *P.brasiliensis* conidia show a higher expression of adhesion molecules during the first 4 days post-challenge. Thus, the intercellular adhesion molecule-1 (ICAM-1) was overexpressed mainly on bronchiolar epithelium, vascular endothelium, pneumocytes and Mφs; the vascular cell adhesion molecule-1 (VCAM-1) was also overexpressed but only in the vascular endothelial cells, while CD18 and Mac-1, two molecules belonging to the β_2 integrin family, were strongly expressed on PMNs and Mφs (González et al., 2005b).

In lungs of mice infected with *P. brasiliensis* conidia, an initial deposition of fibrin-like material was detected after 2 days post-infection. In addition, an increased deposition and rearrangement of the following ECM proteins – laminin, fibronectin, fibrinogen, collagen and proteoglycans – were observed not only at the beginning of infection, but also during the late periods of fungal infection (González et al., 2008c). Interestingly, this increased deposition of ECM proteins in the lungs of infected mice was accompanied by a marked afflux of pro-inflammatory cells (González et al., 2008c).

In addition, *P. brasiliensis* is known to express adhesin-like molecules on its surface that recognize and bind to ECM proteins (Barbosa et al., 2006; González et al., 2005a). More recently, in elegant experiments using antisense technology, the role of a *P. brasiliensis*-adhesin molecule was confirmed when a 32-kDa protein, a putative adhesion member of the haloacid dehalogenase (HAD) superfamily of hydrolases, conferred both adherence capacity to pulmonary human epithelial cells and virulence in a mouse model of infection (Hernández et al., 2010)

The observations described above may suggest that ECM proteins modulate the pathogenesis of PCM by means of two mechanisms: 1) participation in the migration of pro-inflammatory cells into the lungs and 2) serving as a binding protein for *P. brasiliensis* expressing on its surface adhesin-like molecules (receptors). These interactions may serve the fungus both for attachment to host tissue (evading the physical barriers) and dissemination to other organs, contributing in this manner to the establishment of the disease process.

3.2.3 Expression by pulmonary phagocytes of microbicidal molecules

During any infectious process, phagocytic cells are the main effector cells, which upon their activation (e.g., by cytokines), produce microbicidal substances [i.e., degradative enzymes, defensins, lysozymes, reactive oxygen intermediates (ROS) and reactive nitrogen intermediates (RNI)] capable of inhibiting and destroying several pathogens (Nathan & Shiloh, 2000; Newman et al., 2000).

Taking into account that both PMN and Mφs are the principal components of the pulmonary inflammatory infiltrate of mice infected with *P. brasiliensis* conidia, the expression of microbicidal molecules produced by these phagocytic cells in the PCM model was determined. *In vivo* studies failed to detect nitric oxide (NO) production or inducible nitric oxide synthase (iNOS, the enzyme responsible for NO production) during the early days post-challenge in the lungs of mice infected with *P. brasiliensis*. Interestingly, as will be described below, a higher expression of iNOS was observed in the late periods of infection (González et al., 2008d). In additional studies, we observed an increase of *in situ* lysozyme expression (PMN and Mφs) in the lungs of mice infected with *P. brasiliensis* conidia during the first 4 days post-challenge. This expression was accompanied by a decrease in the number of fungal propagules (González et al., 2008), observations suggesting that lysozymes may exert an antifungal effect against *P. brasiliensis*.

Altogether, the above observations led us to propose a description of the initial mechanism triggered by the infection with *P. brasiliensis* conidia:

1. Once the conidia reach the lungs, they adhere to both ECM proteins and epithelial cells through the interaction with adhesins present on their own surface; in addition, the

fungal cells may interact with alveolar Mφs or dendritic cells present on the alveolar space.

2. Once the adhesion process or the cellular interaction takes place, induction of the production of pro-inflammatory cytokines takes place, which in turn stimulates the expression of adhesion molecules with such expression modulating the migration of circulating inflammatory cells into the lung tissue. This event triggers a strong inflammatory process, enhancing cytokine and chemokine production as well as increasing the deposition and rearrangement of ECM proteins.

3. *P. brasiliensis* conidia will experience a transitional process to yeast cells if no inhibitory mechanism intervenes in such process.

4. Once the phagocytes are activated, they will express, or produce, microbicidal molecules capable of destroying the fungus.

5. If the fungus is able to overcome the fungicidal mechanisms exerted by the host's defenses, dissemination to other organs will occur, perhaps using their adhesins to bind to ECM proteins or by producing degradative enzymes able to cleave such ECM proteins. Finally, the disease process will become established.

3.3 Chronic immune responses in the model

The intranasal inoculation of *P. brasiliensis* conidia into BALB/c male mice resulted in a progressive disease characterized by an increase of CFUs in the lungs, with maximal values at the 12th and 16th week's post-infection (Franco et al., 1998). In addition, extrapulmonary dissemination to the spleen (week 4) and liver (week 12) will take place, as indicated by the isolation in culture of the fungus from these organs (McEwen et al., 1987).

Then, during the infectious process corresponding to the chronic stages, different immunological mechanisms such as inflammatory responses, cytokine production, metalloproteinase expression, nitric oxide participation, granuloma formation and, finally, the chronic pulmonary sequelae characterized by fibrosis enter into play, as described below.

3.3.1 Production of cytokines

Additionally, several studies on the cytokines implicated in the chronic stages of experimental PCM have demonstrated, through ELISA assays and the Multiplex system, that from the 4th to the 8th week post-challenge, infected mice exhibited a significant increase in IL-1β, TNF-α, IL-12p40, RANTES, MIG, PDGF-b, IL-13 and TGF-β. Even though these cytokines have been implicated in the formation and maintenance of granuloma, some of them (IL-1β, TNF-α, IL-13 and TGF-β) are also directly involved in fibrosis generation (Franco et al., 1998; Lopera et al., 2011; Naranjo et al., 2011; Wynn, 2007).

Other authors, using both male and female mice in a PCM experimental model, have shown different immune responses that are gender-dependent with high production of Th1 cytokines and T-beta expression by the paracoccin-stimulated cultures of spleen cells from infected female mice; in contrast, cells from infected males produced higher levels of the Th2 cytokines and expressed GATA-3 (Pinzan et al., 2010). These results were confirmed using mice that had been submitted to gonadectomy followed by inverse hormonal reconstitution, where spleen cells derived from castrated males reconstituted with estradiol had produced higher levels of IFN-γ and lower levels of IL-10 than normal males in response to paracoccin stimulus. In contrast, spleen cells from castrated female mice that had been treated with testosterone produced more IL-10 and less IFN-γ than cells from normal females (Pinzan et al., 2010). In conclusion, these results reveal that the sexual hormones had a profound effect on the biology of immune cells, with estradiol favoring protective responses against *P.brasiliensis* infection.

3.3.2 iNOS expression and nitric oxide (NO) production in the lungs

In this PCM pulmonary model, the role of the NO system was determined during the chronic immune response by means of lung biopsies from infected mice. We developed an immunohistochemical stain for iNOS (NOS2) and observed that this enzyme was expressed mainly *in vivo* by the epithelioid histiocytes, with its maximal expression occurring 12 weeks after infection (González et al., 2008d). The expression of iNOS correlated significantly (r=0.77891) with the number of granulomas present in the pulmonary parenchyma (González et al., 2008d), suggesting that at this stage iNOS induction may depend on factors or mechanisms related to the environment in the granuloma (Goldman et al., 1996).

In addition, the *in vivo* administration of aminoguanidine (a highly specific inhibitor of iNOS) to *P. brasiliensis*-infected and noninfected mice induced in the former a significant reduction of their survival in comparison with negative control mice. These results suggest that during the chronic stages (12–17 weeks post-infection), the NO system played an important protective role against fungal infection (González et al., 2008d). This effect has also been observed in a model of latent tuberculosis (Flynn et al., 1998). However, Nascimento et al. (2002) proposed a dual role for nitric oxide in another experimental PCM model, where NOS2-derived NO would be essential for resistance to the fungus, but its overproduction would be associated with susceptibility.

Using NOS2-deficient mice, Livonesi et al. (2009) demonstrated that this enzyme is to be considered as a resistance factor during experimental PCM because it controls fungal proliferation, cytokine production, development of a high inflammatory response and consequently formation of necrosis. Other authors demonstrated that NO has an important role in granuloma modulation, by controlling osteopontin and MMP production, as well as by inducing loose granuloma formation and fungal dissemination, resulting, at later phases, in progression of experimental PCM (Nishikaku et al., 2009). However, iNOS-derived NO seems not to be the sole factor responsible for the immunosuppression observed during the infections caused by *P. brasiliensis*.

3.3.3 Granulomatous inflammation in the lungs during experimental PCM

The granuloma is the histologic hallmark of a variety of infectious and noninfectious processes, including PCM, all of which elicit chronic granulomatous inflammation. The word "granuloma" is derived from the Latin word *granulum*, which means a small particle of grain and, traditionally, is microscopically described as a compact, rounded aggregate of MΦs usually surrounded by a rim of lymphocytes that results in a response to chronic antigenic stimulation. Aggregation of MΦs is the minimum requirement of a granuloma, regardless of whether the lesion also contains necrosis, lymphocytes, plasma cells, or multinucleated giant cells (Mukhopadhyay & Gal, 2010). The granuloma functions both as a niche in which some microorganisms can grow or persist and as an immunologic microenvironment in which cells interact to control and prevent dissemination of the eliciting pathogen (Flynn et al., 2011).

Pulmonary granulomatous inflammation in experimental PCM is a dynamic process that goes from dispersal parenchymal inflammation, to well-defined nodules, from periarterial sheath inflammation to pseudotumoral masses (Figure 2) (Lopera et al., 2011). The lung's area occupied by the inflammatory reaction increases gradually from 8 to 12 weeks after *P.brasiliensis* infection, involving up to 40% of the lung's area. In the following subsections, we will describe the structure and cellular composition of granuloma during the experimental infection; review the formation and maintenance of the granuloma reported in the literature and compare the main features of human and experimental pulmonary histopathology during the course of *P. brasiliensis* infection.

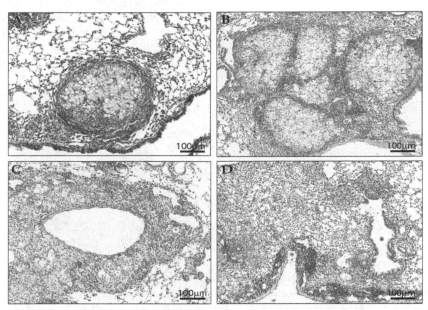

Fig. 2. Pulmonary lesions observed in BALB/c mice infected with *P. brasiliensis* conidia. (A) Well-defined nodules. (B) Confluent granulomas. (C) Periarterial sheath inflammation. (D) Dispersed parenchymal inflammation. H&E stained slides, 10X.

Structure and cellularity of pulmonary lesions: The well-defined granuloma or the nodular pattern corresponds to multiple sphere-like or oval parenchymal granulomas adjacent to terminal bronchioles, about 400 μm in diameter, sometimes isolated but becoming confluent as infection progresses. This is the predominant pattern throughout the infectious process in the lungs of BALB/c mice infected with *P. brasiliensis* conidia. In humans and experimental PCM, the general structure of granuloma consists in two distinct zones: one noncollagenic central zone composed of *P. brasiliensis* yeasts and Mɸs, and one peripheral zone composed by lymphocytes and fibroblastoid-like cells (Kerr et al., 1988). However, the cellularity and pattern of lesions change as infection progresses. A summary of the main structural and cellular changes in the granulomas sequentially observed in the experimental model of PCM is presented below (Lopera et al., 2011).

During the early stages of granuloma development, 4 weeks post-infection in our experimental model, granulomas were composed of a central core or zone of Mɸs and fungi with a frequent and intense infiltration by PMNs, sometimes presenting an apoptotic aspect. Some Mɸs formed multinucleated giant cells. The central zones of the granulomas were surrounded by a fibroblast-like layer expressing concentric layers of reticular fibers with a lesser amount of interstitial collagen. The peripheral zone consisted of a noncontinuous halo of small lymphocytes, at times forming pseudofollicular lymphocyte aggregates. At this time, an intense and diffuse parenchymal inflammation, disposed near or around the granulomas, accompanied the pulmonary response to *P. brasiliensis*.

During the most chronic stages of the infection (8, 12 and 16 weeks), Mφs acquired a xanthomatous aspect, cholesterol crystals appeared in the central zone of the granuloma and a large number of mature plasma cells located at the periphery and mixed with the fibroblastic-like cells were observed. Besides well-defined granulomas, the peak of inflammation (8–12 weeks p.i.) was characterized by periarterial inflammation accompanied by lymphatic dilatation and edema. The cellular infiltrate defined the periarterial inflammatory sheaths with dispersed fungi (Figure 3) and more mature plasmocytes and eosinophils in comparison with the granuloma.

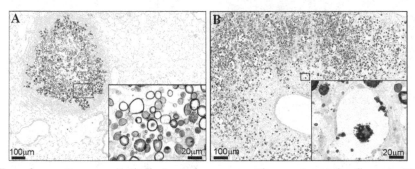

Fig. 3. Fungal aspects as seen in the lesions of a mouse with experimental pulmonary PCM. (A) Nodule full of fungi in the central area (10X), that present multiple-budding yeast cells with varying sizes (insert 100X). (B) Numerous fungi spread all over the periarterial space (10X), several of them presenting a special perifungal space (insert 100X). Grocott's stained slides.

Multiple granulomas fused and formed pseudotumoral masses or "paracoccidioidomas" five to six times larger than nodules (2,000 ± 194 µm in length) were observed in the final period of evaluation (16 weeks p.i.) in this experimental model.

Formation and maintenance of P. brasiliensis-induced granuloma: The mechanisms that drive the migration of cells that will form and maintain the granuloma around *P. brasiliensis* have begun to be explored. However, important differences in the experimental models as concerns the infective propagules (conidia, yeast cells) and the fungal isolates used, as well as the route of inoculation and the experimental host's genetic background, makes conclusions difficult. **Table 1** presents the main results of research that has analyzed the cells and mediators involved in *P. brasiliensis*-induced granulomatous inflammatory response centered on pulmonary findings.

The major biological significance of granuloma is the limitation of the infection to a local area . However, diffuse and loose granulomatous inflammation does not limit infection and is associated with incapacity to control the disease, as shown by the large number of fungal cells and the diminished survival time of infected animals (Livonesi et al., 2008, 2009).

An inflammatory response is necessary for disease control but it is also responsible for the typical immunopathology caused by diseases such as PCM that include tissue necrosis and cavitations in the center of granulomas.

Experimental model	Main results	Reference
Male BALB/c mice infected *i.n.* with 26×10⁶ viable or heat-killed *P.brasiliensis* yeasts; or inoculated with 6.5×10⁶ nonviable fragmented yeast cells	Granuloma formation required viable yeast cells or conidia. Heat-killed *Pb* yeasts or yeast fragments did not induce granuloma formation.	(Bedoya et al., 1986; Cock et al., 2000)
Rats infected *i.p.* with *P.brasiliensis* yeasts	Although most lesions developed in peritoneal cavity, granulomas also appeared in lung. Pulmonary granulomas were less collagenic than those observed in omentum, diaphragm and liver.	(Kerr, et al., 1988)
Male C57Bl/6 mice and IFN-γ and TNF receptor p55-deficient mice infected *i.v.* with 1×10⁶ *P.brasiliensis* yeast cells	IFN-γ and TNF receptor p55-deficient mice were not able to build organized granulomas, presented greater number of fungi and high rates of mortality.	(Souto et al., 2000)
Male C57BL/6 and ICAM-1KO mice infected *i.t.* with 1×10⁶ *Pb* 18 yeast cells	ICAM-1 was required for the early formation of granulomas. In the absence of ICAM-1, granuloma development delayed 60 days vs. 30 days in control mice.	(Moreira et al., 2006)
In vitro granuloma model induced by gp43-coated beads	*In vitro* granuloma formation required B1-cells and Mφs interaction. Mφs alone were not able to migrate to the beads and form granulomas. Soluble gp43 antigen-enhanced granuloma-like structure formation.	(Vigna et al., 2006)
BALB/c and BALB/Xid mice infected *i.t.* with 1×10⁶ *Pb*18 yeast cells	Mice deficient in B1-cells (BALB/Xid mice) exhibited smaller pulmonary granulomas with less fungi and longer survival. Therefore, B1-cells participated in the exacerbation of granulomatous lesions and increased host susceptibility to infection.	(Popi et al., 2008)
C57BL/6 IL-12p40⁻/⁻ and WT mice infected *i.v.* with 1×10⁶ *Pb*18 yeast.	In the absence of the IL-12p40 subunit, involved in both IL-12 and IL-23 formation, mice developed high number of pulmonary granulomas without defined delimitations associated with high number of yeast cells.	(Livonesi et al., 2008)
C57BL/6 iNOS⁻/⁻ and WT mice infected *i.v.* with 1×10⁶ *Pb*18 yeast	iNOS⁻/⁻ mice showed granulomas with high inflammatory response, central necrotic areas, diffuse distribution of cells, incipient reticulin fiber pattern and high number of yeast cells.	(Livonesi et al., 2009)
BALB/c male mice infected *i.n.* with 4×10⁶ *P.brasiliensis* conidia	Extracellular matrix proteins overexpressed and suffered rearrangement process during the course of infection. These ECM proteins localized surrounding the granuloma.	(Gonzalez et al., 2008c)

Abbreviations: *i.n.*: intranasally, *i.p.*: intraperitoneally, *i.t.*: intratracheally *i.v.*: intravenously, *Pb: P. brasiliensis,* WT: wild-type

Table 1. Contribution of cell subsets and molecules in pulmonary granuloma formation following infection with *P. brasiliensis.*

3.3.4 Fibrosis as sequelae of PCM disease

Pulmonary fibrosis is detected in several disorders with known or unknown etiologies (Datta et al., 2011). In this sense, this progressive and prominent complication is also observed in approximately 60% of patients suffering from the chronic form of PCM (Restrepo et al., 2008). Given that the *P. brasiliensis* microniche remains uncharacterized and taking into consideration the prolonged latency observed in PCM, the characteristics of the primary infection have not been defined, and great difficulties have arisen when sequentially evaluating the development of fibrosis attributed to this infection in humans. However, results from the experimental pulmonary PCM model have given convincing evidence as to the progress of this disease (González et al., 2008b).

In contrast with idiopathic pulmonary fibrosis (IPF) for which current research indicates that inflammation is of lesser importance with fibrosis appearing primarily as a disorder of fibroblast proliferation and activation in response to an as yet unknown trigger (Meltzer & Noble, 2008), the development of fibrosis in PCM is a progressive event, resulting from a persistent antigenic stimulus leading to chronic inflammation and establishment of fibrosis mainly located in the perihilar region, the main bronchi and their branches, and the large pulmonary vessels (Restrepo et al., 2011). The functional limitation caused by the development of fibrosis may advance toward cor pulmonale, progressive lung incapacity and finally death (Restrepo et al., 2008; Tobón et al., 2003; Tuder et al., 1985).

The fibrosis process begins with acute injury caused by the interaction of *P. brasiliensis* conidia with ECM proteins and lung epithelial cells; this interaction is followed by chronic granulomatous inflammation with fibroblast proliferation and activation, an increase in ECM proteins predominantly composed of fibronectin, fibrinogen, collagen type I and III, as observed in the surroundings of the granulomas.

These EM proteins contribute to the establishment of fibronodular lesions that continue to advance even after appropriate antifungal therapy with itraconazole, a medication that effectively controls the active stage of this mycosis but does not hinder lung fibrosis (González et al., 2008a, c; Naranjo et al., 2010; Tobón et al., 2003).

Even though patients with chronic PCM show well-established pulmonary lesions at diagnosis, all of them are not in the same stage of infection development, explaining why, although not sequentially, several studies have been able to describe certain histological patterns present during the development of fibrosis in humans. Tuder et al. (1985) described the lungs of 12 patients with chronic PCM in histopathological terms and concluded that chronic pulmonary PCM is a disease that affects both lungs equally and that fibrosis is mainly related to the progressive course of the granulomatous reaction to cicatrization and, to a lesser degree, is probably due to direct induction by the fungi. This study described extensive areas of dense fibrosis close to the hilar region and involved structures such as the bronchi and lymph nodes with fibrosis extending as fibrous septa of variable thickness throughout the lung parenchyma (Tuder et al., 1985).

With the development of HRCT, several studies have been published demonstrating the correlation between histopathological and radiological findings, thus providing a more precise characterization of the pattern and magnitude of the lung abnormalities, as well as better follow-up of patients with chronic pulmonary PCM. In regards to fibrotic findings on chest tomography, this process has been described as thickening of interlobular and alveolar septa, primarily those interconnecting the granulomas (Marchiori et al., 2011). This has been correlated histopathologically with prominent collagen deposition, especially near the hilar regions, comprising lymph nodes, bronchi and the main pulmonary artery branches; additionally, pulmonary architectural alterations were also observed (Funari et al., 1999; Marchiori et al., 2011; Souza et al., 2006).

Notwithstanding, in some patients, fibrosis development has been recorded in the absence of a clearly established granulomatous reaction, thus allowing speculation that the fungus itself might induce an active and higher collagen deposition (Marchiori et al., 2011; Tuder et al., 1985).

In reference to PCM animal models, several have been developed with the purpose of understanding the complete course of the disease; despite differences on the inoculum used (infective forms and concentration), fungal isolates, route of inoculation and host genetic background, the results have made it possible to define certain common phases during the granulomatous inflammation process (Burger et al., 1996; Calich et al., 1985; Da Silva et al., 2009; Xidieh et al., 1999). However, only the murine model of chronic pulmonary PCM in male BALB/c mice induced by the intranasal inoculation of naturally infective conidia has provided a reproducible model to observe in detail not only the characteristics of the inflammatory response induced by *P. brasiliensis* conidia, but also the important components of the PCM residual form (Cock et al., 2000; González et al., 2008a; Restrepo et al., 1992).

In the murine model described above, it was determined that at 4 weeks post-infection, when the granuloma are well shaped, thin fibers of collagen and reticulin became evident, suggesting the beginning of a fibrotic process, which progressed simultaneously with the presence of leukocyte infiltrates surrounding the granuloma (Lopera et al., 2010). After the 8th week post-infection, thick fibers of collagen and reticulin became evident as an indicator of established fibrosis; fibers of both proteins gradually increasing up to 12 weeks post-infection indicated the collagenesis process reaching its highest intensity, with particular involvement of the periarterial space and the surrounding area of the granuloma (Figure 4), whether or not it was confluent. Observations made in the 16th week post-infection revealed a well-established pulmonary fibrosis process (González et al., 2008b, c; Lopera et al., 2010; Naranjo et al., 2010).

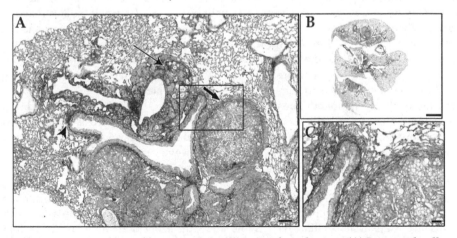

Fig. 4. Characteristics of lung fibrosis in *P. brasiliensis* infected mice. (A) Increased collagen (red fibers) noticed in the periarterial inflammatory reaction (thin arrow), in the periphery of granulomas (thick arrow) and in the bronchial wall (arrow's head). (B) Panoramic view of the entire lung. (C) Detail of collagen fibers deposition in the periphery of a granuloma and around a bronchus. Picrosirius and fast green (PIFG) stained lung sections. (Scale bars: A = 100µm, B = 2mm and C = 30µm).

One of the pathogenic mechanisms involved in the progressive accumulation of collagen and later development of fibrosis could be the disproportion between synthesis and degradation of ECM components such as reticulin and collagen, primarily due to an imbalance among the mediators of matrix degradation, metalloproteinases (MMPs) and their inhibitors (Garcia-de-Alba et al., 2010; Pardo & Selman, 2006). The presence of MMPs, specifically collagenase MMP-1 and gelatinase-A MMP-2, and the tissue inhibitors of MMPs (TIMP-1) was evaluated using immune stain in the murine model of pulmonary PCM. The results indicated that 4 weeks after *P. brasiliensis* intranasal inoculation, 85% of infected mice expressed MMP-1 as MMP-2 and 71% of them expressed TIMP-1, both with moderate intensity; at 16 weeks post-infection, almost all them showed equally positive immune stains to the TIMP-1 and MMPs evaluated, with the difference that close to 37% of them exhibited high stain intensity (Bárcenas et al., 2004). The immune stain was observed on epithelial alveolar cells and alveolar Mφs located in peribronchial tissue, although by immune staining, it was not possible to observe an imbalance between MMPs and TIMP-1. This study suggested that as more collagen becomes deposited, more activity of MMPs and their inhibitors will be present.

Although much remains to be done, the results offered by animal models have contributed greatly to understanding the genesis of the fibrotic process in PCM.

3.3.5 Experimental attempts to control fibrosis

Although currently several antifungal drugs are available for the treatment of PCM, as mentioned above in the diagnosis and treatment sections, the majority of them require prolonged therapies oscillating between 1 and 2 years (Borges-Walmsley et al., 2002). Additionally and even though these antifungal drugs can arrest the progression of the infection by restricting fungal proliferation, the principal sequelae of PCM, pulmonary fibrosis, persists, and it has been observed in both humans and murine models (Naranjo et al., 2010; Tobón et al., 2003). The fibrosis process generates progressive lung incapacity and it is probably a source of *P. brasiliensis* in future relapses of the disease (Borges-Walmsley et al., 2002). For these reasons, the need to search for new drugs or for the implementation of combined therapies has been indicated (Pappas, 2004), including experiments aiming to prevent or at least reduce the appearance of this serious sequela.

According to the recommendations given by the American Thoracic Society, the basic therapy for the treatment of patients suffering from pulmonary fibrosis includes certain immunosuppressive drugs based on the theory that the development of fibrosis is attributable to persistent inflammatory stimulus. However, the effect of using this kind of medication in humans with the chronic form of PCM remains unknown.

Recently, we evaluated the effect of two combined therapies (itraconazole + prednisolone) and (itraconazole + pentoxifylline) on the development of fibrosis using our murine model of pulmonary PCM, which reproduces the human infection from its inception until reaching the chronic form (Naranjo et al., 2011). In this study, the azolic derivative (itraconazole) was used because it is the antifungal treatment of choice for PCM (Restrepo et al., 2011; Shikanai-Yasuda et al., 2006). In reference to the combined itraconazole + prednisolone therapy, the authors reported that although a significant reduction in both granulomatous inflammation and development of fibrosis was observed when this combined therapy was used, once it was ended, the fibrotic process reappeared and progressed over the levels observed when treatment with itraconazole alone was given. On the contrary, the use of itraconazole combined with pentoxifylline, a methylxanthine compound with recognized immune modulatory properties (Inoue et al., 2004; Tong et al., 2004) and antifibrotic effects when acting on fibroblast cells (Fang et al., 2003; Romanelli et al., 1997; Valente et al., 2003), generated good results.

The combined itraconazole + pentoxifylline therapy promptly reduced the granulomatous inflammation and caused a significant and rapid decrease of both thin reticulin and collagen fibers. The most important result was that thick fiber deposition of these proteins, which are considered fibrosis indicators, was reduced to normal levels, as seen in the uninfected mice, and remained low even after the end of the treatment. Considering fungal loads, it was demonstrated that the addition of pentoxifylline to itraconazole treatment did not produce additional deleterious effects on itraconazole antifungal activity; on the contrary, a tendency towards a faster reduction of fungal burdens was observed when the combined therapy was used (Naranjo et al., 2011). These beneficial effects were noted even when such combined therapy was started belatedly at 8 weeks post-infection, a time at which the fibrosis process was already established in the murine model.

The fact that in mice the combined itraconazole + pentoxifylline therapy promptly reduced the development of pulmonary fibrosis to levels lower than those seen with antifungal therapy alone, and that this effect was maintained even after treatment termination, presents a promising advance in the development and establishment of adjunctive immunotherapies for the treatment not only of pulmonary chronic PCM but also of several disorders or chronic infections that lead to the development of fibrosis.

These findings could imply not only a reduction of treatment costs but, more importantly, improvement in the chronic pulmonary PCM patients' quality of life.

4. Pulmonary histopathology in patients with PCM: The counterpart of the experimental infection

Reports on the pathologic features of pulmonary lesions in patients with the chronic adult form of PCM are scarce in the literature. The classical report was published by Tuder et al. (1985), who described five main pathologic aspects in the lungs of 12 patients with PCM as follows:

1. Pneumonic reaction characterized by acute alveolitis with histiocytes, few PMNs, lymphocytes and plasma cells;
2. Early granulomatous formation described as circumscribed epithelioid granulomas with reticulin fibers but with no dense collagen layer surrounding them;
3. Mature and healed granuloma with collagen in their periphery;
4. Mixed pattern (early and mature granuloma in the same pulmonary area);
5. Pulmonary fibrosis.

In addition, the pulmonary lesions could be either diffuse or circumscribed (Machado, 1965).

Most recently, a study that included 23 patients with lung samples obtained by surgical biopsy or at necropsy showed similar pathological features that included alveolar wall and interlobular septal thickening, as determined by the accumulation of inflammatory cells or, less frequently, by fibrosis; filling of the alveolar spaces with inflammatory exudate; granulomas with or without fibrosis; and other evidence of fibrosis, such as architectural distortion and honeycombing. Cavitation secondary to necrosis was also a common finding (Marchiori et al., 2011).

As mentioned before, the PCM experimental animal models revealed a chronic, progressive infection that closely resembled human lesions but that did not reproduce certain histopathological aspects such as cavitated nodules, emphysema and the honeycombing pattern.

5. Radiological aspects of PCM in humans and experimental mice

Conventional HRCT has been applied as a noninvasive tool to evaluate and quantify pulmonary damage occurring in our experimental model of PCM (Lopera et al., 2010). This work has revealed that noninvasive conventional medical x-ray tomography is adequate to follow the sequential lung lesions in experimental PCM in mice. This procedure allowed detection of the main pathological patterns, the differential topographic distribution of the pulmonary lesions in both lungs, and their intensity.

The intensity of the inflammatory reaction, evaluated by histomorphometry, increased until the 12th week of infection, with a subsequent decrease due to the tendency to form predominantly compact and more isolated pseudotumoral masses. This histopathological behavior was also detected by HRCT, as expressed by lung density measures (Hounsfield units, HU) that showed a significant correlation, mainly in the upper or hilar lung region (Figure 5).

When the mice were followed up sequentially, HRCT showed that 80% of them had peribronchial consolidations that persisted throughout the evaluation periods. Pulmonary consolidations were associated with a significant increase in upper lung density as compared with controls, -263 ± 29 vs. -426 ± 8 HU at week 4 ($p<0.001$), -191 ± 25 vs. -403 ± 17 HU at week 8 ($p<0.001$), and -269 ± 43 vs. -445 ± 12 at week 12 ($p<0.001$). At week 16, upper consolidations tended to decrease as well as the corresponding density, -356 ± 33 vs. -466 ± 9 ($p<0.01$).

Histopathological analysis revealed that consolidation, as assessed by HRCT, was equivalent histologically to a confluent granulomatous reaction, while nodules corresponded to individual compact granulomas. During the same period of infection, confluent granulomas formed pseudotumoral masses that obstructed large bronchi. Discrete focal fibrosis was visible gradually around granulomas, but this finding was only evident with histopathology.

Comparing the above results with radiological findings in patients is difficult because the size of lungs, the resolution of the topographer and the protocols used.

In humans, assessment of disease progression and treatment outcome normally includes chest x-rays and then CT studies. At the time of diagnosis and in patients with active disease, chest x-ray revealed interstitial and alveolar-interstitial infiltrates, often bilateral and symmetrical, occasionally confluent, located preferentially in the central and basal areas of the lung (pattern in butterfly wings) (do Valle et al., 1992; Trad et al., 2006). A study of radiological monitoring carried out in 173 patients with chronic PCM reported presence of reticular interstitial infiltrates in 89.3% of the cases and nodular in 54.5%, bilateral alveolar in 45.4%, and mixed (in butterfly wings) in 44.7%. Emphysema was reported in 34.1%, septal lines by 25.7%, pleural thickening by 7.5%. Nine cases (6.8%) presented cavitations and three cases (2.2%) giant nodules or masses (Trad et al., 2006).

CT proved superior to conventional radiographs in demonstrating early interstitial reticular and nodular infiltrates and showed abnormal findings in the majority of patients with chronic pulmonary PCM (more than 93%).

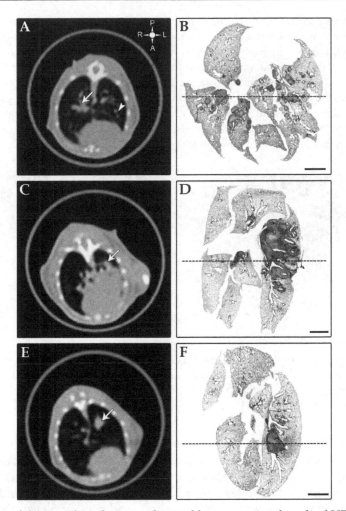

Fig. 5. Patterns of the main lung lesion as detected by conventional medical HRCT and histopathological methods in the experimental mouse PCM model. A, C, E correspond to HRCT images and B, D, F show the corresponding histopathological lesions taken in a coronal plane. The upper right symbol in (A) indicates posterior or dorsal (P), anterior or ventral (A), left (L) and right (R) regions. Dotted lines in B, D and F show an approximated position of the tomographic section. (A) Large nodular lesion represented by a peri-bronquial consolidation (arrow) is located at right hilar region and other left small nodules are indicated by arrowhead. (B) Several nodules with varied sizes. (C) Confluent lesion expressed by left central peri-bronchial consolidation (arrow) extended from the hilum to large area of the parenchyma. (D) Consolidated areas of perivascular and justabronchial granulomatous lesions. (E) Pseudotumoral lesion defining a left central pulmonary mass (arrow). (F) Left central pseudotumoral mass obstructing the bronchus. Scale bar for HRCT images = 1 cm. Scale bar for histopathological images = 2 mm. Adapted from PLoS Negl Trop Dis 4(6): e726. doi:10.1371/journal.pntd.0000726.g005.

The most frequent HRCT findings in patients with pulmonary PCM were ground-glass attenuation areas; small centrilobular, cavitated and large nodules; parenchymal bands; airspace consolidations; interlobular septal thickening; architectural distortion; traction bronchiectasis; paracicatricial emphysema and fibrosis. Most of those HRCT findings concentrated in the periphery and posterior regions involving all lung zones, with slight increased intensity in the middle zones (Funari et al., 1999; Marchiori et al., 2008, 2009; Muniz et al., 2002; Souza et al., 2006). The radiologic patterns described above in patients with pulmonary PCM were dependent on the stage of the disease and on the exclusion or inclusion of patients who had received previous treatment were excluded.

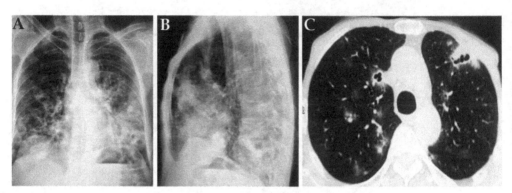

Fig. 6. Radiological findings in a patient with chronic pulmonary PMC at diagnosis. (A, B) Postero-anterior chest and lateral radiographs showing bilateral reticulonodular and ground-glass opacities with cavitations. (C) HRCT shows consolidations, ground glass attenuations and cavitated masses.

6. Final remarks

Infection by *P. brasiliensis* is, no doubt, acquired only in the endemic areas of Central and South America, especially in Brazil. However, as the fungus exhibits the capacity to remain dormant in the tissues of the infected human host for extended periods and is, likewise, able to regain its vitality giving rise to overt disease, one may encounter the mycosis in individuals living in· non-autochthonous areas, distant from those where the primary infection was acquired.

This is why it is imperative to keep informed physicians and other health-related professionals on this endemic mycosis and be prepared to include it among the differential diagnoses of disorders compatible with PCM. A detailed interrogation on the patient's former places of residence or visit should be obtained in order to focus the diagnosis. On the same token, *P. brasiliensis* should be taken into considerations whenever clinical samples and biopsies are being analyzed. It is only through knowledge that the specific diagnosis will be made in these difficult to diagnose non-autochthonous cases.

One of the main aims of this chapter was educational, namely, informing pneumologists and related professionals of the existence of this "tropical" disorder. It should be remembered that *P. brasiliensis* travels along with its host to any part of the world and that this host, now ill, may well be your own patient.

7. References

Albeda, S.M., Smith, C.W. & Ward, P.A. (1994). Adhesion molecules and inflammatory injury. *FASEB J*, Vol.8: 504–512, ISSN 0892-6638.

Bagaggli, E., Franco, M., Bosco, S. de M., Hebeler-Barbosa, F., Trinca, L.A. & Montenegro, M.R. (2003). High frequency of *Paracoccidioides brasiliensis* infection in armadillos (*Dasypus novemcinctus*): an ecological study. *Med Mycol*,Vol. 41, No. 3, pp. 217-223, ISSN 1369-3786.

Barbosa, M. S., Bao, S. N., Andreotti, P. F., de Faria, F. P., Felipe, M. S., dos Santos-Feitosa, L., Mendes-Giannini, M. J. & Soares, C. M. (2006). Glyceraldehyde-3-phosphate dehydrogenase of *Paracoccidioides brasiliensis* is a cell surface protein involved in fungal adhesion to extracellular matrix proteins and interaction with cells. *Infect Immun*, Vol. 74, No. 1, pp. 382–389, ISSN0019-9567.

Bárcenas, C., Cano, L. E., Cock A. M., Martínez, A. R. & Restrepo, A. (2004). Expresión de metaloproteinas y sus inhibidores de tejido en un modelo murino de fibrosis pulmonar. *Med-UNAB*, Vol. 7, No.19, pp. 9-14, ISSN 0123-7047.

Barrozo, L.V., Benard, G., Silva, M.E., Bagagli, E., Marques, S.A. & Mendes, R.P. (2010). First description of a cluster of acute/subacute paracoccidioidomycosis cases and its association with a climatic anomaly. *PLoS Negl Trop Dis*.Vol. 4: e643. ISSN 1935-2735.

Bedoya, V., McEwen, J.G., Tabares, A.M., Jaramillo, F.U. & Restrepo, A. (1986). Pathogenesis of paracoccidioidomycosis: a histopathological study of the experimental murine infection. *Mycopathologia*, Vol. 94, No.3, pp. 133-144, ISSN 0301-486X.

Bellissimo-Rodrigues, F., Machado, A. & Martinez, R. (2011). Paracoccidioidomycosis: epidemiological features of a 1,000 cases series from a hyperendemic area on the Southeast of Brazil. *Am J Trop Med Hyg*, Vol. 85, No.3, pp.546-50. ISSN 0002-9637.

Benard, G., Orii, N. M., Marques, H. H., Mendonça, M., Aquino, M. Z., Campeas, A. E., del Negro, G. B., Durandy, A. & Duarte, A. J. (1994). Severe acute paracoccidioidomycosis in children. *Pediatr Infect Dis J*, Vol. 13, No. 6, pp. 510-515, ISSN 0891-3668.

Benard, G., Kavakama, J., Mendes-Giannini, M. J., Kono, A., Duarte, A. J. & Shikanai-Yasuda, M. A. (2005). Contribution to the natural history of paracoccidioidomycosis: identification of the primary pulmonary infection in the severe acute form of the disease--a case report. *Clin Infect Dis*, Vol. 40, No. 1, pp. e1-4. ISSN1537-6591.

Bethlem, E. P., Capone, D., Maranhao, B., Carvalho, C. R. & Wanke, B. (1999). Paracoccidioidomycosis. *Curr Opin Pulm Med*, Vol.5, No. 5, pp. 319-325, ISSN 1070-5287.

Bialek, R., Ibricevic, A., Aepinus, C., Najvar, L. K., Fothergill, A. W., Knobloch, J. & Graybill, J. R. (2000a). Detection of *Paracoccidioides brasiliensis* in tissue samples by a nested PCR assay. *J Clin Microbiol*, Vol. 38, No. 8, pp. 2940-2942, ISSN0095-1137.

Bialek, R., Ibrecevic, A., Fothergill, A. & Begerow, D. (2000b). Small subunit ribosomal DNA sequences shows *Paracoccidioides brasiliensis* closely related to *Blastomyces dermatitidis*. *J Clin Microbiol*, Vol.38, No. 9, pp. 3190-3193, ISSN0095-1137.

Bittencourt, J.I., de Oliveira R.M. & Coutinho Z.F. (2005). Paracoccidioidomycosis mortality in the State of Parana, Brazil, 1980/1998. *Cad Saude Publica*, Vol. 21, No. 6, pp. 1856 - 1864, ISSN 0102-311X.

Blotta, M. H., Mamoni, R. L., Oliveira, S. J., Nouer, S. A., Papaiordanou, P. M., Goveia,A. & Camargo, Z.P. (1999). Endemic regions of paracoccidioidomycosis in Brazil: a clinical and epidemiologic study of 584 cases in the southeast region. *Am J Trop Med Hyg*, Vol. 61, No. 3, pp. 390-394, ISSN0002-9637.

Bonifaz, A. (2010). Chapter 219: Paracoccidioidomicosis, *in* Bonifaz, A. (ed.), *Micología Médica Básica*, 3rd Ed. McGrow Hill, Mexico, pp. 259-270.

Bonifaz, A., Vázquez-González, D. & Perusquía-Ortiz, A.M. (2011). Endemic systemic mycoses: coccidioidomycosis, histoplasmosis, paracoccidioidomycosis and blastomycosis. *J Dtsch Dermatol Ges*. Vol. 9, No. 9, pp.705-14. ISSN 1610-0387.

Borelli, D. (1972). Some ecological aspects of paracoccidioidomycosis. *Proceedings Panamerican Symposium on Paracoccidioidomycosis*, Washington: Pan American Health Organization, Washington, D:C., PAHO Scientific Publication N° 254, pp. 59-64.

Borges-Walmsley, M. I., Chen, D., Shu, X. & Walmsley, A. R. (2002). The pathobiology of *Paracoccidioides brasiliensis.Trends Microbiol*, Vol. 10, No.2, pp. 80-87, ISSN 0966-842X.

Brummer, E., Restrepo, A., Stevens, D.A., Azzi, R., Gómez, A.G., Hoyos, G., McEwen, J.G., Cano, L.E. & de Bedout, C. (1984). Murine model of paracoccidioidomycosis production of fatal acute pulmonary or chronic pulmonary and disseminated disease. Immunological and pathological observations. *J Exp Pathol*, Vol.1, No. 3, pp. 241-255, ISSN0730-8485.

Brummer, E., Castañeda, E. & Restrepo, A. (1993). Paracoccidioidomycosis: an update. *Clin Microbiol Rev*, Vol. 6, No. 2, pp. 89-117, ISSN 0893-8512.

Buitrago, M.J., Bernal-Martinez, L., Castelli, M.V., Rodríguez-Tudela, J.L. & Cuenca-Estrella, M. (2011). Histoplasmosis and paracoccidioidomycosis in a non-endemic area: a review of cases and diagnosis. *J Travel Med*, Vol.18, No. 1, pp. 26-33, ISSN 1708-8305.

Burger, E., Miyaji, M., Sano, A., Calich, V. L., Nishimura, K. & Lenzi, H. L. (1996). Histopathology of paracoccidioidomycotic infection in athymic and euthymic mice: a sequential study. *Am J Trop Med Hyg*, Vol. 55, No.2, pp. 235-242, ISSN 0002-9637.

Calich, V. L., Singer-Vermes, L. M., Siqueira, A. M. & Burger, E. (1985). Susceptibility and resistance of inbred mice to *Paracoccidioides brasiliensis*. *Br J Exp Pathol*, Vol. 66, No.5, pp. 585-594, ISSN 0007-1021.

Calle, D., Rosero, S., Orozco, L.C., Camargo, D., Castañeda, E. & Restrepo, A. (2001). Paracoccidioidomycosis in Colombia: an ecological study. *Epidemiology Infection*, Vol. 126, No. 2, pp. 309-315, ISSN 0950-2688.

Calvi, S. A., Soares, A. M., Peraçoli, M. T.,Franco, M., Ruiz, R. L. Jr., Marcondes-Machado, J., Fecchio, D., Mattos, M. C. & Mendes, R. P. (2003). Study of bronchoalveolar lavage fluid in paracoccidioidomycosis: cytopathology and alveolar macrophage function in response to gamma interferon; comparison with blood monocytes. *Microbes Infect*, Vol. 5, No. 15, pp. 1373-1379, ISSN 1286-4579.

Campos, M. V., Penna, G. O., Castro, C. N., Morales, M. A., Ferreira, M. S. & Santos, J. B. (2008). Paracoccidioidomycosis at Brasilia's university hospital. *Rev Soc Bras Med Trop*,Vol. 41, No. 2, pp. 169-172, ISSN 0037-8682.

Cano, L.E., Singer-Vermes, L.M., Costa, T.A., Mengel, J.O., Xidieh, C.F., Arruda, C., André, D.C., Vaz, C.A., Burger, E. & Calich, V.L. (2000). Depletion of CD8 (+) T cells *in vivo* impairs host defense of mice resistant and susceptible to pulmonary paracoccidioidomycosis. *Infect Immun*, Vol.68, No. 1, pp. 352-359, ISSN 0019-9567.

Carlos, T. M. & Harlan, J. M. (1990). Membrane proteins involved in phagocyte adherence to endothelium. *Immunol Rev*,Vol. 114, No. 1, pp. 5–27, ISSN 0105-2896.

Caro, E., González, A., Muñoz, C., Urán, M. E., Restrepo, A., Hamilton, A. J. & Cano, L.E. (2008). Recognition of laminin by *Paracoccidioides brasiliensis* conidia: a possible mechanism of adherence to human type II alveolar cells. *Med Mycol*, Vol. 46, No. 8, pp. 795-804, ISSN 1369-3786.

Cock, A. M., Cano, L. E., Vélez, D., Aristizábal, B. H., Trujillo, J. & Restrepo, A. (2000). Fibrotic sequelae in pulmonary paracoccidioidomycosis: histopathological aspects in BALB/c mice infected with viable and non-viable *Paracoccidioides brasiliensis* propagules. *Rev Inst Med Trop Sao Paulo*, Vol. 42, No. 2, pp. 59-66, ISSN 0036-4665.

Coimbra, Jr. C.E., Wanke, B., Santos, R.V., do Valle, A.C., Costa, R.L. & Zancope-Oliveira, R.M. (1994). Paracoccidioidin and histoplasmin sensitivity in Tupi-Monde Amerindian populations from Brazilian Amazonia. *Ann Trop Med Parasitol*, Vol. 88, No. 2, pp. 197-207, ISSN 0003-4983.

Colombo, A. L., Tobón, A., Restrepo, A., Queiroz-Telles, F. & Nucci, M. (2011). Epidemiology of endemic systemic fungal infections in Latin America. *Med Mycol*, Vol. 49, No. 8, pp.785-98. ISSN1460-2709.

Conti-Díaz, I.A. & Calegari L.F. (1979). Paracoccidioidomycosis in Uruguay: its status and current problems. *Bol Oficina Sanit. Panam*, Vol. 86, No. 3, pp. 219–229, ISSN0030-0632.

Conti-Díaz, I. (2007). Point of view on the unknown ecological niche of *Paracoccidioides brasiliensis*. Our hypothesis of 1989: Present status and perspectives. *Rev. Inst. Med. Trop. S. Paulo*, Vol. 49, No. 2, pp. 131-134, ISSN0036-4665.

Coutinho, Z.F., Silva, D., Lazera, M., Petri, V., Oliveira, R.M., Sabroza, P. C. & Wanke, B. (2002). Paracoccidioidomycosis mortality in Brazil (1980-1995). *Cad Saude Publica*, Vol. 18, No. 5, pp. 1441-1454, ISSN 0102-311X.

Da Silva, F. C., Svidzinski, T. I., Patussi, E. V., Cardoso, C. P., De Oliveira Dalalio, M. M. & Hernandes, L. (2009). Morphologic organization of pulmonary granulomas in mice infected with *Paracoccidioides brasiliensis*. *Am J Trop Med Hyg*, Vol. 80, No.5, pp. 798-804, ISSN 1476-1645.

Da Silva, M. B., Marques, A. F., Nosanchuk, J. D., Casadevall, A.,Travassos, L. R. & Taborda, C. P. (2006). Melanin in the dimorphic fungal pathogen *Paracoccidioides brasiliensis*: effects on phagocytosis, intracellular resistance and drug susceptibility. *Microbes Infect*, Vol. 8, No. 1, pp. 197–205, ISSN1286-4579.

Datta, A., Scotton, C. J. & Chambers, R. C. (2011). Novel therapeutic approaches for pulmonary fibrosis. *Br J Pharmacol*, Vol. 163, No.1, pp. 141-72, ISSN 1476-5381.

Defaveri, J., Rexkallah-Iwasso, M.T. & Franco, M.F. (1982). Experimental pulmonary paracoccidioidomycosis in mice: morphology and correlation of lesions with humoral and cellular immune response. *Mycophatologia*, Vol. 77, No. 1, pp. 3–11, ISSN 0301-486X.

Essayag, S.M., Landaeta, M.E., Hartung, C., Magaldi, S., Spencer, L., Suárez, R., García, F. & Pérez, E. (2002). Histopathologic and histochemical characterization of calcified structures in hamsters inoculated with *Paracoccidioides brasiliensis*. *Mycoses*, Vol.45, No.(9-10), pp. 351-357, ISSN0933-7407.

Fang, C. C., Lai, M. N., Chien, C. T., Hung, K. Y., Tsai, C. C., Tsai, T. J. & Hsieh, B. S. (2003). Effects of pentoxifylline on peritoneal fibroblasts and silica-induced peritoneal fibrosis. *Perit Dial Int*, Vol. 23, No.3, pp. 228-36, ISSN 0896-8608.

Fava-Netto, C., De Brito, T. & Lacaz, C.S. (1961). Experimental South American blastomycosis of the guinea pig. *Pathol Microbiol*, Vol. 24, No. 2, pp. 192–206, ISSN0031-2959.

Flynn, J.L., Scanga, C.A., Tanaka, K.E. & Chan, J. (1998). Effects of aminoguanidine on latent murine tuberculosis. *J Immunol*, Vol. 160, No.4 pp. 1796–1803, ISSN 0022-1767.

Flynn, J.L., Chan, J. & Lin, P.L. (2011). Macrophages and control of granulomatous inflammation in tuberculosis. *Mucosal Immunol*, Vol.4, No.3, pp. 271-278, ISSN 1935-3456.

Fornazim, M. C., Balthazar, A., Quagliato, R., Mamoni, R. L., Garcia, C. & Blotta, M. H. S. L. (2003). Evaluation of bronchoalveolar cells in pulmonary paracoccidioidomycosis. *Eur Respir J*, Vol. 22, No. 6, pp. 895–899, ISSN 0903-1936.

Franco, L., Najvar, L., Gómez, B. L., Restrepo, S., Graybill, J. R. & Restrepo, A. (1998). Experimental pulmonary fibrosis induced by *Paracoccidioides brasiliensis* conidia: measurement of local host responses. *Am J Trop Med Hyg*, Vol. 58, No.4, pp. 424-30, ISSN 0002-9637.

Franco, M., Montenegro, M. R., Mendes, R. P., Marques, S. A., Dillon, N. L. & Mota, N. G. (1987). Paracoccidioidomycosis: a recently proposed classification of its clinical forms. *Rev Soc Bras Med Trop*, Vol. 20, No. 2, pp.129-132, ISSN 0037-8682.

Franco, M., Bagagli, E., Scapolio, S. & da Silva Lacaz, C. (2000). A critical analysis of isolation of *Paracoccidioides brasiliensis* from soil. *Med Mycol*, Vol. 38, No. 3, pp. 185-191, ISSN 1369-3786.

Funari, M., Kavakama, J., Shikanai-Yasuda, M. A., Castro, L. G., Bernard, G., Rocha, M. S., Cerri, G. G. & Muller, N. L. (1999). Chronic pulmonary paracoccidioidomycosis (South American blastomycosis): high-resolution CT findings in 41 patients. *AJR Am J Roentgenol*, Vol. 173, No.1, pp. 59-64, ISSN 0361-803X.

Garcia-de-Alba, C., Becerril, C., Ruiz, V., Gonzalez, Y., Reyes, S., Garcia-Alvarez, J., Selman, M. & Pardo, A. (2010). Expression of matrix metalloproteases by fibrocytes: possible role in migration and homing. *Am J Respir Crit Care Med,*Vol. 182, No.9, pp. 1144-52, ISSN 1535-4970.

Gaur, N. K., Klotz, S. A. & Henderson, R. L. (1999). Overexpression of the *Candida albicans* ALA1 gene in *Saccharomyces cerevisiae* results in aggregation following attachment of yeast cells to extracellular matrix proteins, adherence properties similar to those of *Candida albicans*. *Infect Immun*, Vol. 67, No. 11, pp. 6040–6047, ISSN 0019-9567.

Goldman, D., Cho, Y., Zhao, M.L., Casadevall, A. & Lee, S.C. (1996). Expression of inducible nitric oxide synthase in rat pulmonary *Cryptococcus neoformans* granulomas. *Am J Pathol*, Vol. 148, No. 4, pp. 1275–1282, ISSN 0002-9440.

Gomes, E., Wingeter, M. A., & Svidzinski, T. I. (2008) Clinical-radiological dissociation in lung manifestations of paracoccidioidomycosis. *Rev Soc Bras Med Trop*, Vol. 41, No. 5, pp. 454-458, ISSN 1678-9849.

Gomes, G. M., Cisalpino, P. S., Taborda, C. P. & de Camargo, Z. P. (2000). PCR for diagnosis of paracoccidioidomycosis. *J Clin Microbiol*, Vol. 38, No. 9, pp. 3478-3480, ISSN 0095-1137.

Gómez, B. L., Figueroa, J. I., Hamilton, A. J., Diez, S., Rojas, M., Tobón, A. M., Hay, R. J. & Restrepo, A. (1998). Antigenemia in patients with paracoccidioidomycosis: detection of the 87-kilodalton determinant during and after antifungal therapy. *J Clin Microbiol*, Vol. 36, No. 11, pp. 3309-3316, ISSN0095-1137.

Gómez, B.L., Figueroa, J.I., Hamilton, A.J., Ortiz, B., Robledo, M.A., Hay, R.J. & Restrepo, A. (1997). Use of monoclonal antibodies in diagnosis of paracoccidioidomycosis: new strategies for the detection of circulating antigens. *J ClinMicrobiol*, Vol. 35, No. 12, pp. 3278-3283, ISSN 0095-1137.

Gonçalves, A. J., Londero, A. T., Terra, G. M., Rozenbaum, R., Abreu, T. F. & Nogueira, S. A. (1998). Paracoccidioidomycosis in children in the state of Rio de Janeiro (Brazil). Geographic distribution and the study of a "reservarea". *Rev Inst Med Trop São Paulo*, Vol. 40, No. 1, pp. 11-13, ISSN 0036-4665.

González, A., Sahaza, J. H., Ortiz, B. L., Restrepo, A. & Cano, L. E. (2003). Production of pro-inflammatory cytokines during the early stages of experimental *Paracoccidioides brasiliensis* infection. *Med Mycol*, Vol. 41, No. 5, pp. 391-399, ISSN1369-3786.

González, A., Gómez, B. L., Díez, S., Hernández, O., Restrepo, A., Hamilton, A. J. & Cano, L. E. (2005a). Purification and partial characterization of a *Paracoccidioides brasiliensis* protein with capacity to bind to extracellular matrix proteins. *Infect Immun*, Vol. 73, No. 5, pp. 2486-2495, ISSN 0019-9567.

González, A., Lenzi, H. L., Motta, E. M., Caputo, L., Sahaza, J. H., Cock, A. M., Ruiz, A. C., Restrepo, A. & Cano, L. E. (2005b).Expression of adhesion molecules in lungs of mice infected with *Paracoccidioides brasiliensis* conidia. *Microbes Infect*, Vol. 7, No. 4, pp. 666-673, ISSN 1286-4579.

González, A., Caro, E., Muñoz, C., Restrepo, A., Hamilton, A. J. & Cano, L .E. (2008a). *Paracoccidioides brasiliensis* conidia recognize fibronectin and fibrinogen which subsequently participate in adherence to human type II alveolar cells: involvement of a specific adhesin. *Microb Pathog*, Vol. 44, No. 5, pp. 389-401, ISSN 0882-4010.

González, A., Gómez, B. L., Muñoz, C., Aristizábal, B. H., Restrepo, A., Hamilton, A. J. & Cano, L. E. (2008b). Involvement of extracellular matrix proteins in the course of experimental paracoccidioidomycosis. *FEMS Immunol Med Microbiol*, Vol. 53, No. 1, pp. 114-125, ISSN 0928-8244.

González, A., Lenzi, H. L., Motta, E. M., Caputo, L., Restrepo, A., & Cano, L. E. (2008c). Expression and arrangement of extracellular matrix proteins in the lungs of mice infected with *Paracoccidioides brasiliensis* conidia. *Int J Exp Pathol*, Vol. 89, No. 2, pp. 106-116, ISSN 1365-2613.

González, A., Restrepo, A. & Cano, L. E. (2008d). Pulmonary immune responses induced in BALB/c mice by *Paracoccidioides brasiliensis* conidia. *Mycopathologia*, Vol. 165, No. 4-5, pp. 313-330, ISSN 0301-486X.

Hahn, R. C., & Hamdan, J. S. (2000). Effects of amphotericin B and three azole derivatives on the lipids of yeast cells of *Paracoccidioides brasiliensis*. *Antimicrob Agents Chemother*, Vol. 44, No. 7, pp. 1997-2000, ISSN 0066-4804.

Hamacher, J. & Schaberg, T. (1994). Adhesion molecules in lung diseases. *Lung*, Vol. 172, No. 4, pp. 189–213, ISSN 0341-2040.

Hernández, O., Almeida, A. J., González, A., García, A. M., Tamayo, D., Cano, L. E., Restrepo, A. & McEwen, J. G. (2010). A 32-kilodalton hydrolase plays an important role in *Paracoccidioides brasiliensis* adherence to host cells and influences pathogenicity. *Infect Immun*, Vol. 78, No. 12, pp. 5280-5286, ISSN 1098-5522.

Hsu, L.Y., Ng, E.S. & Koh, L.P. (2010). Common and emerging fungal pulmonary infections. *Infect Dis Clin North Am*, Vol. 24, No. 3, pp. 557-577, ISSN 1557-9824.

Iabuki, K. & Montenegro, M.R. (1979). Experimental paracoccidioidomycosis in the Syrian hamster: morphology, ultrastructure and correlation of lesions with presence of specific antigens and serum levels of antibodies. *Mycopathologia*, Vol. 67, No. 3, pp. 131-141, ISSN0301-486X.

Inoue, K., Takano, H., Yanagisawa, R. & Sakurai, M. (2004). Anti-inflammatory Effect of Pentoxifylline. *Chest*, Vol. 126, No.1, pp. 321, ISSN 0012-3692.

Iovannitti, C.A., Finquelievich, J.L., Negroni, R. & Elías-Costa, M.R. (1999). Histopathological evolution of experimental paracoccidioidomycosis in Wistar rats. *Zentralbl Bakteriol*, Vol.289, No. 2, pp. 211-216, ISSN0934-8840.

Izzo, A. A., Lovchik, J. A. & Lipscomb, M. F. (1998). T and B cell independence of endothelial cell adhesion molecule expression in pulmonary granulomatous inflammation. *Am J Respir Cell MolBiol*, Vol. 19, No. 4, pp. 588-597, ISSN 1044-1549.

Kerr, I.B., de Oliveira, P.C. & Lenzi, H.L. (1988). Connective matrix organization in chronic granulomas of experimental paracoccidioidomycosis. *Mycopathologia*, Vol. 103, No.1, pp. 11-20, ISSN 0301-486X.

Koishi, A. C., Vituri, D. F., DionízioFilho, P. S., Sasaki, A. A., Felipe, M. S. & Venancio, E. J. (2010). A semi-nested PCR assay for molecular detection of *Paracoccidioides brasiliensis* in tissue samples. *Rev Soc Bras Med Trop*, Vol. 43, No. 6, pp. 728-730, ISSN 1678-9849.

Lacaz, C. S., Porto, E., Martins, J.E.C., Heins-Vaccari, E.M. & Melo, N.T. (2002). Paracoccidioidomicose, *in* Lacaz C, Porto E, Martins JEC., Heins-Vaccari, E.M., Melo, N.T. (eds.), *Tratado de Micología Médica Lacaz*. 9th ed. Servier. São Paulo, Brazil, pp. 639-729.

Livonesi, M.C., Souto, J.T., Campanelli, A.P., Maffei, C.M., Martinez, R., Rossi, M.A. & Da Silva, J.S. (2008). Deficiency of IL-12p40 subunit determines severe paracoccidioidomycosis in mice. *Med Mycol*, Vol. 46, No.7, pp. 637-646, ISSN 1369-3786.

Livonesi, M.C., Rossi, M.A., de Souto, J.T., Campanelli, A.P., de Sousa, R.L., Maffei, C.M., Ferreira, B.R., Martinez, R. & da Silva, J.S. (2009). Inducible nitric oxide synthase-deficient mice show exacerbated inflammatory process and high production of both Th1 and Th2 cytokines during paracoccidioidomycosis. *Microbes Infect*, Vol. 11, No.1, pp. 123-132, ISSN 1286-4579.

Londero, A. T. (1986). Paracoccidioidomicose: Patogenia, formas clinicas, manifestacões pulmonares e diagnostico. *J Pneumol (Brazil)*, Vol. 12, No. 1, pp. 41-57, ISSN0102-3586.

Londero, A. T., Rios-Gonçalves, A. J., Terra, G. M. & Nogueira, S. A. (1996). Paracoccidioidomycosis in Brazilian children. A critical review (1911-1994). *Arq Bras Med*, Vol. 70, No. 4, pp. 197-203, ISSN.0365-0723 .

Lopera, D., Naranjo, T., Hidalgo, J. M., de Oliveira Pascarelli, B. M., Patiño, J. H., Lenzi, H. L., Restrepo, A. & Cano, L. E. (2010). Pulmonary abnormalities in mice with paracoccidioidomycosis: a sequential study comparing high resolution computed tomography and pathologic findings. *PLoS Negl Trop Dis*, Vol. 4, No.6, pp. e726, ISSN 1935-2735.

Lopera, D., Naranjo, T. W., Cruz, O. G., Restrepo, A., Cano, L. E. & Lenzi, H. L. (2011). Structural and topographic dynamics of pulmonary histopatology and local cytokine profiles in mice infected with *Paracoccidioides brasiliensis* conidia. *PLoS Neglected Tropical Diseases*, Vol.5, No.7, pp. e1232, ISSN 1935-2735.

Machado, J.M.J. & Teixeira G.A. (1965). Das sequelas da blastomicose Sul-Americana. *Hospital*, Vol. 68, No. X, pp.141–147.

Marchiori, E., Escuissato, D.L., Souza, A.S.Jr., Barillo, J.L., Warszawiak, D. & de Souza, A.S. (2008). Computed tomography findings in patients with tracheal paracoccidioidomycosis. *J Comput Assist Tomogr*, Vol. 32, No.5, pp. 788-791, ISSN 1532-3145.

Marchiori, E., Valiante, P.M., Mano, C. M., Zanetti, G., Escuissato, D. L., Souza, A. S. Jr., & Capone, D. (2011). Paracoccidioidomycosis: High-resolution computed tomography-pathologic correlation. *Eur J Radiol*, Vol. 77, No. 1, pp. 80-84, ISSN 1872-7727.

Masinovsky, B., Urdal, D. & Gallatin, W. M. (1990). IL-4 acts synergistically with IL-1 beta to promote lymphocyte adhesión to microvascular endothelium by induction of vascular cell adhesion molecule-1. *J Immunol*, Vol. 145, No. 9, pp. 2886–2895, ISSN0022-1767.

Matute, D. R., Sepulveda,V. E., Quesada, L. M., Goldman, G. H., Taylor, J. W., Restrepo, A. & McEwen, J. G. (2006). Microsatellite analysis of three phylogenetic species of *Paracoccidioides brasiliensis. J Clin Microbiol,* Vol.44, No. 6, pp. 2153-2157, ISSN.

Mayayo, E., Lopez-Aracil, V., Fernandez-Torres, B., Mayayo, R. & Dominguez, M. (2007). Report of an imported cutaneous disseminated case of paracoccidioidomycosis. *Rev Iberoam Micol*, Vol.24, No.1, pp. 44-46, ISSN 1130-1406.

McEwen, J.G., Bedoya, V., Patiño, M.M., Salazar, M.E. & Restrepo, A. (1987). Experimental murine paracoccidioidomycosis induced by the inhalation of conidia. *J Med Vet Mycol*, Vol. 25, No. 3, pp. 165–175, ISSN0268-1218.

McMahon, J. P., Wheat, J., Sobel, M. E., Pasula, R., Downing, J. F. & Martin, W. J. (1995). Murine laminin binds to *Histoplasma capsulatum*. A possible mechanism of dissemination. *J Clin Invest*, Vol. 96, No. 2, pp. 1010-1017, ISSN0021-9738.

Meltzer, E. B. & Noble, P. W. (2008). Idiopathic pulmonary fibrosis. *Orphanet J Rare Dis*, Vol. 3, No. 1, pp. 8, ISSN 1750-1172.

Mendes, R. P. (1994). The gamut of clinical manifestations, *in* Franco, M., Lacaz, C., Restrepo, A., & del Negro, G (eds). *Paracoccidioidomycosis*, CRC Press, Boca Raton, FL, pp. 233–258.

Moreira, A. P., Campanelli, A. P., Cavassani, K. A., Souto, J. T., Ferreira, B. R., Martinez, R., Rossi, M. A. & Silva, J. S. (2006). Intercellular adhesion molecule-1 is required for the early formation of granulomas and participates in the resistance of mice to the infection with the fungus *Paracoccidioides brasiliensis*. *Am J Pathol*, Vol. 169, No. 4, pp. 1270-1281, ISSN0002-9440.

Morejon, K.M., Machado, A.A. & Martinez, R. (2009). Paracoccidioidomycosis in patients infected with and not infected with human immunodeficiency virus: a case-control study. *Am J Trop Med Hyg*, Vol. 80, No. 3, pp. 359-366, ISSN1476-1645.

Moscardi, M.& Franco, M.F. (1980). Experimental paracoccidioidomycosis in mice. I. Immunopathological aspects of intraperitoneal infection. *Rev Inst Med Trop Sao Paulo*, Vol.22, No.6, pp. 286-293, ISSN 0036-4665

Mukhopadhyay, S. & Gal, A.A. (2010). Granulomatous lung disease: an approach to the differential diagnosis. *Arch Pathol Lab Med*, Vol.134, No.5, pp. 667-690, ISSN 1543-2165.

Muniz, M.A., E, M., Magnago, M., Moreira, L.B. & de Almeida Junior, J. (2002). Paracoccidioidomicose pulmonar – aspectos na tomografia computadorizada de alta resolução. *Radiol Bras*, Vol. 35, No.3, pp. 147-154, ISSN 0100-3984

Naranjo, M. S., Trujillo, M., Múnera, M. I., Restrepo, P., Gómez, I., & Restrepo, A. (1990). Treatment of paracoccidioidomycosis with itraconazole. *J Med Vet Mycol*, Vol. 28, No. 1, pp. 67-76, ISSN 0268-1218.

Naranjo, T. W., Lopera, D. E., Diaz-Granados, L. R., Duque, J. J., Restrepo, A. & Cano, L. E. (2010). Histopathologic and immunologic effects of the itraconazole treatment in a murine model of chronic pulmonary paracoccidioidomycosis. *Microbes Infect*, Vol. 12, No.14-15, pp. 1153-62, ISSN 1769-714X.

Naranjo, T. W., Lopera, D. E., Diaz-Granados, L. R., Duque, J. J., Restrepo, A. & Cano, L. E. (2011). Combined itraconazole-pentoxifylline treatment promptly reduces lung fibrosis induced by chronic pulmonary paracoccidioidomycosis in mice. *Pulm Pharmacol Ther*, Vol. 24, No.1, pp. 81-91, ISSN 1522-9629.

Nascimento, F.R.F., Calich, V.L.G., Rodrigues, D. & Russo, M. (2002). Dual role of nitric oxide in paracoccidioidomycosis: essential for resistance but overproduction associated with susceptibility. *J Immunol*, Vol. 168, No.9 , pp. 4593–4600, ISSN 0022-1767.

Nathan, C., & Shiloh, M. U. (2000). Reactive oxygen and nitrogen intermediates in the relationship between mammalian host and microbial pathogens. *Proc Natl Acad Sci USA*, Vol.97, No. 16, pp. 8841-8848, ISSN 0027-8424.

Newman, S. L., Goote, L., Gabay, J. E. & Selsted, M. E. (2000).Identification of constituents of human neutrophil azurophil granules that mediated fungistasis against *Histoplasma capsulatum*. *Infect Immun*, Vol. 68, No. 10, pp. 5668–5672, ISSN0019-9567.

Niño-Vega, G. A., Calcagno, A. M., San-Blas, G., San-Blas, F., Gooday, G. W. & Gow, N. A. (2000). RFLP analysis reveals marked geographical isolation between strains of *Paracoccidioides brasiliensis*. *Med Mycol*, Vol. 38, No. 6, pp. 437-441, ISSN1369-3786.

Nishikaku, A. S., Sanchez-Molina, R. F., Ribeiro, L. C., Scavone, R., Albe, B. P., Silva-Cunha, C. & Burger, E. (2009). Nitric oxide participation in granulomatous response induced by *Paracoccidioides brasiliensis* infection in mice. *Med Microbiol Immunol*, Vol. 198, No. 2, pp.123–135, ISSN 1432-1831.

Nogueira, M. G., Andrade, G. M., & Tonelli, E. (2006). Clinical evolution of paracoccidioidomycosis in 38 children and teenagers. *Mycopathologia*, Vol. 161, No. 2, pp. 73-81, ISSN 0301-486X.

Nucci, M., Colombo, A.L. & Queiroz-Telles, F. (2009). Paracoccidioidomycosis. *Curr Fungal Infect Rep.*, Vol. 3, No. 1, pp. 15-20, ISSN 1936-3761.

Osborn, L., Hession, C., Tizard, R., Vasallo, C., Luhowsky, S., Chi-Rosso, G. & Lobb, R. (1989).Direct expression of vascular cell adhesion molecule-1, a cytokine-induced endotelial protein that binds to lymphocytes. *Cell*, Vol. 59, No. 6, pp. 1203–1211, ISSN0092-8674.

Pappas, P. G. (2004). Immunotherapy for invasive fungal infections: from bench to bedside. *Drug Resist Updat*, Vol. 7, No.1, pp. 3-10, ISSN 1368-7646.

Pardo, A. & Selman, M. (2006). Matrix metalloproteases in aberrant fibrotic tissue remodeling. *Proc Am Thorac Soc*, Vol. 3, No.4, pp. 383-388, ISSN 1546-3222.

Peraçoli, M.T.S., Mota, N.G.S. & Montenegro, M.R. (1982). Experimental paracoccidioidomycosis in the Syrian hamster. Morphology and correlation of lesions with humoral and cell mediated immunity. *Mycopathologia*, Vol. 79, No. 1, pp. 7-17, ISSN0301-486X.

Pereira, R. M., Bucaretchi, F., Barison-Ede, M., Hessel, G. & Tresoldi, A. T. (2004). Paracoccidioidomycosis in children: clinical presentation, follow-up and outcome. *Rev Inst Med Trop São Paulo*, Vol. 46, No. 3, pp. 127-131, ISSN 0036-4665.

Pilewski, J. M. & Albelda, S. M. (1993). Adhesion molecules in the lung. An overview. *Am Rev Respir Dis*, Vol. 148, No. 6, pp. S31–37, ISSN0003-0805.

Pinzan, C.F., Ruas, L.P., Casabona-Fortunato, A.S., Carvalho, F.C. & Roque-Barreira, M. C. (2010). Immunological basis for the gender differences in murine *Paracoccidioides brasiliensis* infection. PLoS ONE, Vol. 5, No. 5, pe10757. ISSN 1932-6203.

Poisson, D., Heitzmann, A., Mille, C., Muckensturm, B., Dromer, F., Dupont, B. & Hocqueloux, L. (2007). *Paracoccidioides brasiliensis* in a brain abscess: First French case. *J Mycol Med*, Vol. 17, pp. 114-118, ISSN1156-5233.

Popi, A.F., Godoy, L.C., Xander, P., Lopes, J.D. & Mariano, M. (2008). B-1 cells facilitate *Paracoccidioides brasiliensis* infection in mice via IL-10 secretion. *Microbes Infect*, Vol.10, No.7, pp. 817-824, ISSN 1286-4579.

Prado, M., da Silva, M. B., Laurenti, R., Travassos, L. R. & Taborda, C. P. (2009). Mortality due to systemic mycoses as a primary cause of death or in association with AIDS in Brazil: a review from 1996 to 2006. *Mem Inst Oswaldo Cruz*, Vol.104, No. 3, pp. 513–521, ISSN 1678-8060.

QuagliatoJr, R., Grangeia, A. T., de Massucio, R. A., De Capitani, E. M., RezendeSde, M. & Balthazar, A. B. (2007). Association between paracoccidioidomycosis and tuberculosis: reality and misdiagnosis. *J Bras Pneumol*, Vol.33, No. 3, pp. 295-300, ISSN 1806-3756.

Ramos, E. S, & Saraiva, L. E. (2008). Paracoccidioidomycosis. *Dermatol Clin*, Vol. 26, No. 2, pp. 257-269, ISSN 0733-8635.

Restrepo, A., McEwen, J.G. & Castañeda, E. (2001). The habitat of *Paracoccidioides brasiliensis*: how far from solving the riddle? *Med Mycol*, Vol. 39, No. 3, pp. 233-241, ISSN 1369-3786.

Restrepo, A., Benard, G., de Castro, C. C., Agudelo, C. A. & Tobón, A. M. (2008). Pulmonary paracoccidioidomycosis. *Semin Respir Crit Care Med*, Vol. 29, No.2, pp. 182-97, ISSN 1069-3424.

Restrepo, A., & Tobón, A.M. (2009). *Paracoccidioides brasiliensis, in* Mandell, G. L., Bennett, J. E., & Dolin, R., (eds), *Mandell, Douglas and Bennett's Principles and Practice of Infectious Diseases, 7th ed.* Elsevier, Philadelphia, pp. 3357-3363.

Restrepo, A., González, A. & Agudelo, C.A. (2011). Chapter 21: Paracoccidioidomycosis, *in*W. Dismukes, C. Kauffman, P. Pappas, J. Sobel (eds): *Essentials of Medical Mycology*, 2nd Ed.: Springer, N.Y, N.Y., pp 367-385.

Restrepo, S., Tobón, A., Trujillo, J. & Restrepo, A. (1992). Development of pulmonary fibrosis in mice during infection with *Paracoccidioides brasiliensis* conidia. *J Med Vet Mycol*, Vol.30, No. 3, pp. 173–184, ISSN0268-1218.

Ricci, G., Mota, F. T., Wakamatsu, A., Serafim, R. C., Borra, R. C. & Franco, M. (2004). Canine paracoccidioidomycosis. *Med Mycol*, Vol.42, No. 4, pp. 379-383, ISSN1369-3786.

Richini-Pereira, V.B., Bosco, S.M.G., Griese, J., Theodoro, R.C., Macoris, S.A.G., Silva, R.J., Barrozo, L., Tavares, P.M.S. & Zancopé-Oliveira, R.M. (2008). Molecular detection of *Paracoccidioides brasiliensis* in road-killed wild animals. *Med Mycol*, Vol.46, No. 1, pp. 35-40, ISSN1369-3786.

Rodrigues, M. L., Dos Reis, G., Puccia, R., Travassos, L. R. & Alviano, C. S. (2003). Cleavage of human fibronectin and other basement membrane-associated proteins by a *Cryptococcus neoformans* serine proteinase. *Microb Pathog*, Vol. 34, No. 2, pp. 65–71, ISSN0882-4010.

Romanelli, R. G., Caligiuri, A., Carloni, V., De Franco, R., Montalto, P., Ceni, E., Casini, A., Gentilini, P. & Pinzani, M. (1997). Effect of pentoxifylline on the degradation of procollagen type I produced by human hepatic stellate cells in response to transforming growth factor-beta 1. *Br J Pharmacol*, Vol. 122, No.6, pp. 1047-54, ISSN 0007-1188.

San-Blas, G., Niño-Vega, G. & Iturriaga, T. (2002). *Paracoccidioides brasiliensis* and paracoccidioidomycosis: Molecular approaches to morphogenesis, diagnosis, epidemiology, taxonomy and genetics. *Med Mycol*, Vol.40, No. 3, pp. 225-242, ISSN1369-3786.

Santo, A.H. (2008). Paracoccidioidomycosis-related mortality trend, state of São Paulo, Brazil: a study using multiple causes of death. *Rev Panam Salud Publica*, Vol.23, No.5, pp. 313-324, ISSN 1020-4989.

Severo, L. C., Roesch, E. W., Oliveira, E. A., Rocha, M. M. & Londero, A. T. (1998). Paracoccidioidomycosis in women. *Rev. Iberoam. Micol.*, Vol. 15, No. 2, pp. 88–89, ISSN1130-1406.

Shankar, J., Restrepo, A., Clemons, K.V. & Stevens, D.A. (2011). Paracoccidioidomycosis: hormones and the resistance of women. *Clinical Microbiology Reviews*, Vol. 24, No. 2, pp. 296-313, ISSN1098-6618.

Shikanai-Yasuda, M. A., Benard, G., Higaki, Y., Del Negro, G. M., Hoo, S., Vaccari, E. H., Gryschek, R. C., Segurado, A. A., Barone, A. A. & Andrade, D. R. (2002). Randomized trial with itraconazole, ketoconazole and sulfadiazine in paracoccidioidomycosis. *Med Mycol*, Vol. 40, No. 4, pp. 411-417, ISSN1369-3786.

Shikanai-Yasuda, M., Queiroz-Telles, F., Poncio, R., Lopes, A. & Moretti, M. (2006). Guideliness in paracoccidioidomycosis. *Rev. Soc. Bras. Med. Trop*, Vol. 39, No.3, pp. 297-310, ISSN 0037-8682.

Shikanai-Yasuda, M. A., Conceição, Y. M., Kono, A., Rivitti, E., Campos, A. F. & Campos, S. V. (2008). Neoplasia and paracoccidioidomycosis. *Mycopathologia*, Vol. 165, No. 4-5, pp. 303-312, ISSN 0301-486X.

Simões, L.B., Marques, S.A. & Bagagli, E. (2004). Distribution of paracoccidioidomycosis: determination of ecologic correlates through spatial analyses. *Med Mycol*, Vol. 42, No. 6, pp. 517-523, ISSN1369-3786.

Soares, A.M., Rezkallah-Iwasso, M.T., Oliveira, S.L., Peraçoli, M.T., Montenegro, M.R. & Musatti, C.C. (2000). Experimental paracoccidioidomycosis in high and low antibody responder mice of Selection IV-A. *Med Mycol.* Vol. 38, No.4, pp. 309-315, ISSN1369-3786.

Souto, J.T., Figueiredo, F., Furlanetto, A., Pfeffer, K., Rossi, M.A. & Silva, J.S. (2000). Interferon-gamma and tumor necrosis factor-alpha determine resistance to *Paracoccidioides brasiliensis* infection in mice. *Am J Pathol*, Vol.156, No.5, pp. 1811-1820, ISSN 0002-9440.

Souza, A.S., Jr., Gasparetto, E.L., Davaus, T., Escuissato, D.L. & Marchiori, E. (2006). High-resolution CT findings of 77 patients with untreated pulmonary paracoccidioidomycosis. *AJR Am J Roentgenol*, Vol. 187, No.5, pp. 1248-1252, ISSN 1546-3141.

Teixeira, M. M., Theodoro, R. C., de Carvalho, M. J., Fernandes, L., Paes, H. C., Hahn, R. C., Mendoza, L., Bagagli, E., San-Blas, G. & Felipe, M. S. (2009). Phylogenetic analysis reveals a high level of speciation in the *Paracoccidioides* genus. *Mol Phylogenet Evol*, Vol. 52, No. 2, pp. 273-283, ISSN1095-9513.

Tobón, A. M., Gómez, I., Franco, L. & Restrepo, A. (1995). Seguimiento post-terapia en pacientes con paracoccidioidomicosis tratados con itraconazol. *Rev Colomb Neumol*, Vol. 7, No. X, pp. 74–78, ISSN0121-5426.

Tobón, A. M., Agudelo, C. A., Osorio, M. L., Alvarez, D. L., Arango, M., Cano, L. E. & Restrepo, A. (2003). Residual pulmonary abnormalities in adult patients with chronic paracoccidioidomycosis: prolonged follow-up after itraconazole therapy. *Clin Infect Dis,* Vol. 37, No. 7, pp. 898-904, ISSN1537-6591.

Tong, Z., Chen, B., Dai, H., Bauer, P. C., Guzman, J. & Costabel, U. (2004). Extrinsic allergic alvcolitis: inhibitory effects of pentoxifylline on cytokine production by alveolar macrophages. *Ann Allergy Asthma Immunol*, Vol. 92, No.2, pp. 234-239, ISSN 1081-1206.

Torrado, E., Castañeda, E., de la Hoz, F. & Restrepo A. (2000). Paracoccidioidomicosis: definición de las áreas endémicas de Colombia. *Biomédica*, Vol.20, No. 4, pp. 327-334, ISSN.0120-4157.

Torres, I., García, A. M., Hernández, O., González, A., McEwen, J. G., Restrepo, A. & Arango, M. (2010). Presence and expression of the mating type locus in *Paracoccidioides brasiliensis* isolates. *Fung Genet Biol*. Vol. 47, No. 4, pp. 373-380, ISSN1096-0937.

Tracey, K. J. & Cerami, A. (1994). Tumor necrosis factor: a pleiotropic cytokine and therapeutic target. *Ann Rev Med*, Vol. 45, No. 1, pp. 491–503, ISSN0066-4219.

Trad, H.S., Trad, C.S., Junior, J.E. & Muglia, V.F. (2006). Revisão radiológica de 173 casos consecutivos de paracoccidioidomicose. *Radiol Bras*, Vol.39, No.3, pp. 175-179, ISSN 0100-3984.

Tuder, R. M., el Ibrahim, R., Godoy, C. E. & De Brito, T. (1985). Pathology of the human pulmonary paracoccidioidomycosis. *Mycopathologia*, Vol. 92, No. 3, pp. 179-188, ISSN0301-486X.

Valente, E. G., Vernet, D., Ferrini, M. G., Qian, A., Rajfer, J. & Gonzalez-Cadavid, N. F. (2003). L-arginine and phosphodiesterase (PDE) inhibitors counteract fibrosis in the Peyronie's fibrotic plaque and related fibroblast cultures. *Nitric Oxide*, Vol. 9, No.4, pp. 229-44, ISSN 1089-8603.

Vigna, A.F., Almeida, S.R., Xander, P., Freymuller, E., Mariano, M. & Lopes, J.D. (2006). Granuloma formation *in vitro* requires B-1 cells and is modulated by *Paracoccidioides brasiliensis* gp43 antigen. *Microbes Infect,* Vol.8, No.3, pp. 589-597, ISSN 1286-4579.

Walker, S. L., Pembroke, A. C., Lucas, S. B. & Vega-Lopez, F. (2008). Paracoccidioidomycosis presenting in the UK. *Br J Dermatol,* Vol. 158, No. 3, pp. 624-626, ISSN0007-0963.

Wasylnka, J. A. & Moore, M. M. (2000). Adhesion of *Aspergillus* species to extracellular matrix proteins: evidence for involvement of negatively charged carbohydrates on the conidial surface. *Infect Immun,* Vol. 68, No. 6, pp. 3377–3384, ISSN0019-9567.

Wynn, T. A. (2007). Common and unique mechanisms regulate fibrosis in various fibroproliferative diseases. *J Clin Invest,* Vol. 117, No.3, pp. 524-529, ISSN 0021-9738.

Xidieh, C. F., Lenzi, H. L., Calich, V. L. & Burger, E. (1999). Influence of the genetic background on the pattern of lesions developed by resistant and susceptible mice infected with *Paracoccidioides brasiliensis. Med Microbiol Immunol,* Vol. 188, No.1, pp. 41-9, ISSN 0300-8584.

Yokomura, I., Iwasaki, Y., Nagata, K., Nakanishi, M., Natsuhara, A., Harada, H., Kubota, Y., Ueda, M., Inaba, T. & Nakagawa, M. (2001). Role of intercellular adhesion molecule 1 in acute lung injury induced by candidemia. *Exp Lung Res,* Vol. 27, No. 5, pp. 417–431, ISSN0190-2148.

Yu, M. L. & Limper, A. H. (1997). *Pneumocystis carinii* induces ICAM-1 expression in lung epithelial cells through a TNF-alpha-mediated mechanism. *Am J Physiol,* Vol. 273, No. 6, pp. L1103–1111, ISSN0002-9513.

6

Inhibition of Adhesion and Invasion of *Pseudomonas aeruginosa* to Lung Epithelial Cells: A Model of Cystic Fibrosis Infection

Ayman M. Noreddin, Ghada Sawy,
Walid Elkhatib, Ehab Noreddin and Atef Shibl
Hampton University,
Hampton, VA,
USA

1. Introduction

Cystic Fibrosis is a lethal autosomal recessive lung disorder resulting from a mutation in the transmembrane conductance regulator (CFTR) protein. The CFTR is a chloride channel encoded by a single gene on chromosome 7. More than 1200 mutations have been identified that result in defective or absent CFTR protein [1]. The most common mutation is ΔF508 (deletion of phenylalanine 508). This deletion leads to a non-functional, misfolded protein that is subsequently degraded [2]. While multiple organ systems are affected, CF is most often characterized by thickened mucus secretions and an inability to clear the lungs [1, 3-4]. In recent decades, improvements in life expectancy were achieved by new methods of antibiotic delivery as well as addition of new treatments to thin lung fluids. An example is the use of DNase to clear the buildup of extracellular DNA that occurs in the CF lung. This also relieves some of the exaggerated inflammatory response that is a characteristic of the CF lung [5].

Over their life time, CF patients experience multiple infections by various pneumonia-causing bacteria [6]. With more patients surviving to adulthood, chronic infections with *Pseudomonas aeruginosa* are coming to the forefront as a leading cause of death [7]. Problems presented by infected CF lung are multi-dimensional; the electrolyte balance and pH of the fluids are abnormal. The mucus is thick and of an alternative composition compared to normal lung and may contribute to colonization with *Pseudomonas aeruginosa* [2, 3, 5]. As such, research is multi-pronged and includes gene therapy to correct the defective protein, amelioration of inflammatory response and thinning of alveolar surface fluids [8, 9]. Significantly, Pseudomonas bacteria colonize the CF lung far easier than normal lung. Normal lung tissue has several naturally occurring defenses that work in concert with commonly prescribed antibiotics for recovery from lung infections [4, 10]. The CF patient appears to lack these natural defenses [1, 7].

Pseudomonas aeruginosa biofilms are difficult to treat due to multi-drug resistance. Many aspects of biofilms from physical structure to genetics and protein expression are under heavy investigation to elucidate the mechanisms by which biofilms develop antibiotic resistance. Within the biofilm matrix, bacteria are well protected from hostile environmental elements and host defenses. Cells in different areas of the biofilm take on various patterns of gene expression, as such; biofilms are described as a community or as functioning similar to a multi-cellular organism [3]. Biofilms develop slowly, destroy surrounding tissue and evade even healthy immune systems. Standard dose antibiotic therapy can reduce biofilm as well as planktonic cells shed from the biofilm, but rarely eradicate the entire biofilm. This allows a cycle of subsequent regrowth and new shedding of planktonic cells which possess altered antibiotic resistance [11]. Some theories describe the heavy matrix, flow channels and oxygen gradients within the biofilm structure as contributing to problems with penetration of antibiotics into the biofilm. Others describe a counteraction of host defenses or alterations in gene and protein expression not only within the biofilm, but also in the CF host [11-13]. In this proposal we will discuss a novel experimental approach to study the pharmacodynamics of antibiotics used to treat *Pseudomonas aeruginosa* biofilms in CF lung versus normal lung.

Pseudomonas aeruginosa is an important human pathogen that can cause a wide range of infectious diseases that are associated with high morbidity and mortality rates [14]. Exposed tissue surfaces lined with epithelia are the most common targets of that pathogen *e.g.* epithelial surface of the eye and airways.

Adhesion of *Pseudomonas aeruginosa* to the airway cellular receptors is the initial event to establish respiratory colonization and infection [12, 15-16]. Interestingly, the affinity of *Pseudomonas aeruginosa* to bind to the inflamed or injured epithelial cells (CF or mechanically ventilated patients) is significantly higher than that to bind normal cell surfaces; thus preventing bacterial adherence may minimize lung pathology for high-risk patients [16].

The exploit of natural compounds, especially carbohydrates, to prevent infection has been considered in lung infectivity studies; since bacteria associated with pneumonia is known to bind the carbohydrate receptors on the pulmonary epithelium [12]. Dextran, a polymer of α (11,16) linked D- glucose (branched at the 3 position), is a widely available polysaccharide that has been used in the *in vitro* and *in vivo* infection models to block the adherence of *Pseudomonas aeruginosa, Hemophilus influenza* and *Staphylococcus aureus* [12, 15]. Berries of *Vaccinium* family (include cranberry) and their extracts that contain a saccharide effective in preventing the attachment of *Escherichia coli* to the uroepithelial receptors are well-known examples as well [12].

Recent studies suggested that many pathogenic organisms have the ability to invade and reside in the host cells during the early stage of infection. The discovery of antibiotic-resistant intracellular *Heamophilus influenzae* in the lung of individuals with Chronic Obstructive Pulmonary Disease (COPD) implicates intracellular bacteria as an important reservoir for the persistent infection [17]. *Pseudomonas aeruginosa* can also survive for up to 24 hours inside the lung epithelium without inducing cytotoxicity and is known to develop resistance to the treatments afterwards [17]. Accordingly, it is equally substantial to combat bacterial adhesion and invasion as a preventive step of the infection as well as the development of bacterial resistance.

It has been reported that some inexpensive natural extracts (e.g. Berries of *Vaccinium* family and dextran) have shown promising anti-adhesion properties with some micro-organisms (e.g. *Escherichia coli*) in the urinary tract infections, therefore, they might worth testing as topical therapeutics for prevention of *Pseudomonas aeruginosa* adhesion and invasion to lung epithelial cells [18-19].

In this study, the efficacy of some natural extracts with potential anti-adhesion properties and their combinations with ciprofloxacin was evaluated as blocking agents for the adhesion and the invasion of *Pseudomonas aeruginosa* PAO1 to A549 lung epithelial cells.

Inhibition of Adhesion and Invasion of Pseudomonas aeruginosa to Lung Epithelial Cells:
A Model of Cystic Fibrosis Infection

135

2. Building CF infection model

Ciprofloxacin and gentamicin sulfate were purchased from Sigma/Aldrich (St. Louis, MO, USA) and their stock solutions were prepared in 0.1N HCl (32 mg/ml) and water (32 mg/ml), respectively, and stored at -80ºC. Before use; the antibiotic dilutions were made in F12-K cell culture medium (Cellgro, Mediatech, Inc, Manassas, VA, USA). Other Cell culture reagents were also obtained from Cellgro, Mediatech Inc. (Manassas, VA, USA). Dextran of molecular weight (MW) 40,000 was provided by Dr. John Brekke (University of Minnesota Duluth, MN, USA). Bacterial culture reagents were obtained from Difco Laboratories (Detroit, MI, USA).

The commercially available *Vaccinium macrocarpon* (cranberries) and *Glycine max* (soybean) were blended and extracted with distilled water (1:1 and 1:3.5, respectively) at room temperature.

Both crude mixtures were left to decant overnight at 4ºC. Their supernatants were then subjected to two steps centrifugation at 4750 rpm for 20 min followed by 12,000 rpm for 10 min. The resultant supernatants were membrane filtered (0.22 µm, Millipore Corp. Billerica, MA). The sterile extracts were then stored at -80ºC in 1ml aliquots till they were used in the adhesion or invasion assays.

The concentrations of the solid contents of such extracts were determined by evaporating the water content at 40ºC and weighing the solid residues until constant weights were achieved.

Pseudomonas aeruginosa strain PAO1 was purchased from American Type Culture Collection (ATCC, Rockville, MD). *P. aeruginosa* PAO1 was grown until achieving the exponential growth phase over 16 hours at 37ºC in Cation Adjusted Muller Hinton Broth (CAMHB) (Sigma-Aldrich, St. Louis. MO) from which 0.5 McFarland (1.5×10^8 CFU/ml) was prepared in F12-K tissue culture medium to initiate adhesion or invasion assays.

A549 lung epithelial cell line was obtained from American Type Culture Collection (ATCC, Rockville, MD). The cells were passed in 75 cm^2 flasks (BD Falcon, San Jose, CA), and then 1.5×10^5 cells were counted using the Hemocytometer and seeded into 12 well tissue culture plates (Becton Dickinson, NJ, USA). The cells were incubated in F12-K medium supplemented with 10% (vol/vol) Fetal Bovine Serum (FBS) at 37ºC in the presence of 5% CO_2 to achieve confluence over 48 hours.

Minimum Inhibitory Concentration (MIC) and Minimum Cytotoxic Concentration (MCC) were two factors controlled the choice of the extract or ciprofloxacin concentrations selected in the adhesion and invasion assays. In order to prevent adhesion or invasion, the bacterial cells need to be alive but incapable of clinging to or intruding into the lung epithelial cells; therefore, sub-MIC had to be determined prior to the assays. On the other hand, the lung cells integrity was kept intact via using sub-MCC of the different tested agents. MICs were determined according to the Clinical and Laboratory Standards Institute (CLSI, M7-A7 and M100-S16, Criteria for *Pseudomonas aeruginosa*). Cytotoxicity of the tested agents against the A549 lung epithelial cell line was determined using crystal violet nuclei staining method as described by Gillies, *et al.* (1986) [10] with minor modifications. Briefly, confluent monolayer of A549 lung epithelial cell was incubated for 2 hrs with 200 µl of two-fold serial dilutions of different tested agents prepared in F12-K Medium, and then the cells were washed twice with phosphate-buffered saline (PBS). After rinsing, the cells were fixed with 1% (vol/vol) gluteraldehyde (Sigma/Aldrich, St. Louis, MO) and stained with 0.1% crystal violet (Fisher Scientific, Pittsburgh, PA) for 15 min. The dye was removed through multiples sterile water rinsing and the absorbed crystal violet was then dissolved with 0.5% (vol/vol) Triton X-100 (Sigma/Aldrich, St. Louis, MO).

Absorbance was measured at λ590 nm using Synergy™2 Microplate Reader (BioTech Instruments, Inc. Vermont, USA). Absorbance data were analyzed using Excel spread sheet and sub-MCCs were determined for different agents.

For SEM analysis, A549 lung epithelial cells were challenged with PAO1 cells for 1 hour, washed 3 times with F12-K medium and subsequently fixed with 5% (vol/vol) gluteraldehyde over 24 hours. The cells were then flushed with sterile deionized water to remove salts and dried before scanning with JSM-6490LV SEM (Peabody, Massachusetts) equipped with a tungsten filament, an accelerating voltages of 15-20 kV and a chamber pressure of 60-70 Pa according to the method described by Carterson *et al* with minor modifications [11]. All infectivity studies were carried out in a sterile class II biological safety cabinet (Sterilgard III Advance, Baker Company, Sanford, Maine, USA) according to the method described Plotkowski, *et al* [12] with some modifications. Initially, the confluent monolayer of A549 lung epithelial cells was incubated with 500µl fresh F12-K cell culture medium (control wells), 500µl of the natural extract or combination solutions (natural extract and ciprofloxacin) in F12-K medium at 37°C for 15 min followed by mixing with 500µl of 0.5 McFarland (1.5 × 10^8 CFU/ml) suspension of *P. aeruginosa* PAO1 prepared in F12-K medium for one minute to achieve homogenous bacterial distribution in Multiwell™ 12-well tissue culture plate (Becton Dickinson, NJ, USA). Ciprofloxacin (0.0625 µg/ml), dextran (50.0 mg/ml), and the aqueous extracts of soybean (42.8 mg/ml), and cranberry (25.4 mg/ml) as well as the combinations of the three later agents with ciprofloxacin were applied as potential anti-adhesion agents in the aforementioned assay. The mixture was incubated at 37°C for 1 hour to establish bacterial adhesion. Each plate had a control well and all experiments were carried out in triplicates.

At the end of the incubation time, cells were gently washed thrice with FBS free F12-K medium to eliminate the non-adhered bacterial cells of *P. aeruginosa* PAO1 and then lysis of the mammalian cells was carried out with 1ml of 1% (vol/vol) tween-20 (Astoria-Pacific, Clackamas, Oregon, USA) at 37°C for 30 min.

After lysis, ten-fold serial dilutions for the *P. aeruginosa* PAO1 suspension in each well followed by plating onto Cation Adjusted Muller Hinton II (CAMHII) agar were carried out. All CAMHII agar plates were incubated at 37°C for 18 hours for determining CFU/ml through viable cell counting for different treatments as well as for the untreated control. Percentage adhesion for each treatment relative to the untreated control was calculated and the averages of triplicate experiments were expressed graphically $\pm$ standard deviations (S.D). Data analysis was carried out using Graphpad prism 5 (GraphPad Software Inc. La Jolla, CA) that utilized One Way Analysis of Variance (ANOVA) followed by Dunnett Multiple Comparison test to determine the significant treatment differences as compared to the untreated control.

Parallel experiments were carried out as described under adhesion assay except for an extra step performed to assess *P. aeruginosa* PAO1 invasion into A549 lung epithelial cells. After 15 min incubation with 500 µL of the drug or the combination solutions in F12-K medium at 37°C, bacterial suspension (500 µL of 0.5 McFarland) was added and mixed with the aforementioned solutions for 1min in Multiwell™ 12-well tissue culture plates. The plates were incubated at 37°C for 2 hours to allow for invasion. Gentamicin exclusion method as described by Fleiszig *et al* [13] was then used to kill the adherent bacterial cells. This step involved washing of the adherent cells with FBS free F12-K medium followed by incubation

Inhibition of Adhesion and Invasion of Pseudomonas aeruginosa to Lung Epithelial Cells:
A Model of Cystic Fibrosis Infection

137

of the infected cells with fresh F12-K medium containing 300µg/ml gentamicin for 1 hour at 37°C. After incubation, the dead bacteria were washed thrice with FBS free F12-K medium and the lung epithelial cells A549 were lysed with 1% (vol/vol) Tween-20 solution to determine the count of internalized *P. aeruginosa* PAO1 cells. The resultant cell suspensions were tenfold serially diluted, plated onto CAMHII agar plates, and incubated as previously described under adhesion assay.

Percentage invasion for each treatment relative to the control was calculated and the averages of triplicate experiments were expressed graphically ± standard deviations (S.D). Data analyses were carried out using Graphpad Prism 5 (GraphPad Software Inc. La Jolla, CA) that utilized the one way ANOVA followed by Dunnett Multiple Comparison adjustment to determine the significance of treatment differences on the invasion of *P. aeruginosa* PAO1 as compared to the control.

Adhesion of *P. aeruginosa* PAO1 to lung epithelial cells A549 was visualized using Scanning Electron Microscopy (SEM). Imaging revealed that *P. aeruginosa* PAO1 could adhere to the lung epithelial cells without disrupting the lung cells morphology (Figure 1).

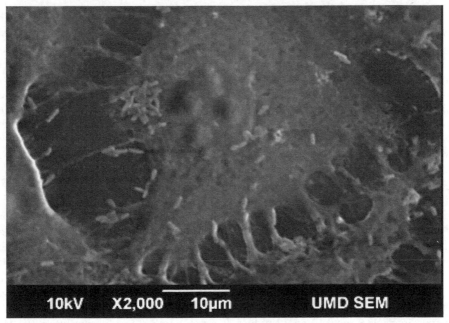

Fig. 1. Scanning Electron Micrograph illustrating the adherence of *Pseudomonas aeruginosa* PAO1 to A549 lung epithelial cells.

The soluble solid ingredients for the applied extracts were determined as described under Materials and Methods and their concentrations were 50.9 mg/ml and 85.7 mg/ml for the aqueous extracts of cranberry, and soybean respectively. Dextran was applied at a concentration level of 50.0 mg/ml.

MIC of ciprofloxacin and natural extracts against *P. aeruginosa* PAO1 and MCC of the same agents on A549 lung epithelial cells were determined according to CLSI criteria and the method described by Gillies *et al.* [10], respectively. The results showed that all the tested natural extracts had relatively high concentrations of MICs against *P. aeruginosa* PAO1 and of MCC on A549 lung epithelial cells (Table 1). These results may indicate that these agents are relatively non-toxic to the A549 lung epithelial cells as well as they cannot inhibit the growth of *P. aeruginosa* PAO1 at the tested concentrations.

Treatment	MIC[a] (μg/ml)	MCC[b] (μg/ml)
Ciprofloxacin	0.125	> 64
Dextran	>10000	>10000
Cranberry Extract	>5090	>5090
Soybean Extract	>8570	>8570

[a]Minimum Inhibitory Concentration
[b]Minimum Cytotoxic Concentration

Table 1. MIC and MCC (μg/ml) values for ciprofloxacin and different natural extracts against *P. aeruginosa* PAO1 and A549 lung epithelial cells, respectively.

Based on the data shown in table (1), sub-MIC and sub-MCC concentrations of both ciprofloxacin and the natural extracts were selected in the adhesion and invasion assays to evaluate their effects, as single agents or in combination with ciprofloxacin, on *P. aeruginosa* PAO1 adhesion and invasion without interfering with the viability of the bacterial or mammalian cells. Accordingly, ciprofloxacin (0.0625 μg/ml), dextran (50.0 mg/ml), cranberry extract (25.5 mg/ml), and soybean extract (42.8 mg/ml) were selected at their subMIC/subMCC for testing the effects of the single treatments on *P. aeruginosa* PAO1 adhesion and invasion to the lung epithelial cells. In combination treatments, the effect of ciprofloxacin (0.0625 μg/ml) on the adhesion and invasion of *P. aeruginosa* PAO1 was assessed with halves of the aforementioned concentrations of the tested single agents.

2.1 Effect of natural extracts and their combinations with ciprofloxacin on the adhesion of *P. aeruginosa* PAO1 to A549 lung epithelial cells

Adhesion of the *P. aeruginosa* PAO1 to the lung epithelial cells was assessed through viable cell counting of the bound bacteria to the cell surface from each independent triplicate experiment and the untreated controls. Adhesion of *P. aeruginosa* PAO1 to A549 lung epithelial cells in the presence of different natural extracts, as single agents and in combination with ciprofloxacin, was expressed as the percentage of adhered bacterial cells to the epithelial cell surface and normalized to that of the untreated controls. In that regard, ciprofloxacin (0.0625 μg/ml), dextran (50.0 mg/ml), cranberry extract (25.5 mg/ml), soybean extract (42.8 mg/ml) could reduce *P. aeruginosa* PAO1 adhesion by 26.3%, 16.4%, 54.5%, and 45%, respectively compared to the untreated control. On the other hand, ciprofloxacin combination with dextran (25.0 mg/ml), cranberry extract (12.7 mg/ml), soybean extract (21.4 mg/ml) could reduce *P. aeruginosa* PAO1 adhesion by 87.5%, 100%, and 72%, respectively as compared to that of the control (Figure 2). Interestingly, combination of ciprofloxacin (0.0625 μg/ml) with cranberry extract (12.7 mg/ml) could completely inhibit the adhesion (0.0%) of *P. aeruginosa* PAO1 to A549 lung epithelial cells. Although dextran was relatively the least effective single anti-adhesion treatment (83.6%±12.1%), it achieved a significant higher effect upon combination with ciprofloxacin (12.5%±4.2%).

Inhibition of Adhesion and Invasion of Pseudomonas aeruginosa to Lung Epithelial Cells:
A Model of Cystic Fibrosis Infection

139

Soybean extract was an effective anti-adhesion agent (55.0%±6.4%) compared to ciprofloxacin (73.7%±2.08%) and their combination could synergistically (28.03%±0.65%) and significantly (P<0.0001) reduce the ability of *P. aeruginosa* PAO1 to adhere to the A549 lung epithelial cells (Figure 2).

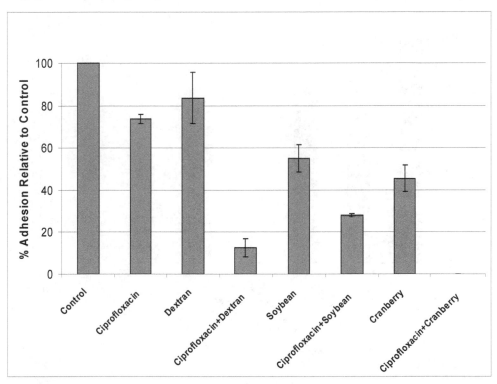

Fig. 2. The effect of different natural extracts alone and in combination with ciprofloxacin on the adhesion of *P. aeruginosa* PAO1 to A549 lung epithelial cells as compared to the untreated control.

2.2 Effect of natural extracts and their combinations with ciprofloxacin on the invasion of *P. aeruginosa* PAO1 to A549 lung epithelial cells

The ability of the adhered bacterial cells to internalize into the lung epithelial cells in the presence of different natural extracts, as single agents or in combination with ciprofloxacin, was assessed through calculation of percentage invasion of *P. aeruginosa* PAO1 from three independent experiments relative to the untreated controls. The results of gentamicin exclusion assay are believed to reflect the count of bacteria that has invaded cells [4, 13] with different treatments. Expectedly, both single cranberry and combination with ciprofloxacin were able to completely abrogate the invasion of *P. aeruginosa* PAO1 to the lung cells (0.0%). Although 45.5%±6.7% of the initial bacterial inoculum was able to bind to the epithelial cells after treatment in the presence of cranberry extract, none of this adhered population was able to penetrate the lung epithelial cells. Following the synergistic effect of cranberry extract, the combination of ciprofloxacin with both of soybean (17.6%±7.12%) and dextran

(11.8%±2.1%) achieved comparable and significant (P<0.0001) anti-invasion effects compared to the control. Similar to the results for the adhesion assay, dextran and soybean were more effective in combination with ciprofloxacin in preventing invasion rather than the single agents (75.5%±2.1%) and (17.6%±11.8%) as shown in figure (3).

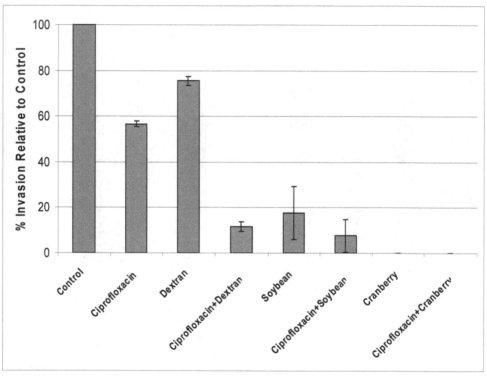

Fig. 3. The effect of different natural extracts alone and in combination with ciprofloxacin on the invasion of P. aeruginosa PAO1 to A549 lung epithelial cells as compared to the untreated control.

3. Discussion

Pseudomonas aeruginosa is a major cause for mortality seen in CF patients [6]. Adhesion and subsequent invasion of that organism to the lung epithelial cells are considered as the initial and substantial steps in the lung infection [5, 14-16]. Once the colonization of the organism is established, it is rarely eradicated. Several strategies have been developed to prevent *P. aeruginosa* infection in CF patients through different antibiotics and immunizations, but were not successful [8, 17-19]; therefore, development of other prophylactic measures as anti-adhesion and anti-invasion approaches is required. Ciprofloxacin, a fluoroquinolone, is considered as an antibiotic of choice for the treatment of the lung infections with *Pseudomonas aeruginosa* [7]. The current study aimed at introducing a new strategy to prevent *Pseudomonas aeruginosa* adhesion and invasion to the lung epithelial cells using different combinations of ciprofloxacin and aqueous extracts from widely available natural

Inhibition of Adhesion and Invasion of Pseudomonas aeruginosa to Lung Epithelial Cells:
A Model of Cystic Fibrosis Infection

141

products such as cranberry, and soybean. Dextran, which has been tested before in many occasions and found to be an effective anti-adhesion agent [2, 8, 11], was tested on that epithelial cell infection model as well to assess its anti-adhesion and anti-invasion activities compared to the other natural products, alone and in combination with ciprofloxacin.

The virulence factors of different *Pseudomonas aeruginosa* strains were attributed either to their direct host cell cytotoxicity or ability to adhere, invade, and survive within the epithelial cells. *P. aeruginosa* PAO1 virulence is categorized under the second types of isolates and invasion of that strain was suggested to contribute to biofilm formation and establishment of chronic lung infections [7]. Interestingly, the binding of *Pseudomonas aeruginosa* to the uninjured epithelial surfaces was found to be minimal. However, the binding ability of the organism increases dramatically in presence of epithelial surface inflammation or injury (such as in CF patients) [6, 20]. Scanning electron microscopy imaging revealed establishment of *P. aeruginosa* PAO1 binding to lung epithelial cells as the first step of *Pseudomonas aeruginosa* infection. Such binding did not affect the cells integrity or morphology (Figure1). Similarly, Fleiszig *et al.* [13] noted that integrity of the infected cells remains unaffected since the strain *P. aeruginosa* PAO1 does not use cytotoxicity as a virulence mechanism against the lung epithelial cells.

In order to exclude the inhibitory effect of ciprofloxacin and the applied natural extracts on *P. aeruginosa* PAO1 and A549 lung epithelial cells, the MICs of ciprofloxacin and the natural extracts against *P. aeruginosa* PAO1 and the MCCs of the same agents were determined to aid selection of the concentrations of different agents that will be tested on the adhesion and invasion models.

Unsurprisingly, the MICs and MCCs values could not be reached within the tested concentration levels for the different natural extracts, which were relatively high compared to ciprofloxacin, indicating that they are relatively non-toxic to the A549 lung epithelial cells as well as to *P. aeruginosa* PAO1. It has been reported that extracts of the natural sources are considered as endless reservoirs of safe and relatively inexpensive bioactive agents [9].

Dextran is a widely available polysaccharide that has been used in clinical settings as plasma expander [2]. It was previously tested as a carbohydrate treatment that blocks the epithelial glycoconjugates and impedes the bacterial legends from binding to pulmonary epithelial cell receptors [2]. Aerosolized dextran has been examined in a mouse infection model to prevent pneumonia caused by *Pseudomonas aeruginosa* and it could significantly reduce the development of pneumonia in the treated group relative to the untreated control animals, being an immuno-stimulant and a sputum rheology enhancer [2].

The combination treatment of dextran with ciprofloxacin disabled the internalization abilities of 85% of the bacterial population that adhered in the control experiments. Application of dextran resulted in an average of 14% reduction in both adhesion and invasion of *P. aeruginosa* PAO1 to the lung epithelia. This reduction is slightly less than that was found by Bryan *et al.* [2] who reported 35% reduction on *P. aeruginosa* PAO1 adhesion to nasal polyp primary culture cells when pretreated with dextran. Factors such as difference in the cell culture type or the experimental conditions may provide an explanation for the disparity in the activities. The same authors proposed that the likely mechanism through which dextran blocks bacterial adhesion was through the non-specific interaction with the epithelial cells; since pre-incubation of *P. aeruginosa* PAO1 with dextran before performing the infection abolished its anti-adhesion properties [2]. Consequently, the inhibitory action of dextran might not only involve *P. aeruginosa* PAO1 adhesion, but also other potential pathogens especially those targeting respiratory epithelia.

To our knowledge, there were no previous studies that reported the utilization of soybean extract as a potential anti-adhesion or anti-invasion treatment. The present study, however, proposes that the aqueous extract of soybean (*Glycine max*) is an additional promising treatment against adhesion and invasion of *P. aeruginosa* PAO1 to the lung epithelial cells. Compared to the control treatment, 28% and 17% of the applied bacterial inoculum were able to adhere and invade the lung epithelial cells, respectively, upon application of soybean extract combination with ciprofloxacin. These results suggest that on average half of the bacterial population that were able to adhere after treatment with soybean extract were not capable to invade the lung epithelial cells

Aqueous extract of cranberry (*Vaccinium macrocarpon*) was by far the most effective anti-adhesion and anti-invasion treatment when used in combination with ciprofloxacin. Cranberry belongs to *Vaccinum* family that has a wide spectrum of *in vitro* antimicrobial activity [21]. Many reports have demonstrated that proanthocyanidines and saccharides of cranberry were able to inhibit adhesion and invasion of some pathogenic microbes *in vitro*, and that cranberry juice clinically prevents urinary tract infection in women by inhibiting *Escherichia coli* adhesion to uroepithelial glycolipid receptors [3, 9]. The activity of the cranberry extract extended to provide protection against resistant strains of *Escherichia coli* by a mechanism that is unlikely to increase the selective pressure associated with antibiotics resistance [3]. Therefore, combining cranberry extract with ciprofloxacin sub-MIC may block the initial steps of infection, adhesion and invasion, as well as minimizing the development of bacterial resistance.

The results of this study may indicate that cranberry extract could turn the adhered bacteria unable to invade the lung epithelial cells since 45% of *P. aeruginosa* PAO1 population that were able to adhere to the lung cells under treatment with cranberry were, simultaneously, incapable of invading those cells and further molecular studies are required to elucidate this interesting point.

In published randomized clinical trial, cranberry juice was found to only affect harmful bacteria leaving normal bacterial flora unaffected; an observation that could suggest the therapeutic benefits of cranberry without having major unexpected side effects [21]. Cranberry juice, capsules and powder were also found to reduce urinary tract infection recurrences as well as the salival counts of the bacteria causing dental carries [21-24].

The significance of proposing the anti-adhesion treatments emanates from the fact that the earlier the establishment of airway infection is prevented the better the expected therapeutic outcome; since the persistence of intracellular bacteria causes sloughing of epithelial cells containing these bacteria and may contribute to spreading of the infection, establishment of the biofilm, rendering the bacterial eradication by the antibiotics difficult and favoring the bacterial endurance in the host airway [7].

In light of these *in vitro* anti-adhesion and anti-invasion effects of the promising natural extracts, further *in vivo* studies are required to explore their putative applications as an alternative strategy to combat the respiratory infections and the potential reduction of the antibiotic resistance rates.

4. Abbreviations

CF: Cystic Fibrosis
COPD: Chronic Obstructive Pulmonary Disease
CAMHB: Cation Adjusted Muller Hinton Broth

MIC: Minimum Inhibitory Concentration
MCC: Minimum Cytotoxic Concentration
CLSI: Clinical and Laboratory Standards Institute
SEM: Scanning Electron Microscopy
ANOVA: Analysis of Variance

5. References

[1] Gambardella S, Biancolella M, D'Apice MR et al. Gene expression profile in CFTR mutated bronchial cell lines.*Clin Exp Med* 2006; 6:157-165.

[2] Soferman R. Immunopathophysiologic mechanisms of cystic fibrosis lung disease. *IMAJ* 2006; 8:44-48.

[3] Singh AP, Chauhan SC, Andrianifahanana M, et al. MUC4 expression is regulated by cystic fibrosis transmembrane conductance regulator in pancreatic adenocarcinoma cells via transcriptional and post-translational mechanisms. *Oncogene* 2007; 26:30-41.

[4] Moskwa P, Lorentzen D, Excoffon KJ, et al. A novel host defense system of airway is defective in cystic fibrosis.*Am J Respir Crit Care Med* 2007; 175:174-183.

[5] Blau H. Cystic fibrosis lung disease: interplay of a microbial microcosm and extremes of inflammation *IMAJ* 2006; 8:58-59.

[6] Bilton D, Henig N, Morrissey B and Golfried MI. Addition of inhaled tobramycin to ciprofloxacin for acute exacerbations of Pseudomonas aeruginosa infection in adult bronchiectasis. *Chest* 2006; 130:1503-1510.

[7] Smyth A. Update on treatment of pulmonary exacerbations in cystic fibrosis *Curr Opin Pulm Med* 2006; 12:440-444.

[8] McLachlan G, Baker A, Tennant P, et al. Optimizing aerosol gene delivery and expression in the ovine lung .*Molecular Therapy* 2007; 15:348-354.

[9] Fischer AC, Smith CL, Cebotaru L, Zhang X, et al. et al. Expression of a truncated cystic fibrosis transmembrane conductance regulator with an AAV5-pseudotyped vector in primates. *Molecular Therapy, 15(4):756-63.*

[10] Delgado MA, Poschet JF, Deretic VI. Nonclassical pathway of Pseudomonas aeruginosa DNA-induced interleukin-8 secretion in cystic fibrosis airway epithelial cells.*Infection and Immunity* 2006; 74(5):2975-2984.

[11] Bavington C, and Page C. Stopping bacterial adhesion: a novel approach to treating infections. Respiration 2005;72: 335-344.

[12] Bryan R, Feldman M, Jawetz SC et al. The effects of aerosolized dextran in a mouse model of *Pseudomonas aeruginosa* pulmonary infection. J Infect Dis 1999;179: 1449-1458.

[13] Howell AB, Vorsa N, Der Marderosian A, Foo LY. Inhibition of the adherence of P-fimbriated *Escherichia coli* to uroepithelial-cell surfaces by proanthocyanidin extracts from cranberries. N Engl J Med 1998;339:1085-1086.

[14] Angus AA, Lee AA, Augustin DK et al. *Pseudomonas aeruginosa* induces membrane blebs in epithelial cells, which are utilized as a niche for intracellular replication and motility. Infect Immun 2008;76:1992-2001.

[15] Imundo L, Barasch J, Prince A, Al-Awqati Q. Cystic fibrosis epithelial cells have a receptor for pathogenic bacteria on their apical surface. Proc Natl Acad Sci U.S.A 1995;92:3019-3023.

[16] Swanson B, Savel R, Szoka F, Sawa T,Wiener-Kronish J. Development of a high throughput *Pseudomonas aeruginosa* epithelial cell adhesion assay. J Microbiol Methods 2003;52:361-366.

[17] Garcia-Medina R, Dunne WM, Singh PK, Brody SL. *Pseudomonas aeruginosa* acquires biofilm-like properties within airway epithelial cells. Infect Immun 2005;73:8298-8305.

[18] Barghouthi S, Guerdoud LM, Speert DP. Inhibition by dextran of *Pseudomonas aeruginosa* adherence to epithelial cells. Am J Respir Crit Care Med 1996;154:1788-1793.

[19] Howell AB, and Foxman B. Cranberry juice and adhesion of antibiotic-resistant uropathogens. JAMA 2002;287:3082-3083.

[20] Gillies RJ, Didier N, Denton M. Determination of cell number in monolayer cultures. Anal Biochem 1986;159:109-113.

[21] Carterson AJ, Honer Bentrup K, Ott CM et al. A549 lung epithelial cells grown as three-dimensional aggregates: alternative tissue culture model for *Pseudomonas aeruginosa* pathogenesis. Infect Immun 2005;73:1129-1140.

[22] Plotkowski MC, Saliba AM, Pereira SH, Cervante MP, Bajolet-Laudinat O. *Pseudomonas aeruginosa* selective adherence to and entry into human endothelial cells. Infect Immun 1994;62:5456-5463.

[23] Fleiszig SM, Zaidi TS, Preston MJ, Grout M, Evans DJ et al. Relationship between cytotoxicity and corneal epithelial cell invasion by clinical isolates of *Pseudomonas aeruginosa*. Infect Immun 1996;64:2288-2294.

[24] Beachey EH. Bacterial adherence: adhesin-receptor interactions mediating the attachment of bacteria to mucosal surface. J Infect Dis 1981;143:325-345.

[25] Kallenius G, Mollby R, Svenson SB, Winberg J. Microbial adhesion and the urinary tract. Lancet 1981;318(8251):866.

[26] Boren T, Falk P, Roth KA, Larson G, Normark S. Attachment of *Helicobacter pylori* to human gastric epithelium mediated by blood group antigens. Science 1993;262:1892-1895.

[27] Speert DP. Prevention of severe lower respiratory infections in patients with cystic fibrosis. Semin Respir Infect 1989;4:266-271.

[28] Pennington JE, Reynolds HY, Wood RE, Robinson RA, Levine AS. Use of a *Pseudomonas Aeruginosa* vaccine in pateints with acute leukemia and cystic fibrosis. Am J Med 1975;58:629-636.

[29] Wood RE, Pennington JE, Reynolds HY. Intranasal administration of a *Pseudomonas* lipopolysaccharide vaccine in cystic fibrosis patients. Pediatr Infect Dis 1983;2:367-369.

[30] Bentzmann S, Roger P, Puchelle E. *Pseudomonas aeruginosa* adherence to remodelling respiratory epithelium. Eur Respir J 1996;9:2145-2150.

[31] Kontiokari T, Salo J, Eerola E, Uhari M. Cranberry juice and bacterial colonization in children: a placebo-controlled randomized trial. Clin Nutr 2005;24:1065-1072.

[32] Weiss EI, Kozlovsky A, Steinberg D, Lev-Dor R, Bar Ness GR. et al. A high molecular mass cranberry constituent reduces mutans streptococci level in saliva and inhibits *in vitro* adhesion to hydroxyapatite. FEMS Microbiol Lett 2004;232:89-92.

[33] Avorn J, Monane M, Gurwitz JH, Glynn RJ, Choodnovskiy I. et al. Reduction of bacteriuria and pyuria after ingestion of cranberry juice. JAMA 1994;271:751-754.

[34] Stothers L. A randomized trial to evaluate effectiveness and cost effectiveness of naturopathic cranberry products as prophylaxis against urinary tract infection in women. Can J Urol 2002;9:1558-1562.

Part 2

Paediatrics

7

Bronchitis in Children

Christian Peiser

*Department for Pediatric Pneumology and Immunology,
Charité, Medical University Berlin,
Germany*

1. Introduction

For a paediatrician, children with bronchitis are part of the daily work. Infections of the respiratory system are the most common reason for children presenting at the doctor´s practice. Almost all infants and younger school children become sick several times a year with a bronchitis. In most cases with the beginning of day nursery or nursery school there is an abrupt accumulation and many parents have the feeling that their child is permanently ill. That bronchitis occurs much more frequently in winter than in summer, as everyone knows from personal experience. The cold air outside and the dry heated air indoors, increases the vulnerability of the mucosa for pathogens. Whether the clinical course of a bronchitis is uncomplicated or associated with a bronchial obstruction, is partly caused by the genetic predisposition of the child. Depending on family history of bronchial asthma and allergies, the risk may be increased many times over. The health damage due to exposure to tobacco smoke is a major point which should not be underestimated.

The following pages describe in the form of a brief overview symptoms and signs of bronchitis in children. The different types and stages of bronchitis are shown. The most common viruses that cause bronchitis are described, in particular the respiratory syncytial virus. One chapter deals with bronchopulmonary dysplasia, an important risk factor for bronchitis in children. Furthermore, some important differential diagnoses are presented, which can become manifest with the typical symptoms of a bronchitis. The laboratory diagnosis with the aim of differentiating between viral and bacterial bronchitis is discussed. Finally, therapeutic options are mentioned.

2. Signs and symptoms of bronchitis in children

2.1 Cough

The main symptom of bronchitis is a cough. At the beginning of the disease it tends to be dry and unproductive. With increasing production of secretion the mucus becomes less viscous, which makes coughing more effective. Some children have such severe coughing attacks that vomiting can be induced. An adequate supply of volume and inhalation therapy with 0.9% NaCl can help to make the mucus more fluid, enabling it to be brought up more easily by coughing. There are medications, usually in the form of so-called cough syrups, which will also assist mucolytic activity. After regression of an acute bronchitis, an unpleasant dry cough can still remain for several days or weeks. This is caused by a transient hyperreactivity of the bronchial system due to the infection-induced inflammation.

2.2 Tachypnoea and dyspnoea

If secreted mucus, an oedema of the bronchial mucosa or a spasm of the bronchial musculature induce bronchial obstruction, tachypnoea and dyspnoea may belong to the acute disorders. Typical clinical signs for dyspnoea are movement of the nostrils, inter- or subcostal retractions, use of accessory respiratory muscles, an upright upper body position, and in the auscultation wheezing and sometimes also rales. In this situation inhalation therapy with bronchodilatatory agents and the systemic administration of steroids may be helpful. Because the expiration is more difficult that the inspiration, an emphysema may be formed due to air trapping. Children with respiratory distress may become anxious and excited, which makes the situation worse. The excitement and anxiety of the parents may also be transferred to the child. In the case of severe respiratory distress, the oxygen saturation in the blood may decrease critically, making oxygen substitution necessary. Measurement of vital parameters and blood gas analyses are standard procedures. The suctioning of secretions and mucus, or the application of respiratory supportive procedures, such as CPAP or intubation and ventilation, should be made immediately possible.

2.3 Pain

Pain in the context of bronchitis can be caused by an inflammatory involvement of the trachea or pleura. In the case of retrosternal pain during coughing, a tracheitis is most probable. Respiratory-dependent, especially in deep inspiration increasing pain, which is localized more laterally in one or both sides of the chest, makes a pleuritis more probable. Especially the dry chafing of inflamed visceral pleura and parietal pleura against each other is very painful. If the child develops shallow breathing to avoid the pain, an insufficient ventilation of the lung may result with the increased risk of a secondary bacterial infection. For this reason, an appropriate analgesia is strongly recommended.

2.4 Fever

Fever is a general clinical sign, which may occur in any infection, including one of the respiratory system. The increase of body temperature is a non-specific symptom and can range from low-grade fever up to hyperpyrexia with acute physical stress for the child. In the case of an infection of the upper respiratory tract, additionally clinical signs (in addition to the cough, tachydyspnea, pain and fever) are sniffing (rhinitis), a sore throat (pharyngitis) and earache (otitis media). Furthermore, swollen and aching cervical lymph nodes are a common local response to the inflammation process.

3. Different types of bronchitis in children

3.1 Acute, complicated, chronic, recurrent

The average duration of an acute bronchitis is about 1 week with the range from ½ week up to 2 weeks. Afterwards a nervous cough may remain for several days or a few weeks. The acute bronchitis has a very high rate of complete recovery; the prognosis is very good. An exception is an acute bronchitis caused by adenovirus; in this case complications in the clinical course or a chronification of the bronchitis are described.

If the symptoms and signs of an acute bronchitis persist for 4 – 6 weeks, we call it complicated bronchitis. If an acute bronchitis is followed by another one, they can be taken for a complicated bronchitis by mistake. Approximately 20% of acute bronchitis has a complicated course. One possible complication is the secondary bacterial superinfection of a primary viral infection. In this case the child needs to be treated with antibiotics. Another possible complication is the transition from bronchitis into bronchopneumonia. In many cases this is detectable by pulmonary auscultation, but to confirm the diagnosis, a chest X-ray is necessary. A primary bacterial bronchitis usually presents clinically as a complicated bronchitis.

Signs and symptoms of a bronchitis persisting for more than 3 months are called chronic bronchitis.

If children repeat lots of acute bronchitis over months, it is called recurrent bronchitis. Mainly children in day nursery or nursery school are affected quite often, because the risk of infection is particularly high there. In the cold seasons bronchitis occurs more frequently compared to the warm seasons.

3.2 Non-obstructive or obstructive

Bronchitis can be associated more or less with bronchial obstruction. The risk of an obstruction depends on the lumen of the inflamed bronchus; the smaller the lumen, the more likely is a clinically relevant obstruction. For this reason, the terms "obstructive bronchitis" and "bronchiolitis" were sometimes used as synonyms. Bronchial obstruction can be caused by the following pathophysiological alterations:

1. The smooth muscles of the bronchus get contracted, which can lead to an acute shortness of breath.
2. The mucosa of the respiratory epithelium is swollen due to the inflammation, which narrows the bronchial lumen.
3. The increased production of mucus clogs the lumen as well. Furthermore, due to the inflammation in the respiratory epithelium, the function of the cilia is reduced, and mucus cannot be transported adequately.

Auscultation of the lung shows wheezing. A so-called silent lung is typical for a severe bronchial obstruction with air trapping and emphysema. In this case the resting expiratory position is shifted to the inspiration, what may create a circulus vitiosus.

3.3 Non-allergic or allergic

Bronchitis is an inflammatory disease of the bronchial mucosa. In most cases the inflammation is caused by an infection. Also allergens may cause an acute or chronic bronchitis, they act mostly as a trigger. The presence of one or more allergies increases the statistical risk for the development of bronchial asthma. Relevant inhalation allergens are dust mites, animal dander, mould fungus and pollen.

As their zoological name "Dermatophagoides" indicates, dust mites feed on epithelia from the skin, of which one person loses about 1.5 grams per day. They are, depending on the type, 0.1 - 0.5 mm in size and they live in normal house dust. They are found in carpets, curtains, upholstered furniture, mattresses, duvets and pillows, stuffed animals etc. The allergen comes from the faeces of the mites. In order to avoid exposure, the following protections should be carried out: the use of an encasing such as a mattress cover, monthly washing of duvets and pillows, occasional freezing of soft toys at -20 °C, followed by rinsing, no long carpets, regular vacuuming and avoidance of dust turbulence.

With regard to animal dander, those species which are most relevant and which human beings have close contact with are especially dogs, cats, guinea pigs, hamsters, horses and birds. The allergen concentration varies within a species, depending on the breed. For this reason it could happen that someone tolerates contact with one cat very well, whereas contact with another cat induces an acute bronchial obstruction. In the case of a clinically relevant allergy against an animal, the contact should be avoided.

The spores of mould fungus can also cause an allergic reaction, like bronchial hyperreactivity or bronchial obstruction. If at home the walls are infested with mould fungus, the house has to be renovated.

Among the pollen, early flowering plants (birch, alder, hazel, willow) and grasses are most relevant. The occurrence of pollen-induced disorders, namely rhinoconjunctivitis and bronchial asthma, are strongly season-dependent and time-limited. On the basis of cross-reactions, for example between birch pollen and apple, in the case of an allergy against birch pollen, an allergic reaction against apple in the form of an oral allergy syndrome may occur. In the case of pollen, allergen avoidance is almost impossible. In order to reduce the intensity of pollen-induced allergy symptoms, desensitization is recommended.

3.4 Special forms: Bronchitis fibroplastica, bronchioloitis obliterans

A special form of bronchitis in childhood is the bronchitis fibroplastica. Older synonyms are fibrinous bronchitis, pseudomembranous bronchitis or Hoffmann's bronchitis. It is characterized by obstruction of the bronchi, usually a lobe or segment, consisting of mucin, which forms large endobronchial casts of rubber-like consistency. Pre-existing pathological conditions, such as bronchial asthma or cystic fibrosis, which are attended by hypersecretion of viscous mucus, may act as triggers. Childhood tuberculosis or primary immunodeficiency seem to be associated with a higher incidence of bronchitis fibroplastica as well. However, exact epidemiological data are still missing. Main symptoms are a cough and dyspnoea, and sometimes pleuritic pain and fever occur. In pulmonary auscultation over the affected area of the lung the breath is quiet or absent; sometimes wheezing or rales can be heard. X-rays of the chest typically show an atelectatic area next to an emphysematic one. The therapy consists in the prompt removal of the sticky casts consisting of mucin via rigid bronchoscopy. If they are not removable, administration of N-acetylcysteine or DNase may be helpful. If a child without known pre-existing diseases falls ill with bronchitis fibro-plastica, additional diagnostic investigations should be carried out: sweat tests, tuberculin tests, allergy tests.

Another special form of bronchitis in children is the bronchiolitis obliterans. An inflammation of the small airways induces a pathologic tissue remodelling with granulations, which obstruct the lumen of the bronchioles. This process may be triggered by infections, inhalation of toxic agents, autoimmune diseases or a chronic rejection after lung transplantation. In the group of long-term survivors after lung transplantation, bronchioltis obliterans is the most frequent cause of death. The clinical signs and symptoms are quite unspecific: a cough and reduced general condition. In pulmonary auscultation the breath is quiet and rales can be heard. The X-ray of the chest eventually shows some infiltration or it looks normal. The disease may begin rapidly or slowly and the clinical course may be progressive or stable. Therapeutic options are a high-dose glucocorticoid administration, and in the case of lung transplantation, an increase in the dosage of the immunosuppressive medication.

4. Different stages of bronchitis in children

4.1 Bronchial hyperreactivity

Bronchial hyperreactivity is a chronic inflammation of the bronchial mucosa with recurrent bronchial obstruction, which may be triggered by infections, allergens or nonspecific stimuli, such as cold air, physical or even emotional stress. The inflammatory activity causes a swelling of the bronchial mucosa with a reduction of the bronchial lumen consecutively. The smaller the lumens are physiologically, such as in infants, the more relevant is its reduction regarding clinical symptoms. Furthermore, inflammation of the bronchial mucosa increases the vulnerability to viruses or bacteria.

To make the diagnosis "bronchial hyperreactivity", an accurate and detailed medical history is the most important step. Additionally, measurement of the lung function may confirm the diagnosis, in particular in the case of a reduced flow in the smaller airways; after administration of a beta-sympathomimetic via inhalation the bronchial obstruction should be reversible, at least partly. The lung function test can be carried out with children who are old enough to participate actively. Furthermore, measurement of the NO-exhalation may be useful to monitor the amount of bronchial inflammation. In some cases it may be helpful to carry out a bronchial provocation test via inhalation of methacholine, histamine or carbachol. Of course, all emergency tools have to be available.

4.2 Bronchitis

Bronchitis is a clinically apparent inflammation of the bronchi, triggered by a bronchial hyprerreactivity, by viruses or bacteria or by allergens. The symptoms (cough, tachypnoea and dyspnoea, pain, fever), the different courses (acute, complicated, chronic, recurrent) and different forms (non-obstructive, obstructive) have been described.

4.3 Bronchiolitis

Bronchiolitis is an inflammation of the smallest bronchi and bronchioles. Due to the small lumens of these airways, swelling of bronchial mucosa may induce severe obstruction quite rapidly, in most cases associated with pulmonary hyperinflation. This can lead to the phenomenon of the so-called silent obstruction, that means barely wheezing, humming or whistling, but fine bubble rales at the end of inspiration. Bronchiolitis is a typical disease of infancy, the age peak is between 4 and 6 months.

4.4 Bronchopneumonia

Bronchopneumonia is a possible course of a complicated bronchitis. Whereas a primary pneumonia normally is localized to one segment or lobe of the lung, in the case of a bronchopneumonia there is a disseminated inflammation from the bronchi down to the alveoli.

4.5 Bronchial asthma

Bronchial asthma is a disease with chronic inflammation of the respiratory system with bronchial hyperreactivity and variable airway obstructions. In many children and adolescents we find a positive family history for asthma and/or allergies. The restriction of the air flow, mainly during the expiration, is caused by spastic contraction of the smooth muscle in the bronchial wall, oedematous swelling of the bronchial mucosa and hypersecretion of viscous mucus. In addition to these pathological mechanisms, a tissue remodelling may take place after bronchial asthma over several years, which makes the airways less elastic. In most cases patients have an allergic bronchial asthma; case of non-allergic asthma and mixed forms are possible as well.

Criteria for the diagnosis of bronchial asthma in children and adolescents are a relative forced ventilation capacity (FEV1/VK) < 75% of age- and gender-related norm and a 15 % increase with prolonged expiratory time, or after inhalation of a short-acting beta-sympathomimetic. A further criterion is a decrease in respiratory resistance (R) > 50% of baseline after inhalation of a short-acting beta-sympathomimetic. If the lung function measurement shows a normal result, but the clinical history is typically for bronchial asthma, then a circadian variability of the measured peak expiratory flow (PEF) > 20% confirms the diagnosis. If the doctor is still in doubt with the diagnosis, a provocation test (for example physical stress or inhalation of metacholine) may be helpful to make the right diagnosis.

The therapy of bronchial asthma is successful if clinical signs and symptoms of the disease are under control, so that the affected children or adolescents feel free from disorders if they are able to partake in sport without any restriction, if there are no side effects of the medications and if no long-term injury will occur. Taken together, if the children or adolescents just have a normal life with this chronic disease. Parts of the therapy are prevention (for example not smoking, either actively or passively, avoidance of allergens, if possible), general procedures (for example participation on training courses of instruction, doing sports, doing physiotherapy), pharmacotherapy and rehabilitation, if it is required. The prescription of drugs should be carried out in accordance with an algorithm, which has various steps depending on the severity of the bronchial asthma and gives the opportunity to step up or step down. Standard drugs in pharmacotherapy of bronchial asthma are low-dose inhaled glucocorticoids and orally administered leukotriene antagonists (additionally or alternatively) for long-term therapy, as well as inhaled short-acting beta-sympatho-mimetics for acute therapy. Because of this treatment, severe asthma attacks have become very rare incidents.

5. Common viruses causing bronchitis in children

Acute bronchitis is almost (in approximately 90%) induced by viruses. The most common ones are respiratory syncytial, parainfluenza-, influenza-, adeno-, rhino-, metapneumo- and human bocavirus. Acute bronchitis, which is induced by bacteria primary, is rare (approximately 10%). In 15% of viral bronchitis a secondary bacterial infection will happen.

5.1 Respiratory syncytial virus (RSV)

It is a member of the family of paramyxoviridae, has a single-stranded RNA and is enveloped. We distinguish two serological groups A and B from each other. The pathogenicity of the virus depends crucially on two glycoproteins on the viral surface: glycoprotein G enables the docking with the host cell, such as pneumocytes, glycoprotein F is responsible for the endocytosis into the cell. The fact that the affected cell undergoes a fusion with neighbouring cells and form syncytia has given the virus its name. Further details of incubation time, infection and clinical signs and symptoms are in the section "Characteristics of RSV infection."

5.2 Parainfluenzavirus

It belongs to the family of paramyxoviridae, has a single-stranded RNA and an envelope. It is (in contrast to the influenza viruses) genetically stable. There are 4 different types. The transmission of the virus proceeds via droplet or smear infection. The incubation period is 3 - 6 days. At the age of 2 years, almost all children have been sick at least once with a parainfluenza infection. In infancy and early childhood parainfluenza virus causes an acute laryngotracheobronchitis with typical croup symptoms.

5.3 Influenzavirus

It is assigned to the family of orthomyxoviridae. It is divided into the 3 types A, B and C, of which A and B are most relevant for infections of humans. The genome of influenza viruses type A and B consists of eight single-stranded RNA segments. This creates a high genetic variability of antigenic drift and antigenic shift, in the case of a dual infection. The eight RNA segments contain the genetic information for 11 proteins, of which one is the neuraminidase. Transmission paths of the virus are aerosols and saliva, as well as contact with contaminated surfaces. The incubation period is 1 - 4 days. Typically we see a high incidence of influenza during the winter months. The epidemic often has its origin in the nursery, kindergarten or school. Because of the high contagiosity, pandemics with high lethality may occur, recently caused by the H1N1 subtype, the so-called "swine flu". In contrast to the common cold, the clinical course of the influenza infection is characterized by significantly reduced general condition, high fever and a much higher complication rate. Children with a disease of the respiratory tract, a heart failure or a deficiency of the immune system have an especially high risk for severe complications. The diagnosis of influenza can be made with a rapid test (usually an Elisa) or by RT-PCR, which is more sensitive and specific, from a nasal or throat swab or corresponding rinse water.

In the case of a severe or complicated clinical course, treatment with an antiviral compound is indicated. In childhood, the neuraminidase inhibitors oseltamivir (oral administration, approved from the first year of life) and zanamivir (inhalation, approved from the fifth year of life) are used. Safety studies were carried out in order to extend the approval of oseltamivir on the first year of life. The vaccination against influenza provides the best protection. Because of the high genetic variability of the virus, the vaccination has to be repeated each year with a current antigen mixture. In addition to the self-protection, the collective protection is of great importance.

5.4 Adenovirus

It is a member of the family of adenoviridae. It is a double-stranded DNA virus with a strong environmental resistance. More than 50 serotypes with various clinical manifestations have been identified so far. The transmission proceeds via droplet or smear infection. The incubation time is between 2 and 10 days. Most adenovirus-induced diseases occur in the age between 6 months and 5 years, usually in the form of a common cold. However, it can lead to complicated clinical courses with severe obstruction, pneumonia or persistent bronchial hyperreactivity for months.

5.5 Rhinovirus

It belongs to the family of picornaviridae, the RNA is single stranded. We know about 100 subtypes; the genetic variability is large. Rhinovirus is transmitted primarily via aerosol. The incubation period is 2 - 5 days. In the first years of life, the incidence of infection with the virus is around 1 - 2 times per year. Whereas in adults rhinovirus infections usually cause a common cold, in infants and small children obstructive bronchitis appear quite often.

5.6 Metapneumovirus

It is a member of the paramyxoviridae, a RNA virus and enveloped. We know 2 subtypes A and B, each with two sub-groups A1 and A2, as well as B1 and B2. Droplet and smear infections are the transmission paths. Incubation time is 4 – 6 days. During the first year of life about one quarter of infants become infected with the metapneumovirus; by the time children start school, almost everyone has had an infection with this ubiquitous virus. Most prevalent symptoms are rhinitis and bronchitis.

5.7 Human bocavirus

The human bocavirus was discovered only in 2005. It belongs to the Parvoviridae family and has a single-stranded DNA. The transmission of the virus proceeds via droplet or smear infection. Accurate epidemiological data are yet to be collected. Clinically, acute respiratory symptoms are most relevant.

6. Characteristics of RSV infection in children

6.1 Risk factors

An RSV infection, which occurs in infancy, may have a severe clinical course. Not only in infancy, but until the age of 5 years, RSV infection may cause disorders of clinical relevance. The majority of children undergo one or more RSV infections during the first 2 years of life, usually without a severe or complicated course. Risk factors for a severe or complicated clinical course are small, narrow airways (this is the reason why infants suffer worse than older children). Boys are affected slightly more often than girls. Another risk factor, which should not be underestimated, is the exposure to tobacco smoke. Furthermore, the family history to allergies has an adverse influence. Pre-term birth or chronic diseases of the lung increase the risk for a complicated course of a RSV infection considerably. We see a seasonal accumulation with endemic-like clusters of RSV infections during the cold autumn and winter months. The transmission occurs by droplet and smear infection. The incubation time is at 3 - 6 days.

6.2 Severity of the clinical course

If the RS virus affects the respiratory epithelium of the smallest bronchi and bronchioles with desquamation of the epithelial cells and oedema of the mucosa, the main symptom is bronchial obstruction. Distal to an obstructed airway, atelectatic areas may be formed, next to emphysematic areas. If this causes a mismatch between ventilation and perfusion, the main symptom is tachydyspnoea with partial or even global respiratory insufficiency. In this case, the infant needs to get hospitalized for oxygen substitution and, if necessary, with respiratory support or even mechanical ventilation. An additional reason for hospitalization is the risk, especially in very young infants, of apnoea and death due to apnoea.

6.3 Diagnosis

The diagnosis can be carried out using a rapid test, which is based on the immunofluorescence method. The inflammation parameters in the blood are only slightly increased. The X-ray of the chest often shows diffuse infiltrations of the lung and a partial reduction of the transmission due to emphysema.

6.4 Limitation of therapeutic options

The therapeutic options are very limited. Because the replication of the RS virus takes place inside the epithelial cells of the lung, bronchodilatatory agents show no positive effect. Treatment with steroids has no effect as well, what is confirmed by meta-analysis. An antiviral therapy with the nucleoside analogue ribavirin is not recommended for the following reasons: firstly, there seems to be no relevant effect; secondly, it is teratogenic and has to be administered via aerosol, which could lead to an exposure of pregnant women who are in contact to the child. There is only one agent with a small, but significant benefit in the case of an RSV bronchitis or bronchiolitis; it is the leukotriene receptor antagonist montelukast. Additionally, supportive therapy, such as inhalation with 0.9% NaCl or decongestant nose drops may be helpful.

6.5 Indications for palivizumab

Palivizumab is a monoclonal antibody against the RS virus. It can be used for passive immunization. It binds to the glycoprotein F, the fusion protein, and thereby prevents the virus entering the cell. During the months with high incidence of RSV infections, palivizumab has to be injected every 4 weeks. Palivizumab is indicated for significant prematurity, bronchopulmonary dysplasia and hemodynamic relevant congenital heart failures. The prophylactic immunization with palivizumab reduces severity and duration of the disease significantly; the hospitalization frequency is halved.

6.6 Recent research on an active immunization

Previous research on an active vaccine, already carried out in the 1960s, was not successful. Currently there are new research activities in this area. A life vaccine against RSV and PIV3 (parainfluenza virus type 3) is in phase 1 / 2 study.

7. Bronchopulmonary dysplasia as a risk factor for bronchitis in children

7.1 Definition and pathophysiology

Today bronchopulmonary dysplasia (BPD) is more relevant than ever. Because of the major advances in neonatology with high survival rates of extremely immature preterm infants, there is an increase of diseases and complications, which are typically associated with prematurity, like BPD. If very preterm infants are born, their lungs are not completely developed, neither structurally nor functionally, especially with respect to the synthesis of surfactant. Because of the respiration prior to maturity, the lung tissue undergoes a fibrotic remodelling process of the alveoli. Prenatal and postnatal factors, such as inflammation, infection, hyperoxia and mechanical ventilation, have an additional adverse effect.

Because the morphological alterations are not visible and the radiological ones do not correlate well with the clinical severity, the BPD is defined by the duration of oxygen supplementation for longer than 28 days. Depending on the amount of oxygen supplementation and the requirement of breathing support, we distinguish mild, moderate and severe BPD.

7.2 Prophylaxis and therapy

The following prophylactic procedures may reduce the severity of BPD: the prenatal anti-inflammatory treatment via administration of beta-dexamethasone to the mother, the so-called "lung maturation", is standard. The application of surfactant as soon as possible is very important. A patent ductus arteriosus with hemodynamic relevance should be treated early, if possible pharmacologically, if necessary via ligature. A protective effect of vitamin A has been demonstrated, although the effect is only minor.

Therapeutic procedures are avoidance of hyperoxia, moderate infusion or even forced diuresis. high-caloric nutrition, gentle ventilation mode, physiotherapy, and in very rare cases, the postnatal application of corticosteroids.

7.3 Prognosis

The BPD also affects the future life of the children: they suffer more frequently with bronchial hyperreactivity and asthma, they have an increased risk for the incidence of respiratory infections, and in the first year of life they are more often hospitalized for acute respiratory problems. Even if they have no symptoms, the measurement of lung function will show worse values.

8. Differential diagnoses of bronchitis in children

8.1 Croup

In distinction from the original diphtheritic croup (which has become very rare thanks to the vaccination), the common croup is a subglottic laryngitis with an inflammatory oedema of the mucosa in the context of a viral infection of the respiratory system. The main prevalence is at the age between 6 months and 6 years. Typically in the late evening or during the night in the cold winter, the affected infants and children get an acute attack with a barking cough, hoarseness, inspiratory stridor and dyspnoea. We divide the croup into 4 different degrees of severity, from just cough and hoarseness without dyspnoea to dramatic dyspnoea with the feeling of combustion.

What are the urgent measures in the case of a croup attack? The first step is to reassure the anxious and excited child. It should be kept in an upright position, in order to allow the use of the thoracal muscles for breathing. The child should be brought into the fresh and cold air, which may reduce the swelling of the respiratory mucosa. If available, a glucocorticoid suppository can be administered by the parents. Prophylactically, a moistening of the air indoors is recommended. In many cases of a moderate croup episode, these easy measures may stabilize the situation, that the parents are able to manage it at home without any professional help. However, in severe cases or in any cases of doubt, the ambulance should be called immediately. The emergency doctor can initiate an inhalation with adrenaline, an oxygen supplementation and an intravenous application of a glucocorticoid. If necessary, the child can be hospitalized and monitored via pulse oximetry. In very rare cases, the sedation of a child (for example with chloral hydrate) is unavoidable. In extreme severe and complicated clinical courses, the treatment of the child at an intensive care unit is recommended.

In the extremely rare case of a diphtheritic croup, the treatment with diphtheria antitoxin has to start immediately. Also extremely rare (thanks to the haemophilus vaccination), a bacterial epiglottitis occurs. But because of its rarity, the risk of misinterpretation as a normal croup is quite high. In contrast to the croup, the epiglottitis usually is associated with high fever, a very poor general condition, a septic clinical course, an increased salivation and dysphagia. An epiglottis is always a peracute emergency. Inspection of the pharynx using a spatula is strictly contraindicated, because the slightest mechanical provocation can induce a complete occlusion of the epiglottis without any possibility for an intubation. Then only cricothyrotomy or tracheostomy can be carried out, to save the life of the child.

8.2 Aspiration

Aspiration of gastric juice or of a foreign body causes coughing. Common foreign bodies are small pieces of an apple or a carrot, half or whole peanuts and all sorts of small parts made of plastic or metal, quite often from the toys, the child has played with. We distinguish between the acute and the chronic foreign body aspiration.

In the case of an acute aspiration the child has an abrupt coughing attack and dyspnoea. Because the beginning of the right main bronchus from the trachea is angulated to a lesser extent compared with the left one, it is preferentially affected. Over the affected side the breath is quiet and wheezing can be heard. Radiologically, a mediastinal shift to the healthy side can be seen.

In contrast to an acute aspiration, which is associated with an abrupt coughing attack and dyspnoea, in the case of a chronic aspiration the clinical symptoms are milder and less severe. In most cases the foreign body is smaller compared to those of an acute aspiration, so that it can slide into a segmental bronchus, settle there and maintain an inflammatory response, which occurs as a chronic cough. This is the reason why chronic aspirations quite often get misinterpreted as a chronic bronchitis of infectious or allergic origin.

For treatment the bronchoscopical removal of the foreign body is necessary, almost always in the form of a rigid bronchoscopy.

8.3 Tuberculosis

In the case of a chronic cough it is important to take the possibility of a pulmonary tuberculosis as a differential diagnosis into account, especially in children who come from high-incidence countries, or if they have had or still have close contact with people coming from such areas. The mycobacterium tuberculosis is transmitted via the aerosols, which comes from coughing people with an open pulmonary tuberculosis. Children are generally less contagious, even if they have an open pulmonary tuberculosis, because there are only a few bacteria in the sputum. This phenomenon is called paucibacillary tuberculosis.

At the slightest suspicion of a tuberculosis infection, an appropriate diagnostic investigation has to be made: next to an accurate medical history and physical examination, immunological tests have to be carried out. These are an intracutanously applied tuberculin test and an IGRA (interferon-gamma release assay) from the blood. The combination of both tests results in an optimal specifity. Additionally, an X-ray from the chest at two levels belongs to the standard diagnostic. The microscopical and microbiological analysis is made from induced sputum or from gastric juice, because children younger than 10 years usually are not able to give sputum spontaneously.

If, in the case of an exposure to tuberculosis, all diagnostic investigations have a negative result, a chemoprophylaxis with isoniazid for 3 months is recommended. If the immunological tests are positive, but the clinical course, the X-ray and the analysis of induced sputum or gastric juice show normal results, then a preventive chemotherapy with either isoniazid as monotherapy for 9 months or alternatively with isoniazid and rifampicin as dual therapy for 4 months should be carried out. If a child has signs or symptoms of a tuberculosis, if pulmonary or extra-pulmonary, a combination therapy with at least 3 tuberculostatic drugs has to be initiated, for example with isoniazid, rifampicin and pyrazinamide. In most cases, after 2 months of treatment the medication can be reduced to an isoniazid/rifampicin - dual therapy. The total duration of the treatment depends on the clinical course and the severity of complication and is at least 6 months. Of course the choice of the tuberculostatic drugs has to be adjusted to possible resistances.

8.4 Cystic fibrosis (CF)

If infants have recurrent obstructive bronchitis with a chronic cough and problems to dissolve the mucus, one differential diagnosis, which has to be taken into account, is CF. Even though it is a rare disease, it is still one of the most common hereditary diseases. The mode of inheritance is autosomal recessive and caused by a mutation in the CFTR (cystic fibrosis transmembrane conductance regulator) - gene, which encodes a chloride ion channel. More than 1500 mutations have been known. The mutation deltaF508 describes the deletion of 3 base pairs, what causes the lack of phenylalanine at position 508 of the protein chain, and is with 70% by far the most frequent one. Depending on the amount of the CFTR defect, there are milder and more severe clinical courses of the disease. Due to the dysfunction of the chloride ion channel, the epithelial fluid film becomes hyperosmolar and the produced mucus gets dyscrinic.

The clinical course is characterized by this problem. Shortly after birth, due to the viscous intestinal secretion, a meconium ileus can be the first complication of a CF. The same problem may occur in later life as distal intestinal obstruction syndrome (DIOS). The most important focus in the progress of the CF is the respiratory system. The viscous sputum cannot be mobilized and brought out adequately, what gives bacteria a good medium for colonization, unfortunately quite often with mucoid pseudomonas aeruginosa and other multi-resistant bacteria. Also pulmonary mycoses (for example an aspergillosis) may occur. These permanent inflammatory processes lead to an irreversible tissue remodelling of the respiratory tract. At the end, atelectatic areaes and emphysematic bullae, insufficient for ventilation or diffusion, replace the normal tissue. Haemoptysis and pneumothoraces are dreaded complications. About 90% of all patients with CF develop an exocrine pancreatic insufficiency with the consequence of an inadequate intestinal absorption of proteins, fats and fat-soluble vitamins, which leads to dystrophy of the affected patients. With further progress of the disease, an endocrine pancreatic insufficiency may occur, which is why about 15% of all patients with CF develop an insulin-dependent diabetes mellitus.

Therapeutical tools are the removal of bronchial secretions by autogenic drainage, physiotherapy, inhalations, mucolysis and ample fluid intake, the antibacterial treatment by intravenous antibiotics, the stimulation of the digestion by dietary fibre enriched food and physical activity, the improvement of the intestinal absorption by replacement of enzymes (porcine pancreas powder) and substitution of vitamins, and the counteraction of dystrophy by high-caloric nutrition.

In the most patients with CF, the life limiting factor is the global respiratory insufficiency. Often, lung transplantation is the only life-prolonging option. Because of the enormous medical progress, especially in the development of new antibiotics, the life expectancy of people with CF increases steadily and rapidly. CF as a disease which occurs exclusively in childhood is part of medical history.

8.5 Primary ciliary dyskinesis

A primary ciliary dyskinesis often causes recurrent bronchitis. It is a genetically determined (usually autosomal recessive) disorder of the respiratory ciliated epithelium and other ciliated cells, resulting in a reduction in mucociliary clearance. Typical clinical symptoms are chronic rhinitis and sinusitis with much secretion, chronic bronchitis with a productive cough and recurrent pneumonia. Additional possible abnormalities are the formation of a hydrocephalus (due to the lack of ciliary motility of the ependymal cells), infertility in male (due to the lack of motility of the sperms) and in female patients (due to the lack of motility of the cilia of the fallopian tube) or a situs inversus (due to the absence of a directed cilia beat during the embryogenesis). A situs inversus occurs in 50% of the patients who are affected by the primary ciliary dyskinesis and it is called Kartagener's syndrome. In the diagnostic investigation of the primary ciliary dyskinesis the measurement of exhaled NO and the analysis of the ciliary function using a light microscope are purposeful tools. For confirmation of the diagnosis, an analysis via an electron microscope is needed. Therapeutic options are physiotherapy, inhalation and antibiotic treatment in the case of bacterial infections.

8.6 Vocal cord dysfunction

The vocal cord dysfunction (VCD) is a functional disorder with an acute spasm of the vocal cords. In most cases school children are affected. A VCD attack can range from a mild dyspnoea to the feeling of suffocation. Fortunately, such episodes are not life threatening, because despite the vocal cord spasm a small air gap still remains. Possible triggers for a VCD attack are coughing, physical exertion, inhalation of cigarette smoke or reflux of gastric juice, postnasal drip syndrome and general stress.

8.7 Gastroesophageal reflux

In the case of a recurrent or chronic cough, of course at first everybody thinks of a disease of the respiratory system. However, a gastroesophageal reflux may also cause such symptoms. Especially in the first months of life, chyme and gastric juice can flow back into the oesophagus and induce an inflammation of the mucosa there. Clinical symptoms may be heartburn, regurgitation, vomiting, feeding problems and finally dystrophia. Further symptoms may be a cough, hoarseness, bronchial obstruction, episodes with apnoea and cyanosis, as well as pneumonia due to aspiration. In order to avoid the gastroesophageal reflux in infants, the nutrition can be thickened and the feeding portions can be reduced by increasing the feeding frequency. In addition, the upper body should be slightly elevated. Potential drugs are antacids or proton pump blockers.

9. Inflammation parameters in the case of bronchitis in children

9.1 C-reactive protein (CRP)

CRP is an annular pentamer with sub-units composed of 206 amino acids each. It is synthesized in the liver and then secreted into the blood. Its concentration in the blood increases within 6 to 48 h in the case of any systemic inflammation. That can be an infectious disease, an immune reaction of non-infectious etiology or large tissue damage. Thus, CRP is an unspecific marker for inflammation and its increase starts with delay. Depending on the laboratory, a plasma concentration up to 0.1 - 1 mg/dl is in the normal range. Concentrations between 1 – 10 mg/dl are typical for mild to moderate concentrations, > 10 mg/dl for severe inflammation. Because of the reasonably long half-life of approximately 24 h, CRP is ideal for the follow-up monitoring of an inflammatory process which can help to evaluate the effectiveness of a treatment.

9.2 Interleukin-6 (IL-6)

IL-6 is a proinflammatory cytokine consisting of 184 amino acids. It is released primarily by monocytes, but also by T-lymphocytes, as well as endothelial and epithelial cells. Infections, non-infectious immunological reactions, tissue hypoxia and trauma induce the release of IL-6 within 6 h. Thus, IL-6 is an unspecific marker for various forms of inflammation as well, but its increase starts much faster. Depending on the laboratory, a plasma concentration up to 10 – 50 ng/l is in the normal range. The half-life in the blood is just a few minutes. Because of this very short half-life, the kinetics shows a narrow peak with the risk of false negative results in the case of measurements outside this peak.

9.3 Complete blood count (CBC)

The CBC may also be helpful in the diagnosis of an inflammation. High increases in the amount of the leucocytes occur in bacterial infections, but also in other inflammatory processes. Like CRP and IL-6, CBC is a non-specific marker of general inflammation. The increase of the leucocytes needs several hours and starts a little bit earlier than the increase of the CRP level. The standard value of the amount of leucocytes depends on the age of life: for adults 4 - 10 / nl, for school children 5 - 15 / nl, for small children 6 - 17,5 / nl and for newborns even 9 - 30 / nl are physiological. The differential blood count shows a reactive shift to the immature leucocytes, because their reinforced presence in the peripheral blood induces an enhanced release of still premature leucocytes from the bone marrow.

9.4 Erythrocyte sedimentation rate (ESR)

The ESR is a very non-specific marker for any kind of inflammation. The pathophysiological mechanisms, which lead to a higher ESR, are as follows: in the case of an inflammatory condition, erythrocytes form aggregates, which have a lower flow resistance compared to the sum of each separate erythrocyte. Furthermore, higher concentrations of acute phase proteins (like CRP), of fibrinogen or of immunoglobulins in the plasma, increase the ESR. It takes several weeks, after an inflammation has taken place, until an increased ESR gets normalized again. Standard value for boys or male adolescents is a sedimentation of 15 mm during 1 h, for girls or female adolescents 20 mm during 1 h.

9.5 Procalcitonin (PCT)

PCT is a protein which is constructed from 116 amino acids. It is produced mainly in the parafollicular C cells of the thyroid gland and in various neuroendocrine cells. Under physiological conditions, it acts as a prohormone of calcitonin. It is known that the release of PCT increases in the case of an infection, which is caused by bacterials, fungi or parasites. In this special condition, PCT is secreted predominantly in cells other the thyroid gland, including leukocytes, adipocytes, myocytes and hepatocytes. Stimuli for the synthesis of PCT in these cells are bacterial endotoxins (lipopolysaccharides = LPS) and cytokines (Interleukin - 1 beta, tumour necrosis factor - alpha). The pathophysiological significance of PCT increase has not yet been clarified. Anyway, there is no effect on the thyroid gland.

The PCT level in the blood increases within 3 h after stimulation by endotoxins or cytokines. The maximum of the PCT level is reached after 8 – 24 h and will be stable for another 24 h. Then the PCT amount will decrease again with a quite long half-life of 20 – 24 h. In healthy individuals, the physiological PCT level is < 0.5 μg/l. Values from 0.5 to 2.0 μg/l are associated with a mild respective moderate systemic infection, values from 2.0 to 10.0 μg/l with a severe systemic infection and values > 10.0 μg/l are in the majority of cases a sign of a sepsis. The amount of PCT correlates with the severity of the infectious disease and the mortality rate. In other very severe diseases, such as multiple trauma, large-scale burning, cardiogenic shock or multiple organ failure, the PCT level increases as well.

PCT remains nearly unaffected in the case of a localized, a viral, an autoimmunological or an allergic inflammation. For this reason it is an excellent marker for the rapid differentiation between viral and bacterial systemic (= antibiotic-requiring) infections.

Furthermore, PCT is well suited for the monitoring of the course of a systemic bacterial infection.

A big advantage of PCT, compared to CRP, CBC and ESR, is its much faster increase, which allows a very early detection of a systemic bacterial infection. Moreover, its predictive value for prediction of sepsis with 0.93 is much better than that of CRP, which is only 0.68. Furthermore, the interference by a therapy with steroids is much lower. One advantage compared to IL-6 is the better biological stability with a much longer half-life, what reduces the risk of false negative results. Additionally, in contrast to IL-6, autoimmunological inflammations do not interfere with PCT.

The measurement of the PCT level in patients with a febrile infection may be helpful to decide whether or not a patient needs an antibiotic treatment. In a clinical study it has been shown that by using a simple algorithm, the knowledge of the PCT level could reduce the administration of antibiotics from 80% previously to 44%.

On the one hand one wants to avoid the "treatment" of a viral infection with antibiotics, on the other hand one wants to assure the start of a required antibiotic therapy in time. Especially newborns and young infants may undergo fulminant clinical courses in the form of severe sepsis, for which reason this age group is very critical, and it is not acceptable to delay the start of an antibiotic treatment. Generally, it seems to be useful to give the measurement of PCT a higher priority than is currently given.

10. Therapeutic concepts for bronchitis in children - pro and contra

In general, a bronchitis may be treated symptomatically, because in most cases it is caused by an viral infection, and there exists no specific treatment. But the importance of the so-called household remedies should not be underestimated: an adequate fluid intake and inhalation of 0.9% NaCl may help to keep the bronchial mucosa moist and to liquefy the mucus. Sage drops may reduce the tussive irritation. The inhalation of essential oils, which are suitable for children, may also help to reduce discomfort, but it should be noted that there is a small risk of sensitization. In addition, there are a number of drugs (some are available in the pharmacy without prescription, some have to be prescribed), which have a reasonably proficient efficacy.

10.1 Sympathomimetic

For the treatment of an acute bronchial obstruction beta 2 - agonists are used, which have a selective effect on the respiratory system, in order to minimize beta 1 – receptor - mediated adverse effects on the heart. The binding of the drug to its receptor activates the adenylyl cyclase whereby ATP is converted to cAMP. That leads to a relaxation of the smooth musculature via a reduction in calcium ion concentration in the cells, and it leads to an inhibition of the release of mediators from mast cells. Generally, short-acting beta 2 - agonists, such as salbutamol, are used. In most cases salbutamol is applied in the form of inhalation, the common dosage is about $\frac{1}{2}$ drop per kg body weight in about 2 ml 0.9% NaCl, administered with an ultrasonic nebulizer. Alternatively, especially en route, 1 – 2 puffs of a spray via a spacer can be used. The frequency of inhalation depends on the severity of bronchial obstruction. 3 - 6 applications in 24 hours are an average frequency during an acute obstructive bronchitis, but it can be increased, if necessary. The oral administration of salbutamol is possible, but because of a lower efficacy and an increase of adverse effects due to a higher intake into the blood this is not recommended as a first choice. Common adverse effects are restlessness, heart palpitations and shakiness. These symptoms are induced by an increased sympathetic activity and can be reduced by reduction of the single dosage or the frequency of administration. In pregnant female adolescents, salbutamol can induces tocolysis via the beta 2 - receptor.

10.2 Anticholinergic

Anticholinergics inhibit acetylcholine due to competition on the muscarinic acetylcholine receptors and antagonize its bronchoconstrictive effect. They were applicated via inhalation. In comparison to the sympathomimetics, their effect is weaker and occurs with a delay. Ipratropium bromide is used most frequently, usually in addition to a beta 2 - agonist, if the sympathomimetic effect is not sufficient. Possible side effects include dry mouth, a bitter taste, tachycardia and arterial hypertension.

10.3 Methylxanthine

The exact mechanism of action of methylxanthines, such as theophylline, is not fully known. Several different mokecularbiological pathways seem to be involved: methylxanthines inhibit the phosphodiesterase, increase intracellular cAMP and antagonize effects on the adenosine receptors. Due to these mechanisms, methylxanthines have bronchodilatatory and anti-inflammatory effects and they stimulate the respiratory centre in the brain stem. They are rarely used, mainly as reserve medication for severe asthma - attacks. Theophylline is then usually given as a continuous infusion. The side effects can be serious: tachycardia, extrasystoles, arterial hypertension, restlessness, insomnia, gastrointestinal disorders or increased diuresis.

10.4 Glucocorticoid

Glucocorticoids induce the secretion of lipocortin, a glycoprotein which inhibits the phospholipase A2 and thereby reduces the release of arachidonic acid. Due to this mechanism, the cyclooxygenase pathway produces less prostaglandins and the lipoxygenase pathway less leukotrienes. Several cytokines, particularly interleukin-1, interleukin-2 and tumour necrosis factor – alpha, are produced in a reduced amount as well. In the peripheral blood the number of monocytes is decreased and also their bactericidal and chemotactic effects, as well as their migration are reduced. All these changes have a non-specific anti-inflammatory effect. Depending on the half-life, glucocorticoids are divided into short-acting (for example cortisone and cortisol), medium-acting (for example prednisone, prednisolone and methyl prednisolone) and long-acting (for example dexamethasone) substances. The systematic administration of glucocorticoids over a short time period may be necessary in the case of an acute severe bronchial obstruction. In infants and young children the application can be carried out in the form of a suppository, which can be done at home by the parents. If a child with an acute severe bronchial obstruction is brought into the emergency room, the intravenous application is part of the standard therapy. The long-term treatment with a glucocoticoid should be done topically, that is via inhalation. Commonly used corticosteroids for an inhalation therapy are budesonide, beclomethasone and fluticasone. The dosages are here in the microgram range; that means, they are by a factor of 100 – 1000 lower than the systemically given dosages. Thereby any side effects are reduced to a minimum. Parents who are afraid of the possible adverse effects of corticoids from long-term treatment should have an informative consultation. If they have the relevant knowledge, then their worries should be placated. If there are local side effects , for example the development of an oral thrush these can arise after inhalation if the mouth is not rinsed with water.

10.5 Leukotriene antagonist

Leukotrienes, products of the arachidonic acid metabolism, are synthesized in mast cells, macrophages, eosinophils and basophils. They have a very strong bronchoconstrictive effect (1000-fold more potent than histamine), induce an oedema of the bronchial mucus via increasing the capillary permeability and increase the production of mucus. Additionally, leukotrienes have a chemotactic influence on inflammatory cells, especially the eosinophils, which sensitizes the nerve fibres occurring in the respiratory tract, resulting in a bronchial hyperreactivity. The most common leukotriene antagonist is montelukast. Because its structure is similar to the leukotriene D4, it acts as a selective competitor at the receptor without the effects mentioned above. Montelukast is used as a long-term anti-inflammatory therapy, often in combination with a topical corticosteroid. Montelukast is administered orally in the evening. The adverse effects that may occur include headache and abdominal pain.

10.6 Mucolytic

Mucolytic respective secretolytic drugs are expectorants. In contrast to secretomotoric drugs, which increase the activity of the ciliated epithelium, expectorants should cause a liquefaction of the bronchial mucus to make it easier to cough it up. Among the mucolytics are acetylcysteine, bromhexin and ambroxol. Acetylcysteine cleaves the disulfide bonds of the mucopolysaccharides. Furthermore, it has an anti-inflammatory effect due to catching free radicals with its reactive SH group. Bromhexin activates enzymes, which cleave the molecules of the mucus and stimulate the glandular cells to increase the mucus production, reduce the viscosity. Ambroxol is a metabolite of bromhexin. In addition to the effects of bromhexin, it stimulates the synthesis of surfacant. Some herbal substances, such as ivy, also belong to mucolytic drugs. Generally, the therapeutic significance of all these so-called cough syrups should not be overestimated. It is much more important that the children drink enough and make inhalations.

10.7 Antitussive

Antitussives reduce the cough by acting on the brain stem. Opiates, like codeine, dihydrocodeine, hydrocodone or noscapine, are the most common drugs against tussive irritation. There are newer substances, such as pentoxiverin, which have the advantage of lacking a sedative effect or an addiction potential. Pentoxiverin is an agonist at the sigma receptor and also acts antagonistically at the muscarinic M1 receptor. Potential side effects are nausea, vomiting and diarrhoea. It is contraindicated in children younger than 2 years because a depressant effect on the respiration cannot be excluded, and in pregnant women because there are no sufficient safety data. However, in childhood antitussives, these should be prescribed only in rare cases with a non-productive cough. Otherwise, if a productive cough is inhibited, the mucus remains in the airways, increasing the risk of secondary bacterial infections with bronchopneumonia.

10.8 Antibiotic

In the case of a bacterial infection treatment with antibiotics is recommended. The choice of the appropriate antibiotic depends on the age of the child, because in different age groups there are different spectra of bacteria. After receiving the antibiogram, the antibiotic therapy can be specified in accordance to sensitivities and resistances of the bacterium. Between community-acquired and nosocomial infections, bacterial spectra differ as well. Sometimes it is not possible to distinguish between a viral and a bacterial infection, since the clinical course and the blood parameters can be quite similar. In this situation it may be that a child will be treated with an antibiotic, although it is just a viral infection with high fever.

10.9 Oxygen supplementation

In the case of severe bronchial obstruction with spasms of the bronchial musculature, with oedema of the bronchial mucosa and production of viscous secretions, ventilation in the airways and diffusion in the alveoli may be disturbed. This can cause a partial (hypoxia, normocapnia) or global (hypoxia, hypercapnia) respiratory insufficiency. If the transcutanously measured oxygen saturation in the blood is too low, the supplementation of oxygen is necessary. Usually the oxygen is supplied via nasal prongs. If small children do not tolerate nasal prongs, a mask can be placed in front of the face, especially during sleep.

In the treatment of premature infants with a respiratory distress syndrome, we have different procedures, because there the toxic effect of oxygen on the immature organs has to be taken into account. Complications caused by oxygen can be BPD, the retinopathy of prematurity and an apoptosis-mediated neurodegeneration. The monitoring of the premature infants should contain a capnometric analysis next to the measurement of the oxygen saturation.

10.10 Physiotherapy

Physiotherapy is required in the case of chronic diseases of the respiratory system (for example cystic fibrosis or primary ciliary dyskinesis), but also in the case of acute pneumological problems (for example the formation of an atelectasis as a complication of pneumonia). The aims of physiotherapy are to attain effective ventilation of all lung sections and an effective drainage of secretion.

10.11 Nasal drops

0.9% NaCl - nose drops are used to moisten and clean the nasal mucosa. Decongestant nose drops (dependent on age 0.25%, 0.5% or 1% xylometazoline) should be given, if the eustachian tube is swollen in response to an infection of the upper airways, in order to guarantee the ventilation of the middle ear. These nose drops should not be given for longer than 7 days, otherwise they could lead to an irreversible damage of the mucosa. A stuffy nose is not a good reason for the application of decongestant nose drops. Depending on the age of the child, a nose spray may be used instead of nose drops.

11. References

Brodzinski H, Ruddy RM. (2009). Review of new and newly discovered respiratory tract viruses in children. *Pediatr Emerg Care*, 25 (5), 51-63, ISSN 0749-5161

Bundesärztekammer (BÄK), Kassenärztliche Bundesvereinigung (KBV), Arbeitsgemeinschaft der Wissenschaftlichen Medizinischen Fachgesellschaften (AWMF). (2011). *Nationale VersorgungsLeitlinie Asthma – Kurzfassung, 2. Auflage. Version 1.3*, available from: http://www.versorgungsleitlinien.de/themen/asthma

Deutsche Gesellschaft für Pädiatrische Infektiologie (DGPI) e. V. (2009). *DGPI Handbuch, Infektionen bei Kindern und Jugendlichen*, Thieme-Verlag, ISBN 978-3-13-144715-9, Stuttgart

Deis JN, Creech CB, Estrada CM, Abramo TJ. (2010). Procalcitonin as a marker of severe bacterial infection in children in the emergency department. *Pediatr Emerg Care*, 26 (1), 51-63, ISSN 0749-5161

Global Initiative for Asthma (GINA). (2010). *Global Strategy for Asthma Management and Prevention*, available from: http://www.ginasthma.org

Mitchell I. (2009). Treatment of RSV bronchiolitis: drugs, antibiotics. *Pediatr Respir Rev*, 10 Suppl 1, 14-15, ISSN 1526-0542

Ramanuja S, Kelkar PS. (2010). The approach to pediatric cough. *Ann Allergy Asthma Immunol*, 105 (1), 3-8

Rieger C, von der Hardt H, Sennhauser FH, Wahn U, Zach M (Eds.). (2004). *Pädiatrische Pneumologie*, Springer-Verlag, ISBN 3-540-43627-8, Berlin

Wainwright C. (2009). Acute viral bronchiolitis in children – a very common condition with few therapeutic options. *Pediatr Respir Rev*, 11, 39-45, ISSN 1526-0542

8

Bronchopulmonary Dysplasia

Shou-Yien Wu[1,2], Sachin Gupta[1],
Chung-Ming Chen[3,4] and Tsu-Fuh Yeh[3,4,5,*]
[1]Division of Neonatology, Dept. of Ped. John Stroger Hospital of Cook County
[2]Rosalind Franklin University of Medicine and Science, Chicago, Illinois
[3]Dept. of Pediatrics
[4]Maternal Child Health Research Center, Taipei Medical University, Taipei
[5]Dept. of Ped. China Medical University, Taichung
[1,2,3]USA
[4,5]Taiwan

1. Introduction

Bronchopulmonary dysplasia (BPD) continues to be the most common and most important complication in preterm infants with RDS. The incidence varies from 20 to 60 % in preterm infants whose weight are < 1500 gram. The presence of BPD is often associated with significant mortality and short term and long term morbidity, including growth failure and neurodevelopment delay.

The exact mechanism and pathogenesis of BPD is not completely understood. However, epidemiology study suggests a changing prevalence and clinical features in recent years. The traditional descriptions of BPD (so call classic or old BPD) are essentially related to lung injuries following mechanical ventilation while the recent description of BPD (new BPD) is probably related more to prematurity of the lungs. The relation between these two types of BPD is not clear. Recent studies indicated that inflammation may play an important role for both the classic and new BPD. Once lung injuries have established, managements are essentially supportive, therefore every effort should be focus on prevention. Proper respiratory care is the most essential in preventing lung injury. Other medications, either to improve the pulmonary function or to reduce the lung inflammation, have been tried with various successes. There is no magic bullet to cure the disease.

2. Definition

The original definition of bronchopulmonary dysplasia by Northway was base on radiological and pathological characteristics in prematurely born infants with respiratory distress syndrome (RDS) who were treated with mechanical ventilation and oxygen supplementation. Subsequently, the definition of BPD was changed to respiratory sequelae in infants requiring oxygen supplementation more than 28 days after birth since BPD may occur in tiny premature infants who have not previously had RDS. This definition was not

---

* Corresponding Author

without debate, because it includes a wide range of infants, i.e. from those ultimately appear to have no residual problems to those with severe BPD. A more practical definition was used: respiratory sequelae in infants who reach term age but are oxygen or mechanical ventilation dependent. The introduction of antenatal steroid prophylaxis, postnatal surfactant treatment caused revolutionary care of premature infants. Nowadays, more extreme low birth weight infants with birth weight < 1000gm and gestation age 23-28 weeks survived, they experienced a mild initial respiratory course, but required a low concentration of oxygen for a long time. In 2001, the United States National Institute of Child Health and Human Development (NICHD) conducted a workshop. A new definition, which categorizes the severity of BPD, was proposed.

2.1 Classic bronchopulmonary dysplasia (Classic BPD)
As described above, the classic BPD was defined as a chronic lung disease occurs in premature infants who had respiratory distress after birth, require oxygen supplementation or mechanical ventilator support at 28 postnatal days or 36 weeks postmenstrual age (PMA). Four stages I, II, III and IV are classified base on radiological findings and associated pathologic changes. Stage I and II describe acute and subacute course of respiratory distress syndrome. Stage III and IV often represent changes associated with chronic lung disease.

Stage I   (2-3 days) is a period of acute RDS. The radiologic picture is similar to RDS.

Stage II (4-10 days) is a period of regeneration. The chest radiograph shows complete opacity of the lung obscuring the heart and lung borders.

Stage III (10-20 days) is a period of transition to chronic disease. The early radiographic changes are replaced by areas of coarse, irregular shaped densities and areas of cyst lesions. Areas of density are caused by interstitial edema or atelectasis due to obstruction of small bronchioles with luminal debris. The cysts represent foci of emphysema.

Stage IV (beyond 1 month) is a period of chronic disease. Chest radiograph shows large cysts and marked fibrosis and edema with areas of consolidation and areas of overinflation.

This definition becomes less relevant in current practice, since the improvement care of RDS, and survival of very tiny babies, classic BPD is uncommonly seen now, instead a new form of BPD (new BPD) is much increased.

2.2 New bronchopulmonary dysplasia (New BPD)
BPD is now defined clinically as a chronic lung disease occurring in premature infants who need for supplemental O_2 for at least 28 days after birth, and its severity is graded according to the oxygen concentration and positive pressure of respiratory support at near term. For gestation age 32 weeks or more, the time of determination varies between 28 days to 56 days before discharge. For gestation age less than 32 week, the time of determination is 36 weeks postmenstrual age 36 weeks. A physiologic test such as pulse oximetry saturation is recommended to confirm the requirement of oxygen supplementation at the time of assessment (Table 1). Again, this definition is made clinically and the incidence of BPD can be various from hospital to hospital.

3. Epidemiology

The incidence of BPD varies among different institutions. This is due to differences in neonatal risk factors among different populations, patient care management and the discrepancies in the definition of BPD. Incidence figures must be interpreted with caution.

Gestation age	< 32 weeks	> 32 weeks
Time point of assessment	36 wk PMA or discharge to home, whichever comes first	28 d to 56 d postnatal age or discharge to home, whichever comes first
Treatment with oxygen > 21% for at least 28 d plus		
Mild BPD	Breathing room air at 36 wk PMA or discharge, whichever comes first	Breathing room air by 56 d postnatal age or discharge, whichever comes first
Moderate BPD	Need for <30% oxygen at 36 PMA or discharge, whichever comes first	Need for < 30% oxygen at 56 d postnatal age or discharge, whichever comes first
Severe BPD	Need for ≥ 30% oxygen and/or positive pressure (PPV or NCPAP) at 36 wk PMA or discharge, whichever comes first	Need for ≥ 30% oxygen and/or positive pressure (PPV or NCPAP) at 56 d postnatal age or discharge, whichever comes first

Adapt from Jobe A. Bancalarie E. Bronchopulmonary Dysplasia. Am J Respir Crit Care Med 2001; 163: 1723-1729.

Table 1. Definition of New Bronchopulmonary Dysplasia: Diagnostic Criteria

For example, better prenatal and postnatal care increase survival of the very tiny infants, more infants who previously would have died now survive and remain oxygen/ventilator dependent at 28 days of age, the overall rate of BPD may increase, but the severity is much less. The denominator may also be different, some reports used all live births of premature infants as denominator; while others used only survived infants.

Parker et al reported the incidence of BPD increased from 10.6% in 1976 through 1980, to 21.7% (981 through 1985), and to 32.9% (1986 through 1990) in very low birth weight neonates (1500 g or less) admitted to a regional newborn care center in USA, while there was concurrent decline of neonatal death during the same periods (26.4%, 18.3%, and 15.9%, respectively). The diagnosis of BPD was given if neonates were treated supplemental oxygen for at least 28 days as a surrogate for oxygen treatment on postnatal day 28.

In 2007, a report from NICHD Neonatal Research Network database of USA shows the survival rate and the incidence of BPD (defined by supplemental O2 at 36 weeks PMA) in infants with birth weight of 501-1500g almost unchanged between1997and 2002. The survival increases slightly (from 84 to 85%) and the incidence of BPD decreases by 1% (from 23 to 22%). Tiny infants have highest rate and severity of BPD: 6% in 1250-1500g; 14%in 1001-1240g; 33% in750-1000g and 46% in 501 to 750g.

Since the release of a consensus statement by the American Academy of Pediatrics and the Canadian Pediatric Society in 2002, the use of postnatal corticosteroid has decreased. There was concern that the decreased use of postnatal steroid might increase the risk of BPD. A recent report from America which includes 77520 premature infants born at ≤32 weeks gestation in California, the overall rate of BPD increased over the decade: 20% in 1997-1999, 24% in 2000-2003 and 25.4% in 2004-2006. The rate of severe BPD also increased significantly: 3.6% 1997-1999, 5.1% in 2000-2003, and 9.5% in 2004-2006.

4. Pathology of bronchopumonary dysplasia

The characteristic changes of classic BPD are airway injury and inflammation, airway epithelial cell metaplasia, and parenchymal fibrosis. In contrast, the characteristic morphology of "new" BPD is disruption of lung development (Figure 1).

4.1 Classic bronchopumonary dysplasia

Four stages are classified according to the severity and anatomic component involved.

Stage I   alveolar and interstitial edema with hyaline membranes, atelectasis, and necrosis of bronchial mucosa are present.

Stage II atelectasis becomes more evident, alternating with areas of emphysema. There is widespread necrosis and repair of bronchial mucosa. Cellular debris fills the airways.

Stage III extensive bronchial and bronchiolar metaplasia and hyperplasia evolve. Areas of emphysema are surrounded by areas of atelectasis, accompanied by massive interstitial edema with thickening of the basement membranes.

Stage IV massive fibrosis of the lung with destruction of alveoli and airways are present. In addition, there is hypertrophy of bronchial smooth muscle and metaplasia of airway mucosa. Finally, there is actual loss of pulmonary arterioles and capillaries and medial muscular hypertrophy of remaining vessels.

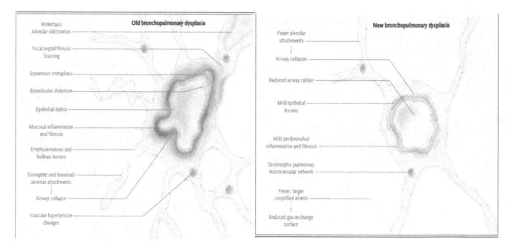

Fig. 1. Airway and Parenchymal Damage in Old and New BPD. „Old" and „new" BPD are two different morphologic outcomes of variable combinations of factors capable of injuring lungs of differing maturity. In old BPD, intense inflammation and disruption of normal pulmonary structures lead to a nonhomogeneous airway and parenchymal disease. In contrast, the main feature of new BDP is diffusely reduced alveolar development, which is associated with a clinically significant loss of surface area for gas excange, with airway injury, inflammation, and fibrosis that are usually milder than in old BPD.
(From Baraldi E., Filippone M. Chronic Lung Disease after Premature Birth. N Engl J M. 2007, 357(8);1951)

4.2 New bronchopulmonary dysplasia

Hislop et al. reported that mechanical ventilation of low birth weight infants leads to fewer alveoli. Husain et al. reported that extremely premature infants (gestation age ranged 24 to 32 weeks) dying of BPD had partial to complete arrest in acinar development whether infants received surfactant treatment or not. The alveolar structures are larger, simplified, and fewer in numbers. The amount of alveolar septal fibrosis is substantially less and tends to be more diffuse in surfactant-treated infants than in infants who did not have surfactant treatment. Coalson studied the autopsy lung specimens from infants who had received both prenatal steroids and surfactant treatment and have found the following findings: enlarged air spaces with minimal alveolization, dysmorphic capillary configuration and variable alveolar wall cellularity and fibrosis. Airway and vascular lesions, when present, tend to be present in infants, who over time develop more severe disease.

5. Pathogenesis

The pathogenesis of BPD is multifactorial. The original concepts of risk factors include: (1) prematurity; (2) respiratory distress; (3) mechanical ventilation; (4) oxygen supplementation. These factors still play an important role in the development of new BPD. However, infection and inflammation, pulmonary edema as result of and patent ductus arteriosus (PDA) or fluid overloading, nutritional deficiencies and genetic factors may also contribute to lung injury. Classic BPD is heavily influenced by injury inflammation and fibrosis; while new primarily is an arrest of development, disorder or delayed modeling and remodeling. (Figure 2)

5.1 Prematurity

Bronchopulmonary dysplasia occurs most commonly in premature infants. Extreme low birth weight infants have a deficiency of surfactant and immature lung parenchyma, compliant chest wall , inadequate respiratory drive and immature antioxidant enzyme system. Most of these infants need supplemental oxygen and assisted ventilation after birth to achieve adequate gas exchange. The functional and structural immaturity increases the risk of lung injury and disruption of normal alveolar development from antenatal and postnatal insults.

Infants born at 23-28 weeks gestation are just beginning to alveolarize the distal saccule of the lung in parallel with the development of the alveolar capillary bed. Alveolar development can be delayed with hypoxia, hyperoxia, inflammations, glucocorticoids, and poor nutrition.

Patent ductus arteriosus (PDA) is present in most ELBW infants. PDA shunt increases pulmonary blood flow, and may result in pulmonary edema. Lung compliance is reduced and lung resistance is increased, creating a need for more vigorous and protracted ventilator support.

5.2 Oxygen toxicity

Inspiration of high oxygen concentration is a major factor in the pathogenesis of BPD, though the precise concentration and duration of oxygen that is toxic to the immature lung has not been established. Any concentration in excess of room air might increase the risk of lung damage when administered over a period of time. Early pulmonary change caused by oxygen toxicity consists of atelectasis, edema, alveolar hemorrhage, inflammation, fibrin deposition, and thickening of alveolar membrane. Continuous high oxygen exposure causes influx of polymorphonuclear leukocytes containing proteolytic enzymes which causes inflammatory reaction and cytotoxic damage.

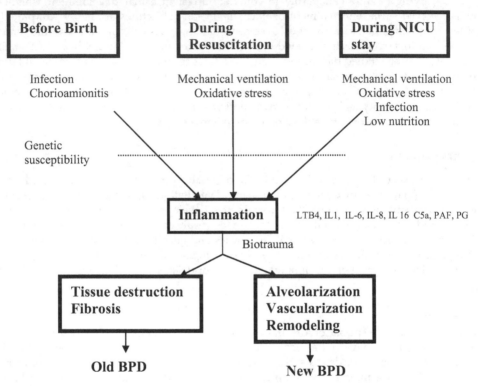

Fig. 2. Pathogenesis of Bronchopulmonary Dysplasia

The fetal lung is exposed to relatively low oxygen tension around 20 to 30 mmHg. Immediately after birth, the arterial oxygen tension climbs to 100 mmHg. The sudden increase of oxygen tension cause substantial oxidative stress. The principle mechanism involves the univalent reduction of molecular oxygen and formation of free oxygen radicals such as superoxide free radical (O_2^-), hydrogen peroxide (H_2O_2), hydroxyl free radical (OH) and singlet oxygen ($^1O_2$). These oxygen free radicals are highly reactive molecules that can cause oxidative damage to lung tissue and trigger the inflammatory reaction. Premature infants have inadequate antioxidant defense system because their antioxidant enzymes such as superoxide dismutase (SOD), catalase (CAT), glutathione peroxidase (GP) are not mature and nutrients deficiencies (vitamin E, vitamin C, beta-carotene, uric acid) are common, thus they are vulnerable to develop lung injury from oxygen toxicity.

5.3 Mechanical ventilation-barotrauma and volutrauma
Barotrauma is the lung injury caused by the pressure used to inflate the lung. The inspiratory pressures needed to inflate the surfactant-deficiency premature lungs often fivefold greater than the physiologic pressure of the normal lung. The alveoli are not

homogenous inflated; some units remain collapsed and require higher pressure to reopen, whereas others become over distended. The resistance of collapsed alveoli to inflate leads to over distension of distal bronchioles during peak inflation and damage of bronchiolar epithelium. These over distension of airways and irregular aeration of alveoli lead to inflammation and release of cytokine.

Barotrauma produces alveolar shear stress, disruption of alveolarization, pulmonary air leak, and release of damaging cytokine and other biologically substances. High ventilator pressure has long been considered as a major cause of BPD, but tissue damage is now more attributed to over-distension of the lung from high tidal volume ventilation (volutrauma). In an animal experiment, Dreyfuss et al. demonstrated the most severe lung injury was seen with high tidal volume with high or low pressure. There were no abnormalities with low volume at high pressure. In clinical settings, however, high pressure usually delivers high volume, which in turn stretches alveolar wall and capillaries.

5.4 Inflammation

Inflammation plays the central role in the development of BPD. Inflammatory reaction may be triggered by factors including infection before or after birth, oxygen free radicals, barotraumas or volutrauma from mechanical ventilation, and pulmonary edema. Neutrophils and macrophages are recruited in the airway and pulmonary tissues. The activated neutrophils adhere to the endothelium of the pulmonary vascular system and thus initiate a sequence of pathogenetic events. Infants who subsequently develop BPD are found to have high concentration of proinflammatory and chemotactic factors in the tracheobronchial aspirate such as leukotrine B_4, interleulcukin-1β, interleukin-8, soluble ICAM-1, anaphylatoxin C5a, platelet aggregation factor and prostaglandin. Pulmonary inflammation affects normal alveolization and angiogenesis, these may further lead to remodeling of developing lung resulting in BPD. Leukotrienes may remain elevated in BPD infants even at 6 months of age and cause bronchoconstrictoin, vasoconstriction, edema, neutrophils chemotaxis and mucus production.

5.5 Prenatal and postnatal infection
5.5.1 Chorioamnionitis

Premature infants who were exposed to maternal chorioamnionitis and required mechanical ventilation after birth have higher incidence of BPD. Proinflammatory mediators IL-1, IL-6 and IL-8 were detected in the early tracheal aspirates from these infants, suggesting lung inflammation occurred before birth. Ureaplasma urealyticum is the most common organism associated with chorioamnionitis. Several studies have suggested an association between Ureaplasma urealyticum tracheal colonization and the development of severe respiratory failure and BPD in very low birth weight infants, but results have not been consistent.

5.5.2 Postnatal infection

Very low birth weight infants with early onset systemic infection or local pneumonia usually present with respiratory signs including cyanosis and apnea which required oxygen therapy or ventilator support. Intubated infants are prone to develop nosocomial infection with deteriorating gas exchange, and are at great risk for development of BPD. The presence of a systemic infection in premature infants was noted to increase the risk of late ductal reopening and failure to respond to medical treatment with indomethacin. Infants with infection and those with PDA had higher levels of 6-ketoprostaglandin F1-α than did control subjects. Levels of tumor necrosis factor-α were also elevated in infants with infection and in those with late PDA. The risk of BPD is enhanced if there is active PDA present at the time of infection.

5.6 Pulmonary edema, patent ductus arteriosus and fluid overloading

Increases pulmonary blood flow from left-to-right shunt blood flow crossing patent ductus arteriosus may result increasing interstitial fluid and pulmonary edema. Pulmonary compliance is reduced and resistance is increased, creating a need for prolonged ventilator support with higher oxygen concentration and ventilation pressure. Clinical evidence suggests that infants with RDS who receive great fluid intake or who do not show a diuretic phase during the first few days of life have a high incidence of BPD. This may be because high fluid intake increases the incidence of PDA. Elevated concentration of myeloperoxidase was noted in the tracheal fluid of infants with PDA, suggesting the increased pulmonary blood flow may result in damage of the pulmonary endothelium and adhesion and migration of polymorphonuclear cells into the lung tissue.

5.7 Nutrition, Vitamin A

Premature infants are undernutrition for days and weeks after birth due to critically ill state, intolerance of enteral feeding and fluid restriction. Sick infants have high caloric demand for growth, increased work of breathing and metabolism. Inadequate nutrition may amplify the lung injury of mechanical ventilation, oxygen toxicity and hinder the repair and recovery course. Vitamin C scavenges free oxygen radicals, as well as it interacts with vitamine E. Vitamin A is important in regulating early lung development and alveolar formation. Vitamin A deficiency may promote chronic lung disease by impairing lung healing, increasing the loss of cilia and squamous-cell metaplasia, increasing susceptibility to infection, and decreasing the number of alveoli.

5.8 Genetics

Studies in VLBW twins demonstrated that BPD status in one twin was a highly significant predictor of BPD in the other twin, irrespective of birth order, Apgar scores and other factors. Monozygotic twins had more BPD and a long duration of hospitalization. Lung development is regulated by a variety of genes that balance between pro- and anti-inflammation, oxygen toxicity, cell injury and death, tissue repair, and infection. Specific genes that are known to be involved in these biologic pathways have been evaluated for their potential contribution to BPD. Approximately half of the initial genetic-association studies have not been replicated.

6. Clinical course

Most infants who develop BPD usually have various degree of respiratory insufficiency resulting from RDS, pneumonia or poor respiratory effort after birth. Oxygen therapy or mechanical support is needed to maintain adequate gas exchange. Their pulmonary condition may show improvement in the first few days but deteriorate later. The pulmonary resistance increases gradually and blood gas shows carbon dioxide retention. Infants require more concentrated oxygen and more ventilator support. The deterioration may be triggered by (1)systemic or local infection; (2) the presence of pulmonary edema associated with PDA, fluid overload or congestive heart failure; (3) severe airway obstruction caused by bronchospasm or tracheobronchomalasia. BPD is often anticipated when mechanical ventilation and oxygen supplementation extend beyond10 to 14 days.

Some infants who have mild or moderate BPD show a slow but steady improvement and wean from support after 28 days old. On the other hand, some deteriorate and ultimately require months of oxygen supply and ventilator support. Respiratory acidosis with high PCO2 greater than 55 mmHg associated with compensated metabolic alkalosis is common. Hypoxemia and hypercarbia result from ventilation-perfusion mismatch and alveolar hypoventilation.

The oxygen requirement decrease gradually as the disease process improves, but it can increase during feeding, physical activity or episode of infection. Intubated infants are easily agitated either because of discomfort or airway obstruction; they are also prone to get nosocomial infection. Growth failure with poor weight gain is common due to insufficient enteral intake and increase work of breathing. Some infants with severe BPD develop pulmonary hypertension, right ventricular hypertrophy and eventually die of right-side heart failure (cor pulmonale).

Radiologic manifestation of mild BPD usually appears normal or mild haziness lung field. Moderate to severe BPD may show hyperinflation, lobar or segmental atelectasis, gas trapping with pulmonary interstitial emphysema (PIE) and increased lung streaking. Fibrosis band and enlarged cyst usually occurs in severe BPD.

Supplemental oxygen and /or ventilator dependent
Recurrent respiratory infection
Lung atelectasis
Gastrointestinal reflux
Aspiration pneumonia
Apnea
Hypertension
Wheezing and bronchospasm
Signs of inappropriate ADH
Signs of pulmonary hypertension and cor-pulmonale
Poor postnatal growth
Increase incidence of sudden infant death
Increase fetal hemoglobin
Neurodevelopmental delay

Table 2. Clinical features associated with BPD

7. Prevention of bronchopulmonary dysplasia

As stated above, the pathogensis of BPD has been linked to immature lung tissue, barotraumas and volutrauma resulting from mechanical ventilation, oxygen injury, and proinflammatory factors. Reduction of the incidence and severity of BPD may be possible through reduction of the causes of BPD. Among many strategies studied in the past, antenatal corticosteroids treatment, postnatal surfactant therapy, and gentle ventilation have been proved to be the most effective methods to target the development of BPD and decrease its severity.

7.1 Pharmacologic agents
7.1.1 Antenatal corticosteroid

Antenatal corticosteroid (ANC) was noted to be the most successful agent in reducing respiratory syndrome and increasing survival in premature infants by Liggins and Howie in 1972. It was not widely used until 1994 when the Consensus Development Conference Statement of National Institute of Health was published. Now women are at risk of preterm birth between 24 and 34 weeks'gestation are routinely given a course of corticosteroid before delivery. A single course of antenatal corticosteroids treatment is associated with an overall reduction of neonatal death, RDS, intraventricular hemorrhage, necrotizing enteritis, respiratory support, intensive care admissions and systemic infections in the first 48hoursof life. Long term follow up study demonstrates improvement of neurodevelopmental outcomes. Steroids accelerate structural maturation and surfactant synthesis of the lung, thus decrease the severity of RDS and BPD. The overall incidence of BPD in the population is not decreased due to increased survival of tiny babies.

Antenatal corticosteroid is most effective if given more than 24 hours after and up to 7 days after administration of the second dose of antenatal corticosteroids. Treatment for less than 24 hours is still associated with better outcome, ANC should be given unless immediately delivery is anticipated or there is evidence corticosteroid will have an adverse effect on the mother. Caution should be exercised when giving corticosteroid therapy to women with systemic infection including tuberculosis and infection.

Betamethasone is the steroid of choice, when available, to be given in a course of two doses of 12mg administered intramuscularly 24 hours apart. An alternative regimen would be four doses of 6mg dexamethasone intramuscularly every 12 hours. Betamethasone is associated with a greater reduction in the risk of death than dexamethasone; it also decreases risk of periventricular leukomalacia which was not found with dexamethasone treatment. Weekly repeat course of ANC reduce the occurrence and severity of RDS, but the short benefits are upset with a reduction in weight and head circumference. Weekly repeat course of ANC are not recommended. Prenatal steroid may decrease airway septation and aveolarization in animal, it is not clear if prenatal steroid itself or the associated increased survival of tiny infant would contribute to the recently high incidence of new BPD.

7.1.2 Postnatal surfactant therapy

The surfactant deficiency lung of premature infants is highly susceptible to lung injury and significant inflammatory reaction. The function of surfactant is to recruit alveoli and prevent atelectasis. Surfactant replacement reduces initial inspired oxygen and ventilation requirements as well as the incidence of respiratory distress syndrome, death, pneumothorax, pulmonary interstitial emphysema and the combined outcome of death or BPD. Combined use of prenatal steroid and postnatal surfactant therapy has proved to have an additive effect in improving lung function. As results of these treatments, the severe classic BPD is rarely seen today.

7.1.3 Methylxanthines

Apnea of prematurity occurs in at least 85 percent of infants who are less than 34 weeks gestation. Widely used treatments include application of continuous positive airway pressure and the prescription of methylxanthines. In fact, methylxanthines – caffeine, theophylline and aminophylline are one of the most common drugs used in premature infants. They inhibit sleepiness-inducing adenosine and improve respiratory drive, reduce the frequency of apnea and the need for mechanical ventilation. Methylxanthines also inhibit TNF-α and leukotriene synthesis, thereby reducing inflammation and innate immunity.

Toxicity with theophylline is more common than with caffeine. Side effects are usually associated with plasma level over 20ug/ml. Serum levels less than 10ug/ml is not beneficial as an aid to wean the ventilator. Because of the narrow range of therapeutic levels of theophylline, caffeine is the drug of choice in the treatment of apnea of prematurity. Davis at el demonstrated an improvement in minute ventilation, an increase in tidal volume, a decrease in lung resistance and improved lung compliance 1 hour following 10 mg/kg of caffeine. In a randomized study by Schmidt et al, infant who received caffeine were less likely to use oxygen at 36 weeks postmenstrual age, and more likely to have ventilator discontinued earlier.

7.1.4 Postnatal corticosteroid

Because inflammation plays a central role in the pathogeneses of BPD, systemic corticosteroids especial dexamethasone have long been used for prevention and treatment of BPD. Lung inflammation is down-regulated by dexamethasone therapy. Dexamethasone is a potent, long acting steroid with almost exclusive glucocorticoid effect. Compared to hydrocortisone, dexamethasone is 25-50 times more potent. The half-life is 36-54 hours. Dexamethasone has been extensively studied in neonatal medicine and has shown to improve pulmonary function, facilitate extubation and decrease the incidence of BPD. However; many associated adverse side effects prevent the routine use of dexamethasone. The short term side effects include hyperglycemia, hypertension, hypertrophic cardiomyopathy, growth failure, GI bleeding and perforation. The risk of GI perforation increases with concomitant indomethacin treatment. There is also a concern of the chronic suppression of the hypothalamic-pituitary-adrenal axis, and long term neurodevelopmental delay.

Striking evidence from multiple studies of the adverse effects of dexamethasone and its long-term neurological effects on preterm infants prompted the American Academy of Pediatrics and the Canadian Pediatric Society to strongly discourage the use of corticosteroids to prevent or treat BPD in 2002. Since the release of this consensus statement, the use of corticosteroids has decreased significant, the incidence and severity of BPD increased significantly during this decade. To each gestation age, the time-related increase in BPD is inversely related to the decrease of dexamethasone use. The decline in use of dexamethasone associated with a concomitant increase in the use hydrocortisone. However, the use of hydrocortisone did not have any impact on the rate and severity of BPD.

7.2 Gentle ventilation

Mechanical ventilation both causes and treats BPD. When used, lowest ventilator setting to obtain adequate ventilation must be applied to minimize the barotrauma-volutrama and oxygen toxicity.

7.2.1 Tidal volume, inspiratory pressure and target range of oxygen saturation

In premature infants with lung disease, functional residual volume is reduced and some parts of alveoli are collapsed. The ideal tidal volume would be that open these collapsed area without over-distend the other areas. In general, initial PIP is set 16-20 cmH$_2$O in order to achieve a tidal volume of 4-6 ml/Kg in ELBW with respiratory failure. Peak inspiratory pressure >20 mmHg is rarely needed. Peak end expiratory pressure is usually set at 4 cmH$_2$O, and short inspiratory time 0.3-0.4 seconds are used.

Oxygen saturation monitored by pulse oximetry offers the most reliable estimate of arterial oxygenation and easy to use. The ranges of oxygen saturation should be targeted between 91 to 95%. Oxygen therapy is very toxic for preterm babies, and maintaining even slightly high oxygen saturation contributes to retinopathy of prematurity and increases the duration of oxygen treatment. The STOP-ROP (Supplemental Therapeutic Oxygen for prethreshold Retinopathy of Prematurity) research group showed that newborn babies who had received oxygen supplementation to maintain saturation at 96-99% presented more pneumonia and a greater incidence of chronic lung disease than did those whose saturation was maintained at 89-94%. The results of the Surfactant, Positive Pressure, and Oxygenation Randomized Trial (SUPPORT) demonstrated that lower target range of oxygenation at 85to 89% did not significantly decrease the combined risk of death or BPD, but it resulted in an increase in mortality.

7.2.2 Permissive hypercarbia

Higher levels of PCO2 45-65 mmHg with pH above 7.20 now are accepted, thus allowing gentle ventilation to minimize lung injury. Early studies suggest that BPD occur more often among newborn infants with PaCO2 below 40mmHg. A randomized, controlled study of NICH Neonatal network demonstrated that mechanical ventilated extremely low birth weight infants who were assigned to minimal ventilation (PCO2 target >52 mm Hg) required less ventilator support at 36 weeks compared with infants with routine ventilation (PCO$_2$ target <48 mm Hg) (1% vs. 16% respectively, p<0.01). Unfortunately, after enrollment of 220 patients, the trial was halted because of unanticipated non-respiratory adverse events related to dexamethasone therapy. The relative risk for death or BPD at 36 weeks in both groups is no difference.

7.2.3 Nasal continuous positive pressure (nCPAP)

Nasal continuous positive pressure supports the breathing through a number of mechanisms: (1). splinting the airway thereby preventing airway obstruction, (2). dilating the airways and reducing resistance to airflow and so diminishing work of breathing, (3) aiding lung expansion and so reducing ventilation perfusion mismatch and improving oxygenation. Nasal CPAP used after extubation can prevent the instability associated with possible respiratory failure and reintubation.

Nasal CPAP, rather than intubation and ventilation, might be started shortly after birth for infants born at 25 to 28weeks' gestation. In the randomized, controlled Continuous Positive Airway Pressure or Intubtion at Birth (COIN) trial, there were fewer days of ventilation in the CPAP group, and a few CPAP infants received oxygen therapy at 28 days, but not at 36 PMA weeks. The early CPAP group did not significantly reduce the rate of death or BPD. Pneumothorax occurs in 6% of the CPAP infants and 3 % in the intubated group. Report from SUPPORT study, infants born 24-28 weeks of gestation, were randomly assigned to intubation and surfactant treatment, or to CPAP treatment initiated in the delivery room. There is no significant difference of death or BPD at 36 weeks. Infants who received CPAP treatment, as compared with infants who received intubation and surfactant treatment, less frequently required intubation or postnatal corticosteroids for BPD, and required fewer days of mechanical ventilation.

The value of early CPAP as a replacement of intubation and ventilation apparently to be established. Surfactant treatment is most effective if given shortly after birth. Tiny infants with respiratory distress receive nCPAP alone after bith may miss the benefit of prophylactic surfactant therapy. In our practice, we intubate these infants soon after birth, give a dose of surfactant treatment, then extubated and change to CPAP support if infants can tolerate, to avoid mechanical ventilation.

8. Management of BPD

Despite of the recent advances of neonatal medicine, little progress has been made in treatment of BPD. Cornerstones of treatment are pulmonary support to maintain optimal oxygen saturation and prevent complications and nutritional support to promote growth. Most patients with mild to moderate BPD gradually improve as healing occurs and lung growth continues. Infants with severe BPD especial who are ventilator dependent are more likely to have acute episodes of pulmonary decompensation secondary due to nosocomial infection, severe airway constriction, pulmonary air leak, increased pulmonary edema and the development of tracheobronchmalacia or cor pulmonale. Physical examination, radiographic survey, laboratory tests and echocardiogram are important in differential diagnosis and guide for specific treatment.

Respiratory support

Infants with established BPD who are ventilator dependent, gentle ventilation are preferred to avoid further lung injury. Oxygen saturation should be kept within 90-95%. Inappropriate low oxygen tension may induce pulmonary vasoconstriction and /or bronchospasm with resultant increase frequency of apnea and hypoxia. Higher PCO2 (55 to 65 mmHg) is accepted if pH is in normal range. Weaning these from mechanical ventilation is difficult and must be accomplished gradually. Caffeine or theophylline are usually used during the weaning phase to stimulate respiratory drive. Nasal CPAP may be applied to infants after extubation.

Infants with BPD who are not on oxygen therapy may experience oxygen desaturation with feeding or physical activity, additional oxygen supply might be need.

Phamacologic agents

Most medications used for treatment of BPD are targeted on one of the following pathophysiologic mechanisms of BPD: (1) bronchopulmonary constriction and airway hyperreactivity, (2) pulmonary edema, (3) airway inflammation, and (4) chronic lung injury and repair.

Bronchodilators

Infants with BPD have increased airway resistance due to peribronchial smooth muscle hypertrophy and airway hyperactivity. Acute bronchospasm in response to hypoxia event could lead to sudden deteriorating pulmonary status. Bronchodilators have been shown to reduce airway resistance, improve lung compliance and increase tidal volume in infants with BPD during acute episodes of bronchospasm. However, their effects are usually short-lived, and many drugs have significant cardiovascular side effects. Inhaled β-2 agonists such as albuterol or levalbuterol have shown to reverse acute episodes of bronchoconstriction and cause few cardiovascular side effects. An initial trial dose can be administered through a meter-dose inhaler with a spacer device or as a nebulized solution. If patients show improvement of gas exchange, the β-2 agonists can be given up to 48hours duration.

Chronic use of β-2 agonists is not recommended since there is no long term benefit in treatment or prevention of BPD in preterm infants. Ipratropium bromide is another anticholinergic preparation that dilates airway.

Methylxanthines are competitive nonselective phosphodiesterase inhibitors, prevent breakdown of cyclic AMP and cyclic GMP. This leads to raise intracellular c-AMP and c-GMP. They also inhibit TNF-α and leukotriene synthesis, thereby reducing inflammation and innate immunity. Methylxanthines are nonselective adenosine receptor antagonists. Adenosine can cause broncho-constriction and potentiate immunologically induced mediator release from lung mast cells. Inhibition of this action will cause bronchodilatation. Theobromine, a metabolic product of caffeine and theophylline, causes vasodilatation and increases urine volume. But methylxanthines are weak bronchodilators with mild diuretic effect, and are infrequently used in the treatment for acute bronchospasm.

Corticosteroid

As discussed above, systemic corticosteroids improve lung function and reduce the need of mechanical ventilation, but because the concern of long term adverse neurological outcome, now this treatment is reserved for infants with severe BPD who cannot be weaned from ventilator support. Dexamethsone with lower dose and shorter duration are usually used to facilitate extubation. A recent pilot study by Yeh et al , has shown that intratracheal instillation of budesonide by using surfactant as vehicle can effectively deliver budesonide to the lung and suppress the lung inflammation and improves pulmonary outcome without significant short term and long term side effects. More studies are needed before it can be recommended.

Nutrition and fluid supply

Adequate nutrition is difficult to achieve in infants with BPD because of high caloric demand, poor tolerance of enteral feeding and restriction of fluid intake. Impaired growth is common in these infants. Malnutrion can delay somatic growth and the development of new alveoli, making successful weaning from ventilator less likely. Infants with poor nutrition are also susceptible to infection. Also, there are special nutrients and vitamins that are frequently deficient in these infants and their lack may increase the risk of lung injury.

Many infants with BPD experience increased energy needs. The reasons for this are not entirely clear; increased work of breathing, catecholamine release due to stress, increased energy requirements for feeding, and the effects of medications probably all play a role. It is not unusual for infants with BPD to require 130 or even 160 Kcal/kg/day to support adequate growth. It may be difficult to provide adequate calories for these infants. They may have ongoing fluid restrictions due to concerns about pulmonary edema. They may experience fatigue with feeding or delayed gastric emptying. Increasing the caloric density of formula or breast milk with a balanced proportion of carbohydrate and fat may be helpful. A high carbohydrate load increases production of CO_2 which may be a concern in infants with respiratory compromise. Excess carbohydrate may also lead to osmotic diarrhea. Excess dietary fat may delay gastric emptying and exacerbate gastroesopageal reflux.

Diuretics

Infants with chronic lung disease tend to retain interstitial fluid which results in increased respiratory distress, increase in oxygen requirement, increase in ventilator settings, hypoxemia and hypercarbia. Diuretics mobilize fluid, improve lung compliance and decrease resistance.

Furosemide

Furosemide is the most commonly used diuretic. It is a potent and rapid acting loop diuretic. It can be used orally and intravenously. The main benefit of the intravenous route is a quick response.

Mechanism of Action: At the ascending loop of Henle, furosemide inhibits active reabsorption of chloride resulting in lower sodium and water reabsorption. It also acts against antidiuretic hormones, and increases urine aldosterone excretion. Furosemide decreases left ventricular filling pressure by increasing venous capacitance. Furosemide helps in chronic lung disease by both diuretic and vasculature effects.

Adverse effects: Main adverse effects of chronic furosemide therapy are hypercalciuria, nephrocalcinosis and hypochloremia. Electrolytes should be monitored carefully. Ototoxicity is related to plasma concentration and is usually reversible after cessation of therapy. Other side effects include: osteopenia, cholelithiasis, displacement of bilirubin and hyperparathyroidism.

According to Cochrane review in preterm infants < 3 weeks of age with BPD, intravenous furosemide administration has either inconsistent effects or no detectable effect. In infants less than 3 weeks of age with BPD, a single intravenous dose of 1 mg/kg of furosemide transiently improves pulmonary mechanics. Chronic enteral or intravenous furosemide administration improves both oxygenation and pulmonary mechanics. The Cochrane review concluded that there is little evidence to support any benefit of fu- rosemide administration with respect to ven- tilatory support, length of hospital stay, survival or long-term outcome. Accordingly, routine or sustained uses of systemic loop diuretics in infants with BPD cannot be recommended.

Inhaled furosemide has been shown to transiently improve pulmonary function. No long-term outcomes have been studied. More trials are needed before this delivery method can be recommended for routine use.

Thiazide Diuretics

Thiazides work by inhibiting sodium reabsorption in the distal tubule. In contrast to furosemide, thiazides decrease calcium excretion.

Potassium Sparing Diuretic

Spironolactone is a competitive antagonist of aldosterone. It is a weak diuretic and is usually given in combination with thiazides. There are very few randomized control trials. By Cochrane reviewer's opinion, in infants less than 3 weeks of age with BPD, chronic administration of thiazide and spironolactone improves lung compliance at four weeks of treatment and reduces need for furosemide. Only one study showed long-term benefits such as decreased rates of death and artificial ventilation.

Diuretics				
Drug	Site of Action	Route	Onset	Dose
Furosemide	Loop diuretic	IV PO	15-30 min 30-60 min	1 mg/kg/dose 1-3 mg/kg/dose
Hydrochlorothiazide	Distal tubule	PO	1-2 hrs	2-4 mg/kg/day
Spironolactone	Aldosterone antagonist	PO	3-5 days	1.5-3 mg/kg/day

Table 3.

Inhaled Nitric Oxide (INO)

INO decreases pulmonary vascular resistance and improves oxygenation. It is pro- posed that INO will improve oxygenation, improve ventilation and will decrease respiratory support. Side effects include methemoglobinemia and direct pulmonary injury if excessive INO is used

Studies on INO were done with different doses, started at different ages, different durations of treatment, and in infants whose characteristics were different among the studies. INO was approved by FDA to term and near-term infants. AAP Committee on Fetus and Newborn recommended that centers that provide INO therapy should provide comprehensive long-term medical and neurodevelopment follow-up and should establish prospective data collection for treatment time, course, toxic effects, treatment failure, use of alternative therapies, and outcomes.

A systematic review which included 11 studies failed to show a significant benefit of INO on BPD. Cochrane database for systematic review by Keith J Barrington in 2006 concluded: INO as rescue therapy for the very ill ventilated preterm infant does not appear to be effective, and may increase the risk of severe IVH. Later use of INO to prevent BPD also does not appear to be effective. Early routine use of INO in mildly sick preterm infants may decrease serious brain injury, and may improve survival without BPD. Further studies are needed.

Antioxidants

Free radical and oxidant stress cause dam- age to DNA, cell membrane, protein and lipids. Free radicals are produced by many mechanisms such as mitochondrial electron transport chain, prostaglandin metabolism, ischemia-reperfusion, hypoxia, neutrophil and macrophage activations, and endothelial cell hypoxanthine-xanthine oxidation. There is a balance between free radical production and clearing by the antioxidant system. The antioxidant defense system includes enzymatic components such as Co-Zn superoxide dismutase (SOD) glutathione peroxidase, and a non-enzymatic components such as glutathione, selenium, zinc, vitamin E and vitamin C. Preterm infants have an immature antioxidant defense system, and are highly exposed to oxidant stress, therefore prone to get tissue damage. Many antioxidant agents have been tried to treat or prevent BPD in new-born. These include:

Vitamin E: Tocopherol is a fat-soluble, anti- oxidant and it decreases reactive oxygen species The American Academy of Pediatrics Committee on Nutrition has recommended daily supplementation of 5-25 IU of vitamin E in preterm infants. Supplementing very low birth weight infants with vitamin E as an anti- oxidant agent has been proposed for pre- venting or limiting retinopathy of prematurity, intracranial hemorrhage, and chronic lung disease. In clinical trials, vitamin E supplementation did not affect the incidence of BPD. Vitamin E supplementation significantly increased the risk for necrotizing enterocolitis and sepsis.

Superoxide dismutase: Intra-tracheal ad- ministration of CuZn SOD in preterm infants did not reduce BPD. It decreased the need for asthma medications, emergency department visits and hospitalizations during the one year follow-up.Rosenfeld et al showed that radiologic evidence, clinical signs of BPD and days of CPAP were less in patients treated with SOD, and no side effects were observed. Cochrane database concluded that there is insufficient evidence that super- oxide dismutase is efficient in preventing chronic lung disease of prematurity, but it is well-tolerated, and has no serious adverse effects.

N acetyl cysteine (NAC): NAC is a precursor of cysteine, which is essential in Glutathione synthesis. Glutathione is a non- enzymatic antioxidant. NAC treatment in preterm infants did not prevent BPD or death, and did not improve lung function at discharge from the hospital .

Allopurinol: Allopurinol is inhibitor of xanthine oxidase, an enzyme which generates superoxide radicals. It did not decrease BPD in preterm infants of 24-32 weeks' gestation.

Metaltonin: Metaltonin is a hormone that is found in all biological organisms, and is a potent free radical scavenger. Melatonin treatment reduced the proinflammatory cytokines (IL-6, IL-8 and tumor necrosis factor (TNF)-alpha), and improved the clinical out- come in mechanically ventilated newborns with respiratory distress.

Vitamin A: Vitamin A is very important for the health of epithelial tissues. It reduces ciliary loss, and is associated with increased alveoli. In animals studies, vitamin A deficiency has been associated with necrotizing tracheobronchiolitis and squamous metaplasia the changes akin to BPD. Very low birth weight infants are known to have low vitamin levels.

There have been several studies looking at vitamin A in the prevention of BPD. The largest study by Tyson et al showed significant decrease (from 62% to 55%) in combined outcome of death or chronic lung disease.

Meta-analysis also revealed similar results.

A follow-up study did not show any untoward outcome at 18 to 22 months of age. Many units routinely use vitamin A for prevention of BPD. Five thousand IU of Vitamin A has to be given by tri-weekly intramuscular injections for four weeks. In one study it was given by oral route but was not effective in preventing BPD. Intravenous emulsion preparation needs to be studied by randomized control trials.

Cimetidine: In animal studies, lung injury as result of induction of cytochrome P450 by oxygen exposure may result in the release of free radical oxidants and arachidonic acid metabolites, that can be reduced by cimetidine. In study by Cotton et al of infants weighing less than 1250 grams who were mechanically ventilated and required oxygen, Cimetidine had no significant effect on the severity of respira tory insufficiency at 10 day postnatal age, and did not affect the tracheal aspirate levels of inflammatory markers or arachidonic acid metabolites.

Azithromycin: A macrolid antibiotic, azithromycin, acts act as a free radical scavenger, inhibits cytokines, and inhibits neutrophil chemotaxis. In a study by Bal- lard HO et al on extremely premature infants requiring mechanical ventilation, azithromycin did not affect mortality, incidence of BPD and days on ventilator.

Alpha-1 protease inhibitor (A1PI): Matrix Metalloproteinase is a member of a family of extracellular enzymes that are essential in proteolysis activity against extra cellular matrix proteins such as collagen, elastic lamina and fibronectin. These enzymes are produced by variety of cells such as fibro- blasts, osteoblasts, macrophages, monocytes and neutrophils. These enzymes are essential in growth, tissue remodeling, angiogenesis and wound healing. If the balance between activation and inhibition of this enzymes is disturbed, many pathological conditions can occur such as bronchopulmonary dysplasia. In a study by Stiskal JA et al, the incidence of CLD in survivors was lower in infants treated with intravenous A1PI as compared with a placebo group, but the difference was not statistically significant. The incidence of pulmonary hemorrhage was lower in the treated group.

Thyroxine, did not reduce the incidence of BPD. Estradiol and progesterone hormonal replacements were studied in 83 infants, but did not show decrease in incidence of BPD.

9. Conclusion

BPD is disease of multi-etiology. A large number of extremely preterm infants who survive are developing BPD, but the severity of the lung damage is considerably less than that observed in the classic form of BPD. Because most of these infants have only mild initial respiratory distress and, therefore, do not receive aggressive ventilation, other factors must be involved in the pathogenesis of this new, milder type of BPD. Clinical and epidemiological data strongly suggest that infections, either prenatal or postnatal, and the presence of PDA are major factors in the development of BPD. For this reason, efforts to prevent BPD in extremely low-birth weight infants should include an aggressive approach in the prevention and effective treatment of infections and PDA. BPD has long term adverse pulmonary and neurodevelopment outcome. Steroids usage for treatment of BPD also has been shown to have adverse neurodevelopment. Available data are sometime conflicting and inconclusive; clinicians must use their own clinical judgment to balance the adverse effects of BP D with the potential adverse effects of steroids for each individual patient.. Very low birth weight infants who remain on mechanical ventilation after 1 to 2 weeks of age are at very high risk of developing BPD . When considering corticosteroid therapy for such an infant, clinicians might conclude that the risks of a short course of glucocorticoid therapy is warranted . This individualized decision should be made in conjunction with the infant's parents. Other treatment and management are largely been supportive and most of them have no long term benefits. A recent pilot study from Yeh et al indicated that intratracheal instillation of budesonide using surfactant as vehicle can effectively deliver budesonide into the lungs and can significantly suppress lung inflammation, improve pulmonary outcome and without immediate and long term adverse effect.. More studies are needed to prove this. Until that time, proper respiratory care and avoidance of NICU infection are the most important steps leading to lower incidence of BPD.

10. Acknowledgements

Supports in Part from National Health Research Institute (NHRI-EX-100-9818PI) Taiwan

11. References

Aaltonen R., Vahlberg T., Lehtonen L., Alanen A. Ureaplasma urealyticum: no independent role in the pathogenesis of bronchopulmonary dysplasia. *Acta Obstet Gynecol Scand* 2006;85(11):1354–1359.

Abele-Horn M., Genzel-Boroviczeny O., Uhlig T., Zimmermann A., Peters J., Scholz M. Ureaplasma urealyticum colonization and bronchopulmonary dysplasia: a comparative prospective multicentre study. *Eur J Pediatr* 1998;157(12):1004–1011.

ACOG Committee opinion committee on obstetric practice antenatal corticosteroid therapy for Fetal Maturation. October 1998 Number 210.

American Academy of Pediatrics, Committee on Fetus and Newborn. Postnatal corticosteroids totreat or prevent chronic lung disease in preterm infants. *Pediatrics* 2002;109(2):330 –338

Baraldi E, Filippone M, Chronic lung disease after premature birth. *N Engl J Med* 2007; 357:1946-55

Baud O, Foix-L'Helias L, Kaminski M et al, Audibert F, Jarreau PH, Papiernik E, Huon C, Lepercq J, Dehan M, Lacaze-Masmonteil T. Antenatal glucocorticoid treatment and cystic periventricular leukomalacia in very premature infants. *N Engl J Med* 1999; 341(16):1190-6.

Bhandari V, Gruen J R. The Genomics of Bronchopulmonary Dysplasia. *NeoReviews* Aug 2007; 8: e336 - e344.

Capers CC, Ward ES, Murphy JEetal. Use of theophylline in neonate as an aid to ventilator weaning. *Ther Drug Monit* 1992; 14 (6):471-4.

Carlo WA, Stark AR, Wright LL, et al. Minimal ventilation to prevent bronchopulmonary dysplasia in extremely-low-birth-weight infants. *J Pediatr* 2002 Sep;141(3):370-4.

Clark RH, Gerstmann DR, Jobe AH, et al. Lung injury in neonates: causes, strategies for prevention and long-term consequences. *J Pediatr* 2001;139:478-86

Coalson JJ : Pathology of Bronchopulmonary Dysplasia. *Semin Perinatol* 30:179-184

Coalson JJ, Winter V, deLemos RA. Decreased alveolarization in baboon survivors with bronchopulmonary dysplasia. *Am J Respir Crit Care Med* 1995;152:640–646

Davis JM, Bhutani VK, Stefano JL, Fox WW et al. Changes in pulmonary mechanics following caffeine administration in infants with bronchopulmonary dysplasia. *Pediatr Pumlonol* 1989;6 (1) 49-52.

Denjean A, Paris-Llado J, Zupan V, et al: Inhaled salbutamol and beclomethasone for preventing broncho-pulmonary dysplasia: a randomized double-blind study. *Eur J Pediatr* 157:926-931, 1998

Engle WA, and the Committee on Fetus and Newborn the American Academy of Pediatrics. Surfactant-Replacement Therapy for Respiratory Distress in the Preterm and Term Neonate. *Pediatr* 2008;121(2):419-432

Fanaroff AA, Stoll BJ, Wright LL, Carlo WA, Ehrenkranz RA, Stark AR, et al. Trends in neonatal morbidity and mortality for very low birth weight infants. *Am J Obstet Gynecol* 2007;196:147.e1-8.

Garland JS, Buck RK, Allred EN, Leviton A. Hypocarbia before surfactant therapy appears to increase bronchopulmonary dysplasia risk in infants with respiratory distress syndrome. *Arch Pediatr Adolesc Med* 1995;149:617-22.

Gonzalez A, Sosenko IRS, Chandar J, et al. Influence of infection on patent ductus arteriosus and chronic lung disease in premature infants weighting 1000 grams or less. *J Pediatr* 1996;128:470–478

Gronec P, Reuss D, Gotze-Speer B. Speer C.P.The effects of dexamethasone on chemotactic activity and inflammatory mediators intracheobroncheal aspirates of preterm infants at risk for chronic lung disease. *J Pedistr* 1993; 122:938-944

Groneck P, Speer CP. Inflammatory mediators and BPD. *Arch Dis Child Fetal Neonatal Ed* 1995; 73:F1-3

Hansen T., Corbet A. Chronic lung disease- Bronchopulmonary dysplasia. In Taeusch, Ballard and Avery (ed) Schaffer & Avery's Diseases of The Newborn. 6th ed. Saunders, 1991, p519

Hislop AA, Wigglesworth JS, Desai R, Aber V. The effects of preterm delivery and mechanical ventilation on human lung growth. *Early Hum Dev* 1987;15:147– 64

Hussain NA, Siddiqui NH, Stocker JR. Pathology of arrested acinar development in postsurfactant bronchopulmonary dysplasia. *Hum Pathol* 1998;29:710–717.

Jobe A, Ikegami M. Mechanisms initiating lung injury in the preterm. *Early Hum Dev* 1998;53:81–94

Jobe A. Bancalarie E. Bronchopulmonary dysplasia. *Am J Respir Crit Care Med* 2001; 163: 1723-1729.

Khilfeh M, Agrawal V, Yeh TF. Pharmacological treatment and prevention of chronic lung disease in preterm infants,*www.neonatologytoday.net/newsletters/nt-apr10.pdf*

Kraybill EN, Runyan DK, Bose CL, Khan JH. Risk factors for chronic lung disease in infants with birth weight of 751 to 1000 grams. *J Pediatr.* 1989;115:115-20.

Kuo HT, Lin HC, Tsai CH, Chouc IC, Yeh TF. A follow-up study of preterm infants given budesonide using surfactant as a vehicle to prevent chronic lung disease in preterm infants. J Pediatr. 2010 Apr;156(4):537-41. Epub 2010 Feb 6.

Lee B.H., Stoll BJ, McDonald SA, Higgins RD, Adverse Neonatal Outcomes Associated With Antenatal Dexamethasone Versus Antenatal Betamethasone . *Pediatrics* 2006;117;1503-1510

Liggins GC, Howie RN. A controlled trial of antepartum glucocorticoid treatment for prevention of the respiratory distress syndrome in premature infants. *Pediatrics* 1972;50:515-525

NIH Consensus Statement Effect of Corticosteroids for Fetal Maturation on Perinatal Outcomes 1994 Feb 28-Mar 2;12(2):1-24

Northway WH Jr, Rosan RC, Porter DY. Pulmonary disease following respirator therapy of hyaline membrane disease: Bronchopulmonary dysplasia. *N Engl J Med* 1967;276:357

Parker RA, Lindstrom DP, Cotton RB. Evidence from twin study implies possible genetic susceptibility to bronchopulmonary dysplasia. *Semin Perinatol* 1996;20 :206 –209

Parker RA, Lindstrom DP, Cotton RB. Improved survival accounts for aost, but not all, of the increase in bronchopulmonary dysplasia. *Pediatrics* 1992;90:663-668

RCOG Green-top Guideline No. 7. October, 2010 Antenatal Corticosteroids to Reduce Neonatal Morbidity and Mortality.

Rhen T,Cidlowski J. Antiinflammatory action of glucocorticoids-new mechanisms for old drugs. *N Engl J Med* 2005;353:1711-23

Schelonka R.L., Katz B., Waites K.B., Benjamin D.K. Critical appraisal of the role of Ureaplasma in the development of bronchopulmonary dysplasia with metaanalytic techniques. *Pediatr Infect Dis J* 2005;24(12):1033–1039

Schmidt B, Roberts RS, Davis P et al. Caffeine therapy for apnea of prematurity. *N Engl J Med* 2006; 354

Schmit B, Roberts RS, Davis Pet al. Long-Term effects of Caffeine therapy for apnea of prematurity. *N Engl j Med* 2007 357 (19) 1893-902

Shinwell E, Lerner-Geva, Lusky A, Reichman B. Less postnatal steroids, more bronchopulmonary dysplasia: a population-based study in very low birthweight infants. *Arch Dis Child Fetal Neonatal Ed.* 2007;92(1):F30-F33

Speer CP. Inflammation and bronchopulmonary dysplasia: a continuous story. *Semin Fetal Neonat Med* 2006; 11(5):354-362

Speer CP. New insights into the pathogenesis of pulmonary inflammation in preterm infants. *Biol Neonate* 2001;79:205–209

Stark AR, Carlo WA, Tyson JE, et al. Adverse effects of early dexamethasone in extremely-low-birth-weight infants: National Institute of Child Health and Human Development Neonatal Research Network. *N Engl J Med* 2001;344:95-101

SUPPORT Study Group of the Eunice Kennedy Shriver NICHD Neonatal Research Network. Early CPAP versus surfactant in extremely preterm infants. *N Engl J Med* 2010;362:1970-9.

SUPPORT Study Group of the Eunice Kennedy Shriver NICHD Neonatal Research Network. Target ranges of oxygen saturation in extremely preterm infants. *N Engl J Med* 2010;362:1959-69.

Tyson JE, Wright LL, Oh W, et al. Vitamin A supplementation for extremely-low-birth-weight infants. National Institute of Child Health and Human Development Neonatal Research Network. *N Engl J Med* 1999; 340:1962.

Van Marter LJ, Dammann O, Allred EN, et al. Chorioamnionitis, mechanical ventilation and postnatal sepsis as modulators of chronic lung disease in preterm infants. *J Pediatr* 2002;140:171-176

Van Marter LJ, et al. Hydration during the first days of life and the risk of bronchopulmonary dysplasia inlow birth weight infants. *J Pediatr* 1990;116:942

van Waarde W.M., Brus F., Okken A., Kimpen J.L. Ureaplasma urealyticum colonization, prematurity and bronchopulmonary dysplasia. *Eur Respir J* 1997;10(4):886-890

Varsila E, Hallman M, Venge P, et al. Closure of patent dutus arteriosus dereases pulmonary myeloperoxidase in premature infants with respiratory distress syndrome. and the risk of bronchopulmonary dysplasia in low birth premature infants with respiratory distress syndrome. *Biol Noonate* 1995;67:167-171 (20): 2112-21.

Watterberg K, Scott SM. Evidence of Early Adrenal Insufficiency in Babies Who Develop Bronchopulmonary Dysplasia. *Pediatrics* 1995; 95: 120-125

Watterberg KL, Demers LM, Scott SM, Murphy S. Chorioamnionitis and early lung inflammation in infants in whom bronchopulmonary dysplasia develops. *Pediatrics* 1996; 97: 210-215.

Watterberg KL, Gerdes JS, Gifford KL, Lin HM. Prophylaxis against early adrenal insufficiency to prevent chronic lung disease in premature infants. *Pediatrics* 1999;104 :1258 -1263.

Wu SY, Joseph T, Medha Kamat , Suma Pyaty Tsu-Fuh Yeh TF. Postnatal corticosteroid to prevent or treat chronic lung disease in preterm infants. *www.neonatologytoday.net/newsletters/nt-nov09.pdf*

Yeh TF, J. Lin YJ, HuangC C, Chen,Y J, Lin CH, Hong C. Lin HC, Hsieh WS, Lien YJ. Early Dexamethasone Therapy in Preterm Infants: A Follow-up Study. *Pediatrics* May 1998; 101: e7

Yeh TF, Lin YJ, Hsieh WS, Lin HC, Lin CH, Chen JY, Kao HA, Chien CH. Early postnatal dexamethasone therapy for the prevention of chronic lung disease in preterm Infants with respiratory distress syndrome: A multi-centers clinical trial. *Pediatrics* 1997; 100: e3

Yeh TF, Lin YJ, Lin HC, et al. Outcomes at school age after postnatal dexamethasone therapy for lung disease of prematurity. *N Engl J Med* 2004;350: 1304-13

Yeh TF, Torre JA, Rastogi A, Anyebuno MA, Pildes RS Early postnatal dexamethasone therapy in premature infants with severe respiratory distress syndrome: a double-blind, controlled study. *J Pediatr* 1990; 117:273-282

Yoder B, Harrison M, Clark R. Time-Related changes in steriod use and bronchopulmonary
    dysplasia in preterm infants. *Pediatrics* 2009;124: 673-679

Yeh TF, Lin H C, Chang C H., Wu T S, Su B H, Tsai C L, Pyati S, Tsai C H. Early
    Intratracheal Instillation of Budesonide Using Surfactant as a Vehicle to Prevent
    Chronic Lung Disease in Preterm Infants: A Pilot Study. Pediatrics 121 (5) e1-e9,
    May, 2008.

9

Bronchopulmonary Dysplasia: The Role of Oxidative Stress

Jean-Claude Lavoie and Ibrahim Mohamed
Université de Montréal
Canada

1. Introduction

One of the critical and chronic complications of preterm birth is bronchopulmonary dysplasia (BPD). The incidence of BPD is high, ranging from 40% to 70% of infants born before 28 completed weeks' gestation (Stoll et al., 2010). The disease is characterized by impaired alveolar and vascular maturation, with long-term consequences on a number of systems including neurodevelopment. Risk factors for BPD include gestational age at birth, sex, inflammation and/or infection, oxygen supplementation, mechanical ventilation, and parenteral nutrition. Although the etiology of BPD is not well understood, risk factors are all associated with oxidative stress. A modulation of the redox environment is believed to play a major role in the pathogenesis of BPD.

This chapter will start by describing BPD, and then focus on the molecules involved in oxidative stress, the aim being that a better understanding favours more effective clinical intervention. Each of the risk factors in turn will be discussed according to the implied redox modifications occurring during BPD development.

2. Description of BPD

2.1 Historical perspective

Prior to the era of mechanical ventilation, few infants of very low birth weight (less than 1500 g) survived, and neonatal mortality for extremely low birth weight infants (less than 1000 g) exceeded 90% (Behrman et al., 1971). Most survivors required little or no oxygen supplementation initially but later deteriorated to requirements of up to 40% in order to prevent cyanosis. On radiography, findings included microcystic changes as well as varying degrees of hyperinflation and flattening of the diaphragm. Some infants recovered spontaneously over weeks to months but others died, with postmortem examination revealing hyperaeration and reduced alveolar septa. Wilson and Mikity in 1960 were the first to describe this chronic pulmonary syndrome, in a case report of five very small preterm survivors (Wilson & Mikity, 1960). At that time, assisted ventilation was not used in preterm infants. An additional 29 babies with Wilson–Mikity syndrome (WMS) were identified at the same medical institution in 1969 (Hodgman et al., 1969), and many other cases worldwide.

After the introduction of mechanical ventilation to manage respiratory distress syndrome in the mid-1960s, reports began to appear of radiographic and pathological abnormalities that seemed to result from exposure to high concentrations of oxygen and mechanical ventilation. In 1967, Northway et al. coined the term "bronchopulmonary dysplasia" to describe findings of pulmonary complications following respiratory therapy for hyaline membrane disease (Northway et al., 1967). Northway et al. believed the critical factor to be exposure to an inspired oxygen concentration > 80% for longer than 150 hours.

The 1990s saw major changes in both obstetric and neonatal care for preterm labour, with surfactant administration and assisted ventilation. The outcome of most preterm infants improved in the first half of the decade, particularly for infants with very low birth weight, who benefitted from decreased mortality and morbidity (Horbar et al., 2002). Following these changes, classical BPD, which occurred as a result of injury to the immature lung, became less common. Chronic lung disease in preterm infants became increasingly attributable to the response of the immature lung to early air breathing rather than to damage from barotrauma or oxygen toxicity. In 1999, Jobe described the "new" BPD as occurring in immature infants who did not have extensive lung disease soon after birth (Jobe, 1999). Jobe attributed the "new" BPD to pulmonary anomalies resulting from an inhibition of alveolar and vascular development (Jobe, 1999).

2.2 Clinical definitions
With the change in clinical presentation over time, a variety of definitions of BPD have been used in the literature.

i.   **Original criteria for BPD**: A U.S. National Institutes of Health (NIH) workshop held in 1979 proposed to define BPD as a "continued oxygen dependency during the first 28 days plus compatible clinical and radiographic changes" (Natl Inst Health Consens Dev Conf Summ, 1979).

ii. **Traditional definition**: Instead of the original definition, Shennan et al. (1988) suggested a more accurate predictor of BPD to be, "the requirement for additional oxygen at a corrected postnatal gestational age of 36 weeks in infants born with a birth weight of less than 1,500 g". This definition appears to also predict pulmonary outcome among infants with the "new" BPD (Davis et al., 2002).

iii. **Severity definition**: Participants at a joint U.S. National Institute of Child Health & Human Development (NICHD)-National Heart, Lung, and Blood Institute (NHLBI) workshop defined mild, moderate and severe BPD according to both 28 days' and 36 weeks' criteria (Jobe & Bancalari, 2001). Mild BPD was defined as the need for supplemental oxygen at 28 days after birth but not at 36 weeks' postmenstrual age (PMA); moderate BPD, the need for supplemental oxygen at 28 days and at a fraction of inspired oxygen (FiO_2) < 0.30 at 36 weeks' PMA; and severe BPD, the need for supplemental oxygen at 28 days and, at 36 weeks' PMA, the need for mechanical ventilation and/or FiO_2 > 0.30. In a validation study, the NICHD–NHLBI workshop definitions accurately predicted pulmonary outcomes including percent of patients needing treatment with pulmonary medications and rehospitalization for pulmonary causes (Ehrenkranz et al., 2005).

iv. **Physiological definition**: An inherent limitation of all previous definitions is that the need for oxygen is determined by individual physicians rather than on the basis of a physiologic assessment. The assumption that the criteria on which the decision to administer oxygen is uniform and applied similarly across institutions is erroneous because there is no consensus in the literature, neonatologists have widely divergent practices regarding oxygen-saturation targets. Indeed, published literature cites acceptable saturation ranges from 84% to 98% (Garg et al., 1988; Moyer-Mileur et al., 1996; Sekar & Duke, 1991; Walsh, 2003; Zanardo et al., 1995). Accordingly, the physiological definition determined BPD at 36 weeks of correct age as follows: 1) In all infants treated with mechanical ventilation, continuous positive airway pressure, or supplemental oxygen at $FiO_2 > 0.30$, without additional testing; 2) If the $FiO_2 < 0.30$, infants are to be gradually weaned to room air, in a timed stepwise fashion; those who cannot maintain an $SaO_2 \geq 88\%$ are diagnosed with BPD, unless they pass a timed, continuously monitored oxygen reduction test. An oxygen saturation 80% to 87% for 5 minutes, or < 80% for 1 minute, indicates BPD. If all SaO_2 measurements over 15 minutes $\geq 96\%$, or if instead, all SaO_2 measurements in a 60-minute period > 88%, the infant is deemed not to have BPD (Walsh et al., 2003).

To evaluate the impact of the physiological definition on BPD rates, 1598 consecutively born preterm infants (birth weight 501–1249 g) in hospital at 36 weeks' PMA were prospectively assessed and assigned an outcome using both the clinical and physiological definitions of BPD. The NICHD neonatal network centers demonstrated that many babies who, according to the nursing staff, required oxygen were able to maintain an $SaO_2 > 90\%$ on room air. Though 560 (35%) had clinical BPD (oxygen use at 36 weeks), only 398 (25%) had physiological BPD (as defined above) (Walsh et al., 2004).

2.3 Structural lung changes

As described by Northway et al. (1967), the histological features of classical BPD included prominent interstitial fibrosis, alveolar overdistention alternating with regions of atelectasis, and airway abnormalities such as squamous metaplasia and excessive muscularization. On the other hand, the "new" BPD shows histological features consistent with developmental arrest and impaired alveolar development (Husain et al., 1998): alveoli are fewer in number and larger in diameter than normal; the fibrosis, squamous metaplasia and excessive airway muscularization seen in classical BPD are conspicuously absent; airway and microvascular growth are affected. A short comparative study by Bhatt et al. (2001) found decreased levels of vascular endothelial growth factor (VEGF) and angiogenic receptors Flt-1 and Tie-2 in infants who died from BPD vs. from other causes. The authors concluded that the lungs from infants with BPD showed abnormal development of alveolar microvessels (abnormal placement in the alveolar septa) and that the capillaries were frequently dilated, changes attributable to low VEGF and associated receptors (Bhatt et al., 2000, 2001). Controls were five children born at term who died at a mean of 3.4 ± 1.3 days, whereas the five BPD subjects were born at 27 ± 2 weeks' gestation, received $FiO_2 > 0.5$ during 37 ± 33 days, and died at 65 ± 34 days.

2.4 Epidemiology

BPD remains the most prevalent and one of the most serious long-term sequelae of preterm birth (Fanaroff et al., 2007). There is considerable variation in reported rates, however, depending upon the centre. Among 4213 infants born in 2003 at 24–31 weeks' gestation in 10 different European regions, the rate of BPD (oxygen requirement at 36 weeks' PMA) was anywhere from 10.5% to 21.5% (Zeitlin et al., 2008).

A 2010 NICHD Neonatal Research Network report on neonatal outcomes of extremely preterm infants assessed 9575 infants born at extremely low gestational ages (22–28 weeks) and very low birth weights (401–1500 g) at network centers between January 1, 2003 and December 31, 2007. Including babies with mild BPD (oxygen therapy for 28 days but use of room air at 36 weeks), the incidence of BPD as determined by the severity-based definition was 68%; traditional definition, 42%; physiologic definition, 40% (Stoll et al., 2010).

2.5 Demographic factors

Factors linked to BPD include: 1) low gestational age at birth (Kraybill et al., 1989; Darlow & Horwood, 1992; Antonucci et al., 2004; Ambalavanan & Novak, 2003), 2) low birth weight (Darlow & Horwood, 1992; Hakulinenet al., 1988; Avery et al., 1987; Ambalavanan et al., 2008), 3) growth restriction (small for gestational age) (Durrmeyer X et al., 2011; Lal Mk et al., 2003; Zeitlin J et al., 2010), 4) male sex (Kraybill et al., 1989; Darlow & Horwood, 1992; Ambalavanan & Novak, 2003; Avery et al., 1987), and 5) white race (Avery et al., 1987; Palta et al., 1991). In a recent cohort, BPD affected 85% of infants born at 22 weeks' gestation vs. 23% of those born at 28 weeks' (Stoll et al., 2010). Furthermore, of the infants affected by BPD in a large American study which included over 9.5 million very low birth weight infants between 1993 and 2006, 59.3% were male while 40.7% were female (male : female ratio = 1.46 : 1) (Stroustrup & Trasande, 2010).

2.6 Impact of perinatal lung injury later in life

Preterm infants with BPD commonly develop impaired health, neurodevelopment, and quality of life later on in childhood. Often noted are: 1) increased risk of postneonatal mortality (Van Marter, 2009), 2) higher rates of rehospitalization (Jeng et al., 2008), 3) long-term pulmonary impairments (Broström et al., 2010) such as asthma (Baraldi et al., 2009) and emphysema (Wong et al., 2008), 4) failure to thrive (Theile et al., 2011), and 5) cognitive impairment (Anderson & Doyle, 2006), cerebral palsy (Koo KY et al 2010; Majnemer et al., 2000), and global neurodevelopmental deficits (Short EJ et al, 2003).

3. The preterm lung: Set-up for injury

Human lung development proceeds in five regulated stages: embryonic (3–7 weeks' gestation), pseudoglandular (7–17 weeks'), canalicular (17–27 weeks'), saccular (28–36 weeks') and alveolar and microvascular maturation (36 weeks' gestation to at least 2 years after birth). The lungs of preterm infants born at 24–28 weeks' gestation are in the late canalicular or early saccular stages and therefore cannot support efficient gas exchange. Branching and expansion of air spaces to form saccules and thinning of mesenchyme occur later in gestation, as do the formation of alveoli and the synthesis of surfactant by type II alveolar cells which only commence in late gestation. Any injury to the lung at the early stages of development can potentially alter the developmental process, leading to long-term pulmonary sequelae (Chakraborty et al., 2010).

Whereas fetal development is predicated on a hypoxic environment, at birth the oxidative load is sharply increased. At the same time, oxygen demands increase abruptly. The baby born at term easily adapts to this transition in most cases but for the preterm infant, the intra- to extra-uterine transition is not without risks. Among the reasons why the preterm infant is more likely to experience oxidative injury than more mature newborns and older children are the following: 1) intracellular defences against oxidative stress are still poorly developed; 2) the preterm infant is often, for various reasons, exposed to high concentrations of supplemental oxygen; and 3) the fetus and premature infant are also susceptible to inflammation and infection that may lead to increased oxidative stress (Saugstad, 2010).

It may therefore be instructive to look at some of the molecules implicated in oxidative stress, while drawing parallels with the corresponding processes in BPD. This added insight will contribute to delimiting specific sources of oxidant molecules that may contribute to the development of BPD, a topic we will explore later in the chapter in relation to BPD risk factors.

4. Oxidative stress

In utero, the arterial pressure of oxygen (PaO_2) is close to 30 mm Hg. After birth, with the baby breathing in ambient air, the PaO_2 rises to 75 mm Hg. This greater oxygen load increases the concentration of dissolved oxygen available for oxidative phosphorylation in the mitochondria, organelles that release 1-3% of oxygen in the form of reactive oxygen species (ROS).

Inspired oxygen (O_2) is a diatomic molecule with two free electrons ($\bullet O\text{-}O\bullet$). This molecule has the highest half-cell reduction potential (E_{hc}) *in vivo* (E_{hc} for the $\frac{1}{2}O_2/H_2O$ couple = 0.816 V). Consequently, dissolved O_2 readily accepts an electron ($\bullet$) from donors such as polyunsaturated fatty acids or ascorbic acid, generating the free radical superoxide anion ($\bullet O\text{-}O\bullet\bullet$ or $O_2\bullet^-$). This transformation of O_2 into $O_2\bullet^-$ is spontaneous, generating the oxidized form of vitamin C (dehydroascorbate, DHA) and/or the by-products of fatty acid oxidation (lipid peroxides, aldehydes such as malondialdehyde or 4-hydroxy-2-nonenal (HNE), or isoprostanes). The reaction may also be catalyzed by nicotinamide adenine dinucleotide phosphate (NADPH) oxidase. Thus, the inspiration of diatomic oxygen leads to an increase in the cellular concentration of free radicals ($O_2\bullet$) as well as free O_2, which will contribute to metabolic regulation by hydroxylation of several biologically active molecules. For instance, O_2 is essential for the degradation of hypoxia-inducible factor-1α (HIF-1α); HIF-1α activates transcription of the gene encoding VEGF, an important growth factor for angiogenesis. This process is impaired in BPD (Husain et al., 1998; Bhatt et al., 2000, 2001). Figure 1 shows a number of oxidative-reduction (redox) reactions of interest.

4.1 Superoxide anion

The dismutation of the superoxide anion ($O_2\bullet^-$) into O_2 and H_2O_2 (2 $\bullet O\text{-}O\bullet\bullet$ + 2H$^+\rightarrow$ $\bullet O\text{-}O\bullet$ + H$\bullet\bullet O\text{-}O\bullet\bullet$H) may be either spontaneous or catalyzed by a superoxide dismutase (SOD). In preterm infants, the pulmonary activity of SOD is suspected to be immature. As reported by Lee Frank in several animal species (mice, hamster, rat, guinea pig), the pulmonary activity of SOD, catalase, and glutathione peroxidase are only 10-15% of that in term babies, in preterm newborns < 32 weeks of human-equivalent gestation (Frank & Sosenko, 1987a, 1987b; Frank, 1991). As a result, the levels of $O_2\bullet^-$ may be higher in preterm than term neonates. Furthermore, the oxidant property of $O_2\bullet^-$ is not related to the attraction of an electron from a common antioxidant such as ascorbate, but to the donation of an electron to a free transition metal such as ferric iron (Fe^{3+}) in a Haber-Weiss reaction ($O_2\bullet^-$ + Fe^{3+} $\rightarrow$ O_2 + Fe^{2+}). The resulting ferrous ion (Fe^{2+}) from this reaction reacts rapidly with hydrogen peroxide (H_2O_2) in a Fenton reaction to generate Fe^{3+}, OH$^-$ and $\bullet$OH. This hydroxyl radical ($\bullet$OH) is among the most reactive of molecules, leading to the oxidation of proteins, lipids and DNAs. Therefore, high oxygen supplementation coupled with low SOD activity add to oxidative stress, and this may be evidenced by an increase in the by-products of lipid peroxidation (lipid peroxides, malondialdehyde, HNE, alkanes such as ethane and pentane, and isoprostanes) and/or of protein oxidation (carbonyl compounds, o-dityrosine). Newborn infants receiving O_2 supplementation have demonstrably elevated levels of markers of oxidative stress such as exhaled ethane and pentane (Nycyk et al., 1998; Pitkanen et al., 1990), serum HNE (Ogihara et al., 1999), F_{2a}-isoprostanes in tracheal aspirate (Cotton et al., 1996) or in plasma (Ahola et al., 2004), protein-carbonyl in bronchoalveolar fluid (Gladstone & Levine et al., 1994) or o-dityrosine in urine (Kelly & Lubec, 1995; Lubec et al., 1997). It has been suggested that some of these markers may be higher in the first few days of life in preterm infants who will develop BPD as compared to those who will not (Gladstone & Levine et al., 1994; Hodgman et al., 1969). Hence, reducing the $O_2^{\bullet-}$ levels in preterm neonates has been a seductive approach to BPD prevention. Indeed, a randomized study of human recombinant SOD administered intratracheally in the first 24 hours to preterm infants at high risk (birth weight 600-1200g) has been associated with a lower incidence of respiratory illnesses such as wheezing, asthma and pulmonary infections (Davis et al., 1993; Davis et al., 2003).

4.2 Hydrogen peroxide
As noted in Figure 1, H_2O_2 is generated following high oxygen supplementation. Chemically, H_2O_2 is a relatively stable molecule that can diffuse passively through cell membranes. Its oxidation reactions occur in two ways, one by accepting an electron from ferrous iron (Fe^{2+}) to generate the free radical hydroxyl ($\bullet OH$), the other by oxidizing sulfhydryl or thiol groups (R-SH) on protein. By its high affinity for thiol, H_2O_2 is considered an important player in the regulation of several metabolic pathways (Winterbourn & Hampton, 2008). Of interest to BPD, H_2O_2 can activate nuclear factor kappa B (NF-kB) (Flohé et al., 1997; Haddad, 2002; Haddad & Land, 2000; Takada et al., 2003), upregulating the transcription of genes encoding pro-inflammatory cytokines (Randell et al., 1990). H_2O_2 also contributes to the stability of HIF-1α (Bonello et al., 2007; Chen Y Shi, 2008; Haddad, 2002; López-Lázaro, 2006; Simon, 2006), a transcription factor involved in angiogenesis. It is therefore important that the intracellular level of H_2O_2 be tightly regulated.

The intracellular concentration of H_2O_2 depends on the balance between production from the dismutation of superoxide anions catalyzed by manganese superoxide dismutase (MnSOD) (Buettner et al., 2006), and detoxification by catalase and/or glutathione peroxidase. Catalase has a high catalytic activity but relative low affinity for H_2O_2 (K_m of 1.1 M) (Jones & Suggett, 1968), whereas glutathione peroxidase has a K_m close to 1 µM (Flohéa & Branda, 1969). With the exception of erythrocytes (Gaetani et al., 1996), catalase is present in peroxisomes and mitochondria. Glutathione peroxidase, however, is present in the cytosol, where it is an efficient regulator of the intracellular level of H_2O_2. Reduction of H_2O_2 by glutathione peroxidase implies a conversion of glutathione (GSH) to its disulfide form (GSSG). The cell exerts tight control over the intracellular concentrations of GSH and GSSG in order to maintain the appropriate redox environment for the various cellular processes to occur efficiently. Indeed, the redox potential is a component of the Gibbs free energy equation that predicts the feasibility of a chemical reaction. Several biochemical pathways are dependent on the intracellular redox potential, including NF-κB activation and HIF-1α levels as discussed earlier (Bonello et al., 2007; Chen & Shi, 2008; Haddad et al., 2000; Haddad & Land, 2000; Land & Wilson, 2005; López-Lázaro, 2006; Roy et al., 2008). In the presence of a large peroxide load or sustained generation of peroxides, the formation of GSSG can exceed the capacity of glutathione reductase to recycle it into GSH, and the redox potential will change to a more oxidized state.

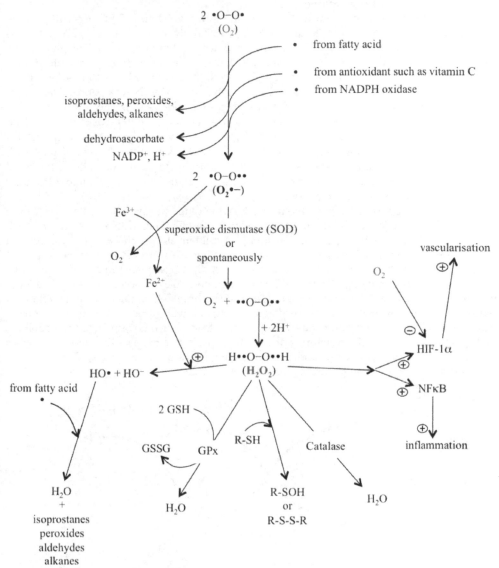

Fig. 1. Relationship between oxidant molecules and endogenous antioxidant defences.

Oxygen (O_2) supplementation as well as hydrogen peroxide (H_2O_2) from parenteral nutrition can lead to modulation of: 1) transcription factors such as hypoxia-inducible factor-1α (HIF-1 α) and nuclear factor kappa B (NF-κB), important players in the pathogenesis of BPD; 2) levels of oxidative stress markers (isoprostanes, peroxides, lipid aldehydes, alkanes); 3) activity of thiol-sensitive proteins (R-SH); and 4) redox potential of glutathione (GSH), as influenced by glutathione peroxidase (GPx) and the intracellular concentrations of reduced (GSH) and oxidized (GSSG) glutathione.

4.3 Redox potential of glutathione

The redox potential is dependent of the concentration of GSH and GSSG according to the Nernst equation: $\Delta E = \Delta E° \cdot (RT/nF) \cdot \log ([GSH]^2/[GSSG])$ (Schafer & Buettner, 2001). In cells extracted from the endotracheal aspirate of intubated newborns, the level of glutathione increases with gestational age and female sex, being lower in preterm and male infants (Lavoie & Chessex, 1997). The sex is a significant risk factor for BPD, as BPD affects more boys than girls (Ambalavanan et al., 2008; Ambalavanan & Novak, 2003; Darlow & Horwood, 1992; Kraybill et al., 1989; Stroustrup & Trasande, 2010). The low glutathione concentration measured in preterm newborns (Lavoie & Chessex, 1997) is associated with an oxidized redox potential. Low blood level of glutathione were also reported in preterm neonates with chronic lung disease (White et al., 1994). Recently, Chessex et al. (2010) demonstrated a correlation between BPD severity in preterm infants (26 ± 1 weeks' gestation) and blood redox potential measured one week after birth: the more oxidized the redox potential, more severe the disease.

As previously reported (Schafer & Buettner, 2001), the redox potential acts as a switch for a number of metabolic pathways, inducing cellular proliferation, differentiation or death (apoptosis) (Figure 2). During organ development, cells must pass through the various cell cycle stages in order to allow for continued remodelling. This process is essential to proper lung development (Bruce et al., 1999; Luyet et al., 2000). Consequently, the redox potential must also cycle continuously (Figure 3). The proliferation phase is accompanied by a higher metabolic rate leading to increased generation of ROS. These ROS in turn favour a shift of the redox potential toward a more oxidized status, inducing the differentiation phase. Alternatively, the oxidized status may 1) induce apoptosis, which favours tissue remodelling, and 2) activate redox-sensitive factors inducing the transcription of genes that encode enzymes involved in glutathione synthesis and GSSG recycling (glutathione reductase). This last event will shift the redox potential toward a more reduced state, beginning a new cell cycle.

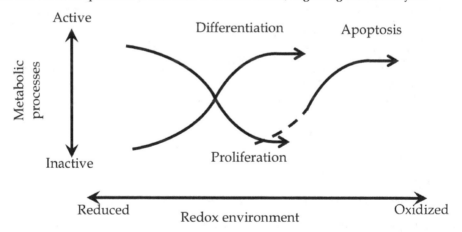

Fig. 2. The redox environment influences metabolic processes.
By modulation from a more reduced to a more oxidized state, the redox environment allows activation and inactivation of various metabolic processes controlling the cell cycle. A reduced state favours cellular proliferation whereas an oxidized state favours differentiation. A more oxidized state will also induce cell death by apoptosis. (Adapted from Schafer FQ et al., 2001)

The link between redox potential and BPD can be explained by an exacerbated apoptosis rate caused by an abnormally elevated redox potential (Luyet et al., 2000). Lung samples from premature baboons with BPD (Das et al., 2004) showed a large number of apoptotic events. In newborn guinea pigs given parenteral nutrition for 4 days, the alveolar count was 20% lower when the nutritive solution was infused without light protection, peroxide concentration being higher in light-exposed solutions (Section 5.2 below) (Lavoie et al., 2004, 2005, 2008). On histology, 30% of alveolar cells were in an apoptotic state (Lavoie et al., 2004). During normal alveolar development, however, about 10% of cells die by apoptosis (Luyet et al., 2000), in order to thin the septa between alveoli for more efficient gas exchange (Bruce et al., 1999; Luyet et al., 2000).

Various factors may contribute to a shift in redox potential to a more oxidized state (Figure 3, dashed line). An induced or sustained oxidized status favours the apoptosis process, leading to a loss of tissue such as observed in BPD (Das et al., 2004; Lavoie et al., 2004, 2005, 2008). In preterm infants, these factors are oxygen supplementation, parenteral nutrition (containing peroxides), and inflammation.

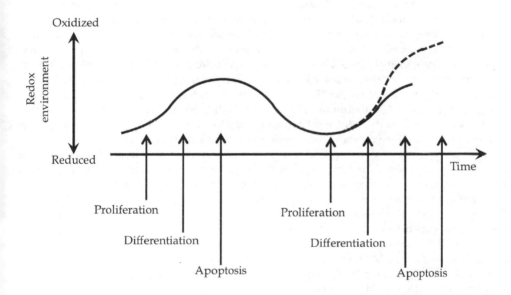

Fig. 3. The redox environment as a function of time.

A normal oscillation of the redox environment occurs over time, between a more reduced and a more oxidized state. As the environmental redox potential changes, pulmonary development is supported by cell proliferation, differentiation, and controlled apoptotic events. An excessively oxidized redox environment, such as that caused by oxidative stress, will favour an apoptotic phase, leading to loss of cells and impaired development.

5. Sources of oxidant molecules in BPD

Oxygen supplementation and parenteral nutrition are exogenous sources of oxidant molecules affecting the preterm neonate. Inflammation, however, is an endogenous source of oxidants and its role is complex. Indeed, inflammation can either be a source or consequence of oxidative stress. In this section, we will analyze each of these sources for their potential role in BPD.

5.1 Oxygen supplementation

Oxygen supplementation increases ROS generation in the lungs. For this reason, and because of the potential effect of oxidative stress on the development of BPD, it has been hypothesized that high O_2 concentration in inspired air is linked to the development of BPD in preterm neonates (Northway et al., 1967). This hypothesis is supported by animal studies. In rats, exposure to 95% O_2 during the first week of life resulted in a 13% reduction in pulmonary alveolar surface area at 40 days (Randell et al., 1990). However, the impact of oxygen has recently been questioned. Although major clinical advances such as the use of surfactant and continuous positive airway pressure (CPAP) have led to a reduction in oxygen supplementation, their impact on lessening the incidence of BPD has been only about 3% per year between 1993 and 2006, for a global reduction of 30% in 13 years (Stroustrup & Trasande, 2010). This relatively weak contribution was confirmed by studies in newborn preterm baboons, where a reduction in the fraction of inspired oxygen (FiO_2) from 80-100% to 21-50% had no significant impact on the levels of fibrosis and alveolar hypoplasia (Coalson et al., 1995, 1999). Similarly, a 2010 study of 1316 human infants born at less than 28 weeks' gestation reported a non-significant effect of ventilation strategy leading to a lower oxygen saturation (85-89% versus 91-95%) on the incidence of BPD (SUPPORT Study Group, 2010). Furthermore, The use of high-dose antioxidants scavenging free radicals (vitamins C and E) did not have any protective effect against alveolar hypoplasia (Berger et al., 1998). Free radicals were therefore not the major player in BPD.

If higher O_2 in inspired air could lead to a greater cellular concentration of H_2O_2 that is not quenched by vitamins C or E, the apparently weak effect of oxygen supplementation on BPD development must be explainable by another source of oxidant molecules masking the impact of O_2. It is noteworthy that the major risk factor for BPD is gestational age; the lower the age, the greater the incidence of BPD. Coincidentally, the more premature the infant, the greater is his dependence on parenteral nutrition. A 2011 study showed that preterm infants developing BPD received more parenteral than enteral nutrition (Wemhöner et al., 2011). In the various studies on BPD, including those in baboons, the gestation ages of the subjects were such that the infants likely required parenteral nutritive support, a major source of ROS and particularly of H_2O_2 (Laborie et al., 1998; Lavoie et al., 1997). In itself, parenteral nutrition may be sufficient to induce the development of BPD. In fact, however, it is highly probable that both parenteral nutrition and oxygen supplementation induce oxidative stress, by both increasing the intracellular concentration of H_2O_2 and modifying the redox potential of glutathione (Chessex et al., 2010).

5.2 Parenteral nutrition

Parenteral nutrition consists of the intravenous administration of a solution containing amino acids, dextrose, electrolytes, vitamins and lipids. Parenteral nutrition is essential for the nutritional support of the preterm infant, bypassing a gastrointestinal system whose immaturity severely limits the natural feeding process. Although parenteral nutrition is sufficient to support growth in the child, the instability of the nutrients in solution favours the generation of undesirable molecules. The admixture of redox-sensitive elements such as amino acids (tryptophan, tyrosine and others), polyunsaturated fatty acids, and vitamin C, in the presence of a strong oxidizing molecule such as dissolved oxygen, will induce oxidation of the nutrients and the formation of their consequent derivatives. For instance, peroxidation of omega-6 polyunsaturated fatty acids will yield lipid hydroperoxides and HNE (Massarenti et al., 2004; Silvers et al., 2001), while vitamin C and dissolved oxygen will produce H_2O_2 (Laborie et al., 1998; Lavoie et al., 1997). As vitamin C is the most powerful antioxidant found in parenteral nutrition, the main source of peroxides in parenteral nutrition would appear to be the multivitamin preparation (Laborie et al., 1998; Lavoie et al., 1997). Furthermore, this solution contains riboflavin, a photosensitive molecule. In the presence of light, photoexcited riboflavin catalyzes a peroxide-producing reaction (Laborie et al., 1998). The simple act of adequately shielding parenteral nutrition solutions from ambient light halved the concentration of peroxides in the infused solution (Chessex et al., 2001; Laborie et al., 1998, 1999, 2000; Lavoie et al., 1997, 2007) as well as in the urine of preterm infants (Bassiouny et al., 2009; Chessex et al., 2001). Adequate photoprotection of parenteral nutrition has also been reported to reduce the incidence of chronic lung disease (Bassiouny et al., 2009) or BPD (Chessex et al., 2007) in premature infants.

As administered in neonatal units, without adequate photoprotection, parenteral nutritive solutions are contaminated with several molecules having the potential to perturb the redox status of the lung, i.e. lipid hydroperoxides (Silvers et al., 2001), HNE (personal communication of Lavoie JC, 2011), ascorbylperoxide (Lavoie et al., 2004; Maghdessian et al., 2010), and H_2O_2 (Laborie et al., 1998; Lavoie et al., 1997; Silvers et al., 2001). All these molecules are detoxified by the glutathione system. Since glutathione levels are low in preterm infants (Lavoie & Chessex, 1997), these molecules can conceivably overwhelm the glutathione system, allowing the redox potential to shift toward an oxidized state. Infusion of parenteral nutrition without light protection for 4 days in newborn guinea pigs was associated with: 1) a loss of glutathione (Lavoie et al., 2000), 2) a more oxidized glutathione redox potential (Lavoie et al., 2008), and 3) a lower alveolar count (Lavoie et al., 2004, 2005, 2008), as compared to animals infused with a fully photoprotected solution. A recent study demonstrated that the blood glutathione redox potential measured in 7-day-old preterm infants (26 ± 1 weeks' gestation) was correlated with the severity of BPD; a more oxidized status was measured in the most severe cases (Chessex et al., 2010). Therefore, current knowledge suggests that each oxidant molecule affecting the glutathione system, whether from oxygen supplementation or from parenteral nutrition, may contribute to the development of BPD.

5.3 Inflammation
The third major risk factor for BPD is inflammation, a significant source of ROS (Federico et al., 2007; Pereda et al., 2006). Several pro-inflammatory cytokines have been detected in aspirated fluids from infants with BPD, the concentration increasing as a function of assisted ventilation duration and level of oxygen supplementation (Bose et al., 2008). As previously demonstrated, exposure to high amounts of O_2 favours the production of H_2O_2, a known activator of transcription factor NF-κB (Flohé et al., 1997; Haddad, 2002; Haddad & Land, 2000; Takada et al., 2003), which in turn upregulates the expression of several pro-

inflammatory cytokine genes (Federico et al., 2007; Pereda et al., 2006). The oxygen-cytokine connection was further supported by research showing that oxygen supplementation induced an inflammatory response in preterm infants (Lavoie et al., 2010). The association between BPD and inflammation may therefore be explained by an initial oxidative stress followed by a local increase in H_2O_2 concentration. However, other researchers have argued that an inflammatory process independent of the variation in inspired oxygen concentration could also induce BPD, for example chorioamnionitis (Gien & Kinsella, 2011). Paananen R et al (2009) reported that elevated plasma concentrations of IL-6, a pro-inflammatory cytokine, and IL-10, an anti-inflammatory cytokine, on the first day of life were indicative of greater BPD risk, independently of previous exposure to chorioamnionitis (39% of the 128 preterm neonates in the cohort had had chorioamnionitis; incidence of BPD in cohort, 25%). The lack of correlation between an initial inflammatory process and BPD development was confirmed in 2010 in a study investigating the association between chorioamnionitis and BPD (Prendergast, et al., 2010). From the 71 preterm infants developing BPD, 41 had been exposed to chorioamnionitis and/or funisitis. Their results, however, showed a significant correlation between the severity of BPD and gestational age or birth weight. Thus, endogenous infection does not seem to be connected to the development of BPD while cytokines are, underlining a possible implication of oxidative stress early in life.

6. Strategies for prevention/treatment

Under the hypothesis that glutathione, by its very involvement in the cellular redox environment, could be a key player in BPD development, one strategy to prevent BPD development or reduce its severity would be to preserve or increase the intracellular concentration of glutathione. It is noteworthy that the low levels of glutathione observed in preterm infants (Lavoie & Chessex, 1997) are not due to a defective enzymatic process. Indeed, GSH synthesis is very active, even in newborns of 26 weeks' gestation (Lavoie & Chessex, 1998). The defect comes rather from the immaturity of the cellular transport system of cysteine (Lavoie et al., 2002), an amino acid whose low intracellular availability limits the synthesis of glutathione (Deneke & Fanburg, 1989). This fact may explain the failure of intravenous administration of N-acetylcysteine to prevent the development of BPD in extremely low birth weight newborns (Ahola et al., 2003).

If it is difficult to increase the intracellular concentration of glutathione, one must at least prevent its consumption by reducing oxidative stress. This can be partly achieved by monitoring blood oxygen saturation levels to prevent excessive oxygen supplementation. Prevention of inflammation will help as well. However, limiting peroxide contamination in parenteral nutrition is essential. Though photoprotection of the solution may be difficult to institute in the clinical setting, the process must be initiated in the pharmacy department at the time of compounding and continued until bedside. New nutritive strategies leading to improvements in the nutritive quality of parenteral products, reducing the oxidation of nutrients and preventing the generation of oxidant molecules, will have a positive impact on the incidence of BPD.

7. Conclusions/perspectives

Presently, no therapy exists for BPD (Gien & Kinsella, 2011) and its prevention is difficult. The etiology is multifactorial. This chapter focused on the part played by oxidative stress, in particular the glutathione redox potential. While a number of oxidant sources can contribute to the shift in redox potential toward a more oxidized state, several BPD-related factors were found to have an impact, among them oxygen supplementation, parenteral nutrition, and inflammation. Modification of even one of these factors may decrease the incidence of BPD, but the best practice remains to administer a combination of new measures, as suggested by Geary C et al. (2008), including early use of surfactant and nasal continuous positive airway pressure for ventilatory support, as well as lowered oxygen saturation targets and better nutritive support. It is remarkable that all associations between biochemical markers and BPD have been observed with parameters measured in the first days of life (Ahola et al., 2004; Geary et al., 2008; Gladstone & Levine, 1994; Lavoie et al., 2008; Ogihara et al., 1999; Pitkanen et al., 1990; Welty, 2001). The first week of life, in both infants and animal models, seems be a critical window during which all efforts to reduce oxidative stress must be pursued.

8. Acknowledgements

The authors are grateful to Danielle Buch, medical writer/editor at the Applied Clinical Research Unit of the Sainte-Justine Research Centre, for editing of this chapter.

9. References

Ahola T, Lapatto R, Raivio KO, Selander B, Stigson L, Jonsson B, Jonsbo F, Esberg G, Stôvring S, Kjartansson S, Stiris T, Lossius K, Virkola K, Fellman V. 2003. N-acetylcysteine does not prevent bronchopulmonary dysplasia in immature infants: a randomized controlled trial. J Pediatr 143:713-719.

Ahola T, Fellman V, Kjellemer I, Raivio KO, Lapatto R. 2004. Plasma 8-Isoprostane Is Increased in Preterm Infants Who Develop Bronchopulmonary Dysplasia or Periventricular Leukomalacia. Pediatr Res 56: 88–93.

Ambalavanan N, Novak ZE. 2003. Peptide Growth Factors in Tracheal Aspirates of Mechanically Ventilated Preterm Neonates. Pediatr Res 53: 240–244.

Ambalavanan N, Van Meurs KP, Perritt R, Carlo WA, Ehrenkranz RA, Stevenson DK, Lemons JA, Poole WK, Higgins RD; NICHD Neonatal Research Network, Bethesda, MD. 2008. Predictors of death or bronchopulmonary dysplasia in preterm infants with respiratory failure. J Perinatol 28:420-426.

Anderson PJ, Doyle LW. 2006. Neurodevelopmental outcome of bronchopulmonary dysplasia. Semin Perinatol 30:227-232.

Antonucci R, Contu P, Porcella A, Atzeni C, Chiappe S. 2004. Intrauterine smoke exposure: a new risk factor for bronchopulmonary dysplasia? J Perinat Med 32:272-277.

Avery ME, Tooley WH, Keller JB, Hurd SS, Bryan MH, Cotton RB, Epstein MF, Fitzhardinge PM, Hansen CB, Hansen TN, et al. 1987. Is chronic lung disease in low birth weight infants preventable? A survey of eight centers. Pediatrics 79:26-30.

Baraldi E, Carraro S, Filippone M. 2009. Bronchopulmonary dysplasia: definitions and long-term respiratory outcome. Early Hum Dev 85:S1-S3.

Bassiouny MR, Almarsafawy H, bdel-Hady H, Nasef N, Hammad TA, Aly H. 2009. A randomized controlled trial on parenteral nutrition, oxidative stress, and chronic lung diseases in preterm infants. J Pediatr Gastroenterol Nutr 48:363-369.

Behrman RE, Babson GS, Lessel R. 1971. Fetal and neonatal mortality in white middle class infants. Mortality risks by gestational age and weight. Am J Dis Child 121:486-489.

Berger TM, Frei B, Rifai N, Avery ME, Suh J, Yoder BA, et al. 1998. Early high dose antioxidant vitamins do not prevent bronchopulmonary dysplasia in premature baboons exposed to prolonged hyperoxia: a pilot study. Pediatr Res 43:719-726.

Bhatt AJ, Pryhuber GS, Huyck H, Watkins RH, Metlay LA, Maniscalco WM. 2001. Disrupted Pulmonary Vasculature and Decreased Vascular Endothelial Growth Factor, Flt-1, and TIE-2 in Human Infants Dying with Bronchopulmonary Dysplasia. Am J respir Crit Care Med 164:1971-1980.

Bhatt AJ, Amin SB, Chess PR, Watkins RH, Maniscalco WM. 2000. Expression of Vascular Endothelial Growth Factor and Flk-1 in Developing and Glucocorticoid-Treated Mouse Lung. Pediatr Res 47 :606-613.

Bonello S, Zähringer C, BelAiba RS, Djordjevic T, Hess J, Michiels C, KietzmannT , Görlach A. 2007. Reactive Oxygen Species Activate the HIF-1α Promoter Via a Functional NFκB Site. Arterioscler Thromb Vasc Biol 27:755-761.

Bose CL, Dammann CEL, Laughon MM. 2008. Bronchopulmonary dysplasia and inflammatory biomarkers in the premature neonate. Arch Dis Child Fetal Neonatal Ed 93:F455-F461.

Broström EB, Thunqvist P, Adenfelt G, Borling E, Katz-Salamon M. 2010. Obstructive lung disease in children with mild to severe BPD. Respir Med 104:362-370.

Bruce MC, Honaker CE and Cross RJ. 1999. Lung fibroblasts undergo apoptosis following alveolarization. Am J Respir Cell Mol Biol 20:228-236.

Buettner GR, Ng CF, Wang M, Rodgers VG, Schafer FQ. 2006. A new paradigm: manganese superoxide dismutase influences the production of H2O2 in cells and thereby their biological state. Free Radic Biol Med 41:1338-1350.

Chakraborty M, McGreal EP, Kotecha S. 2010. Acute lung injury in preterm newborn infants: mechanisms and management. Paediatr Respir Rev 11:162-170.

Chen H, Shi H. 2008. A reducing environment stabilizes HIF-2α in SH-SY5Y cells under hypoxic conditions. FEBS Lett 582:3899–3902.

Chessex P, Laborie S, Lavoie JC, Rouleau T. 2001. Photoprotection of solutions of parenteral nutrition decreases the infused load as well as the urinary excretion of peroxides in premature infants. Semin Perinatol 25:55-59.

Chessex P, Harrison A, Khashu M, Lavoie JC. 2007. In preterm neonates, is the risk of developing bronchopulmonary dysplasia influenced by the failure to protect total parenteral nutrition from exposure to ambient light? J Pediatr 151:213-214.

Chessex P, Watson C, Kaczala G, Rouleau T, Lavoie ME, Friel J, Lavoie JC. 2010. Determinants of oxidant stress in extremely low birth weight premature infants. Free Radic Biol Med 49:1380-6.

Coalson JJ, Winter V, DeLemos RA. 1995. Decreased alveolarization in baboon survivors with bronchopulmonary dysplasia. Am J Respir Crit Care Med 152:640-646.

Coalson JJ, Winter VT, Siler-Khodr T, Yoder BA. 1999. Neonatal chronic lung disease in extremely immature baboons. Am J Respir Crit Care Med 160:1333-1346.

Cotton RB, Morrow JD, Hazinski TA, Roberts LJ, Law AB, Steele S. 1996. F2-isoprostanes (F2-I) in tracheobronchial aspirate fluid (TBAF) indicate association between increased FiO2 and lipid peroxidation in the lungs of premature infants. *Pediatr Res* 39: 329A.

Darlow BA, Horwood LJ. 1992. Chronic lung disease in very low birthweight infants: a prospective population-based study. J Paediatr Child Health 28:301-305.

Das KC, Ravi D, Holland W. 2004. Increased apoptosis and expression of p21 and p53 in premature infant baboon model of bronchopulmonary dysplasia. Antioxid Redox Signal 6:109-116.

Davis JM, Rosenfeld WN, Sanders RJ, et al. 1993. Prophylactic effects of recombinant human superoxide dismutase in neonatal lung injury. J Appl Physiol 74:2234-2241.

Davis PG, Thorpe K, Roberts R, Schmidt B, Doyle LW, Kirpalani H, Trial of Indomethacin Prophylaxis in Preterms (TIPP) Investigators. 2002. Evaluating "old" definitions for the "new" bronchopulmonary dysplasia. J Pediatr 140:555-560.

Davis JM, Parad RB, Michele T, et al. 2003. Pulmonary outcome at one year corrected age in premature infants treated at birth with recombinant CuZn superoxide dismutase. Pediatrics 111:469-476.

Deneke SM, Fanburg BL. 1989. Regulation of cellular glutathione. Am J Physiol 257:L163-L173.

Durrmeyer X, Kayem G, Sinico M, Dassieu G, Danan C, Decobert F. 2011. Perinatal Risk Factors for Bronchopulmonary Dysplasia in Extremely Low Gestational Age Infants: A Pregnancy Disorder-Based Approach. J Pediatr Oct 31. [Epub ahead of print]

Egreteau L, Pauchard JY, Semama DS, Matis J, Liska A, Romeo B, Cneude F, Hamon I, Truffert P. 2001. Chronic oxygen dependency in infants born at less than 32 weeks' gestation: incidence and risk factors. Pediatrics 108:E26.

Ehrenkranz RA, Walsh MC, Vohr BR, Jobe AH, Wright LL, Fanaroff AA, Wrage LA, Poole K. 2005. Validation of the National Institutes of Health Consensus Definition of Bronchopulmonary Dysplasia. Pediatrics 116:1353-1360.

Fanaroff AA, Stoll BJ, Wright LL, et al; NICHD Neonatal Research Network. 2007. Trends in neonatal morbidity and mortality for very low birthweight infants. Am J Obstet Gynecol 196: 147.e1-8.

Federico A, Morgillo F, Tuccillo C, Ciardiello F, Loguercio C. 2007. Chronic inflammation and oxidative stress in human carcinogenesis. Int J Cancer 121:2381-2386.

Floréa L, Branda I. 1969. Kinetics of glutathione peroxidase. Biochim Biophys Acta (BBA) – Enzymology 191:541-549.

Flohé L, Brigelius-Flohé R, Saliou C, Traber MG, Packer L. 1997. Redox regulation of NF-kappa B activation. Free Radic Biol Med 22:1115-1126.

Frank L, Sosenko IR. 1987a. Prenatal development of lung antioxidant enzymes in four species. J Pediatr 110:106-110.

Frank L, Sosenko IR. 1987b. Development of lung antioxidant enzyme system in late gestation: possible implications for the prematurely born infant. J Pediatr 110:9-14.

Frank L. 1991. Developmental aspects of experimental pulmonary oxygen toxicity. Free Radic Biol Med 11:463-494.

Gaetani GF, Ferraris AM, Rolfo M, Mangerini R, Arena S, Kirkman HN. 1996. Predominant role of catalase in the disposal of hydrogen peroxide within human érythrocytes. Blood 87:1595-1599.

Garg M, Kurzner SI, Bautista DB, Keens TG. 1988. Clinically unsuspected hypoxia during sleep and feeding in infants with bronchopulmonary dysplasia. Pediatrics 81:635-642.

Geary C, Caskey M, Fonseca R, Malloy M. 2008. Decreased incidence of bronchopulmonary dysplasia after early management changes, including surfactant and nasal continuous positive airway pressure treatment at delivery, lowered oxygen saturation goals, and early amino acid administration: a historical cohort study. Pediatrics 121:89-96.

Gien J, Kinsella JP. 2011. Pathogenesis and treatment of bronchopulmonary dysplasia. Current Opinion in Pediatrics 23:305-313.

Gladstone IM, Levine RL. 1994. Oxidation of proteins in neonatal lungs. Pediatrics 93:764-768.

Haddad JJ. 2002. Oxygen-sensing mechanisms and the regulation of redox-responsive transcription factors in development and pathophysiology. Respir Res 3:26.

Haddad JJE, Land SC. 2000. O2-evoked regulation of HIF-1a and NF-kB in périnatal lung epithelium requires glutathione biosynthesis. Am J Physiol Lung Cell Mol Physiol 278:L492-L503.

Haddad JJE, Olver RE, Land SC. 2000. Antioxidant/Pro-oxidant Equilibrium Regulates HIF-1α and NF-κB Redox Sensitivity. Evidence For Inhibition By Glutathione Oxidation In Alveolar Epithelial Cells J Biol Chem 275:21130-21139.

Hakulinen A, Heinonen K, Jokela V, Kiekara O. 1988. Occurrence, predictive factors and associated morbidity of bronchopulmonary dysplasia in a preterm birth cohort. J Perinat Med 16:437-446.

Hodgman JE, Mikity VG, Tatter D, Cleland RS. 1969. Chronic respiratory distress in the premature infant. Wilson-Mikity syndrome. Pediatrics 44:179-195.

Horbar JD, Badger GJ, Carpenter JH, Fanaroff AA, Kilpatrick S, LaCorte M, Phibbs R, Soll RF; Members of the Vermont Oxford Network. 2002. Trends in mortality and morbidity for very low birth weight infants, 1991-1999. Pediatrics 110:143-151.

Husain AN, Siddiqui NH, Stocker JT. 1998. Pathology of arrested acinar development in postsurfactant bronchopulmonary dysplasia. Hum Pathol 29:710-717.

Jeng SF, Hsu CH, Tsao PN, Chou HC, Lee WT, Kao HA, Hung HY, Chang JH, Chiu NC, Hsieh WS. 2008. Bronchopulmonary dysplasia predicts adverse developmental and clinical outcomes in very-low-birthweight infants. Dev Med Child Neurol 50:51-57.

Jobe AH. 1999. The New BPD: An Arrest of Lung Development. Pediatr Res 46:641-643.

Jobe AH, Bancalari E. 2001. Bronchopulmonary Dysplasia. Am J Respir Crit Care Med 163:1723-1729.

Jones P, Suggett A. 1968. The Catalase-Hydrogen Peroxide System. Kinetics Of Catalatic Action At High Substrate Concentrations. Biochem J 110 :617-620.

Kelly FJ, Lubec G. 1995. Hyperoxic injury of immature guinea pig lung is mediated via hydroxyl radicals. Pediatr Res 38: 786-791.

Kraybill EN, Runyan DK, Bose CL, Khan JH. 1989. Risk factors for chronic lung disease in infants with birth weights of 751 to 1000 grams. J Pediatr 115:115-120.

Koo KY, Kim JE, Lee SM, Namgung R, Park MS, Park KI, Lee C. 2010. Effect of severe neonatal morbidities on long term outcome in extremely low birth weight infants. Korean J Pediatr 53:694-700.

Laborie S, Lavoie JC, Chessex P. 1998. Paradoxical role of ascorbic acid and riboflavin in solutions of total parenteral nutrition: implication in photoinduced peroxide generation. Pediatr Res 43:601-606.

Laborie S, Lavoie JC, Pineault M, Chessex P. 1999. Protecting solutions of parenteral nutrition from peroxidation. JPEN J Parenter Enteral Nutr 23:104-108.

Laborie S, Lavoie JC, Pineault M, Chessex P. 2000. Contribution of multivitamins, air, and light in the generation of peroxides in adult and neonatal parenteral nutrition solutions. Ann Pharmacother 34:440-445.

Lal MK, Manktelow BN, Draper ES and Field DJ. 2003. Chronic lung disease of prematurity and intrauterine growth retardation: a population-based study. Pediatrics 111:483–487.

Land SC, Wilson SM. 2005. Redox Regulation of Lung Development and Perinatal Lung Epithelial Function. Antioxidants & Redox Signaling 7:92-107.

Lavoie JC, Belanger S, Spalinger M, Chessex P. 1997. Admixture of a multivitamin preparation to parenteral nutrition: the major contributor to in vitro generation of peroxides. Pediatrics 99:E6.

Lavoie JC, Chessex P. 1997. Gender and maturation affect glutathione status in human neonatal tissues. Free Radic Biol Med 23:648-657.

Lavoie JC, Chessex P. 1998. Development of glutathione synthesis and gamma-glutamyltranspeptidase activities in tissues from newborn infants. Free Radic Biol Med 24:994-1001.

Lavoie JC, Laborie S, Rouleau T, Spalinger M, Chessex P. 2000. Peroxide-like oxidant response in lungs of newborn guinea pigs following the parenteral infusion of a multivitamin preparation. Biochem Pharmacol 60 :1297-1303.

Lavoie JC, Rouleau T, Truttmann AC, Chessex P. 2002. Postnatal gender-dependent maturation of cellular cysteine uptake. Free Radic Res 36:811-817.

Lavoie JC, Chessex P, Rouleau T, Migneault D, Comte B. 2004. Light-induced byproducts of vitamin C in multivitamin solutions. Clin Chem 50:135-140.

Lavoie JC, Rouleau T, Chessex P. 2004. Interaction between ascorbate and light-exposed riboflavin induces lung remodelling. J Pharm Exp Ther 311: 634-639.

Lavoie JC, Rouleau T, Chessex P. 2005. Effect of coadministration of parenteral multivitamins with the lipid emulsion on lung remodeling in an animal model of TPN. Pediatr Pulmonol 40:53-56.

Lavoie JC, Rouleau T, Tsopmo A, Friel J, Chessex P. 2007. Influence of lung oxidant and antioxidant status on alveolarization: role of light-exposed TPN. Free Radic Biol Med 45:572-577.

Lavoie JC, Rouleau T, Tsopmo A, Friel J, Chessex P. 2008. Influence of lung oxidant and antioxidant status on alveolarization: role of light-exposed total parenteral nutrition. Free Radic Biol Med 45:572-577.

Lavoie P, Lavoie JC, Watson C, Rouleau T, Chang BA, Chessex P. 2010. Inflammatory response in preterm infants is induced early in life by oxygen and modulated by TPN. Pediatr Res 68:248-51.

López-Lázaro M. 2006. HIF-1: hypoxia-inducible factor or dysoxia-inducible factor? FASEB J 20:828–832.

Lubec G, Widness JA, Hayde M, Menzel D, Pollack A. 1997. Hydroxyl radical generation in oxygen treated infants. Pediatrics 100: 200-204.

Luyet C, Burri PH and Schittny JC. 2000. Pre- and postnatal lung development, maturation, and plasticity. Suppression of cell proliferation and programmed cell death by dexamethasone during postnatal lung development. Am. J Physiol Lung Cell Mol Physiol 282:L477-L483.

Maghdessian R, Cote F, Rouleau T, Ouadda AB, Levy E, Lavoie JC. 2010. Ascorbylperoxide contaminating parenteral nutrition perturbs the lipid metabolism in newborn guinea pig. J Pharmacol Exp Ther 334:278-284.

Majnemer A, Riley P, Shevell M, Birnbaum R, Greenstone H, Coates AL. 2000. Severe bronchopulmonary dysplasia increases risk for later neurological and motor sequelae in preterm survivors. Dev Med Child Neurol. 42:53-60.

Massarenti P, Biasi F, de FA, Pauletto D, Rocca G, Silli B, et al. 2004. 4-Hydroxynonenal is markedly higher in patients on a standard long-term home parenteral nutrition. Free Radic Res 38:73-80.

Moyer-Mileur LJ, Nielson DW, Pfeffer KD, Witte MK, Chapman DL. 1996. Eliminating sleep-associated hypoxemia improves growth in infants with bronchopulmonary dysplasia. Pediatrics 98:779-783.

Natl Inst Health Consens Dev Conf Summ. 1979. Antenatal diagnosis. Sponsored by the National Institute of Child Health and Human Development 2:11-15.

Northway WH Jr, Rosan RC, Porter DY. 1967. Pulmonary disease following respirator therapy of hyaline-membrane disease. Bronchopulmonary dysplasia. N Engl J Med 276:357-368.

Nycyk JA, Drury JA, Cooke RWI. 1998. Breath pentane as a marker for lipid peroxidation and adverse outcome in preterm infants. Arch Dis Child Fetal Neonatal Ed 79: F67–F69.

Ogihara T, Hirano K, Morinobu T, Kim HS, Hiroi M, Ogihara H, Tamai H. 1999. Raised concentration of aldehyde lipid peroxidation products in premature infants with chronic lung disease. Arch Dis Child Fetal Neonatal Ed 80: F21–F25.

Paananen R, Husa AK, Vuolteenaho R, et al. 2009. Blood cytokines during the perinatal period in very preterm infants: relationship of inflammatory response and bronchopulmonary dysplasia. J Pediatr 154:39–43.

Palta M, Gabbert D, Weinstein MR, Peters ME. 1991. Multivariate assessment of traditional risk factors for chronic lung disease in very low birth weight neonates. The Newborn Lung Project. J Pediatr. 119:285-292.

Pereda J, Sabater L, Aparisi L, Escobar J, Sandoval J, Viña J, López-Rodas G, Sastre J. 2006. Interaction between cytokines and oxidative stress in acute pancreatitis. Curr Med Chem 13:2775-2787.

Pitkanen OM, Hallman M, Andersson SM. 1990. Correlation of free oxygen radical-induced lipid peroxidation with outcome in very low birthweight infants. J Pediatr 116: 760-764.

Prendergast M, May C, Broughton S, Pollina E, Milner AD, Rafferty GF, Greenough A. 2010. Chorioamnionitis, lung function and bronchopulmonary dysplasia in prematurely born infants. Arch Dis Child Fetal Neonatal Ed 96:F270-F274.

Randell SH, Mercer RR, Young SL. 1990. Neonatal hyperoxia alters the pulmonary alveolar and capillary structure of 40-day-old rats. Am J Pathol 136:1259-1266.

Roy S, Khanna S, Sen CK. 2008. Redox regulation of the VEGF signaling path and tissue vascularization: Hydrogen peroxide, the common link between physical exercise and cutaneous wound Healing. Free Radic Biol Med 44:180-192.

Saugstad OD. 2010. Oxygen and oxidative stress in bronchopulmonary dysplasia. J Perinat Med 38:571-577.

Schafer FQ, Buettner GR. 2001. Redox environment of the cell as viewed through the redox state of the glutathione disulfide/glutathionne couple. *Free Radic Biol Med* 30:1191-1212

Sekar KC, Duke JC. 1991. Sleep apnea and hypoxemia in recently weaned premature infants with and without bronchopulmonary dysplasia. Pediatr Pulmonol 10:112-116.

Shennan AT, Dunn MS, Ohlsson A, Lennox K, Hoskins EM. 1988. Abnormal pulmonary outcomes in premature infants: prediction from oxygen requirement in the neonatal period. Pediatrics 82:527-523.

Short EJ, Klein NK, Lewis BA, Fulton S, Eisengart S, Kercsmar C, Baley J, Singer LT. 2003. Cognitive and academic consequences of bronchopulmonary dysplasia and very low birth weight: 8-year-old outcomes. Pediatrics 112:e359.

Silvers KM, Darlow BA, Winterbourn CC. 2001. Lipid peroxide and hydrogen peroxide formation in parenteral nutrition solutions containing multivitamins. JPEN J Parenter Enteral Nutr 25, 14-17.

Simon MC. 2006. Mitochondrial reactive oxygen species are required for hypoxic HIF alphastabilization. Adv Exp Med Biol 588:165-170.

Stoll BJ, Hansen NI, Bell EF, Shankaran S, Laptook AR, Walsh MC, hale EC, Newman NS, Schibler K, Carlo WA, Kennedy KA, Poindexter BB, Finer NN, Ehrenkranz RA, Duara S, Sanchez PJ, O'Shea M, Goldberg RN, Van Meurs KP, Faix RG, Phelps DL, Freantz ID, Watterberg KL, Saha S, Das A, Higgins RD, Eunice Kennedy Shriver National Institute of Child Health and Human Development Neonatal Research Network. 2010. Neonatal Outcomes of Extremely Preterm Infants From the NICHD NeonatalResearch Network. Pediatrics 126;443-456.

Stroustrup A, Trasande L. 2010. Epidemiological Characteristics and Resource Use in Neonates With Bronchopulmonary Dysplasia: 1993 -2006. Pediatrics 126:e291-e297.

SUPPORT Study Group of the Eunice Kennedy Shriver NICHD Neonatal Research Network, Finer NN, Carlo WA, Walsh MC, Rich W, Gantz MG, et al. 2010. Early CPAP versus surfactant in extremely preterm infants. N Engl J Med 362:1970-1979.

Takada Y, Mukhopadhyay A, Kundu GC, Mahabeleshwar GH, Singh S, Aggarwal BB. 2003. Hydrogen peroxide activates NF-kappa B through tyrosine phosphorylation of I kappa B alpha and serine phosphorylation of p65: evidence for the involvement of I kappa B alpha kinase and Syk protein-tyrosine kinase. J Biol Chem 278:24233-24241.

Theile AR, Radmacher PG, Anschutz TW, Davis DW, Adamkin DH. 2011. Nutritional strategies and growth in extremely low birth weight infants with bronchopulmonary dysplasia over the past 10 years. J Perinatol May 26 [Epub ahead of print].

Van Marter LJ. 2009. Epidemiology of bronchopulmonary dysplasia. Semin Fetal Neonatal Med. 14:358-366.

Walsh MC, Wilson-Costello D, Zadell A, Newman N, Fanaroff A. 2003. Safety, Reliability, and Validity of a Physiologic Definition of Bronchopulmonary Dysplasia. J Perinatology 23, 451-456.

Walsh MC, Yao Q, Gettner P, Hale E, Collins M, Hensman A, Everette R, Peters N, Miller N, Muran G, Auten K, Newman N, Rowan G, Grisby C, Arnell K, Miller L, Ball B,

McDavid G; National Institute of Child Health and Human Development Neonatal Research Network, 2004. Impact of a Physiologic Definition on Bronchopulmonary Dysplasia Rates. Pediatrics 114:1305–1311.

Welty SE. 2001. Is There a Role for Antioxidant Therapy in Bronchopulmonary Dysplasia? J. Nutr 131: 947S–950S.

Wemhöner A, Ortner D, Tschirch E, Strasak A, Rüdiger M. 2011. Nutrition of preterm infants in relation to bronchopulmonary dysplasia. BMC Pulmonary Medicine 11:7.

White CW, Stabler SP, Allen RH, Moreland S, Rosenberg AA. 1994. Plasma cysteine concentrations in infants with respiratory distress. J Pediatr 125:769-777.

Wilson MG, Mikity VG. 1960. A new form of respiratory disease in premature infants. AMA J Dis Child 99:489-499.

Winterbourn CC, Hampton MB. 2008. Thiol chemistry and specificity in redox signaling. Free Radic Biol Med 45:549-561.

Wong PM, Lees AN, Louw J, Lee FY, French N, Gain K, Murray CP, Wilson A, Chambers DC. 2008. Emphysema in young adult survivors of moderate-to-severe bronchopulmonary dysplasia. Eur Respir J 32:321-328.

Zanardo V, Trevisanuto D, Dani C, Bottos M, Guglielmi A, Cantarutti F. 1995. Oxygen saturation in premature neonates with bronchopulmonary dysplasia in a hammock. Biol Neonate 67:54-58.

Zeitlin J, Draper ES, Kollée L, Milligan D, Boerch K, Agostino R, Gortner L, Van Reempts P, Chabernaud JL, Gadzinowski J, Bréart G, Papiernik E; MOSAIC research group. 2008. Differences in rates and short-term outcome of live births before 32 weeks of gestation in Europe in 2003: results from the MOSAIC cohort. Pediatrics 121:e936-e944.

Permissions

The contributors of this book come from diverse backgrounds, making this book a truly international effort. This book will bring forth new frontiers with its revolutionizing research information and detailed analysis of the nascent developments around the world.

We would like to thank Professor E.M. Irusen, for lending his expertise to make the book truly unique. He has played a crucial role in the development of this book. Without his invaluable contribution this book wouldn't have been possible. He has made vital efforts to compile up to date information on the varied aspects of this subject to make this book a valuable addition to the collection of many professionals and students.

This book was conceptualized with the vision of imparting up-to-date information and advanced data in this field. To ensure the same, a matchless editorial board was set up. Every individual on the board went through rigorous rounds of assessment to prove their worth. After which they invested a large part of their time researching and compiling the most relevant data for our readers. Conferences and sessions were held from time to time between the editorial board and the contributing authors to present the data in the most comprehensible form. The editorial team has worked tirelessly to provide valuable and valid information to help people across the globe.

Every chapter published in this book has been scrutinized by our experts. Their significance has been extensively debated. The topics covered herein carry significant findings which will fuel the growth of the discipline. They may even be implemented as practical applications or may be referred to as a beginning point for another development. Chapters in this book were first published by InTech; hereby published with permission under the Creative Commons Attribution License or equivalent.

The editorial board has been involved in producing this book since its inception. They have spent rigorous hours researching and exploring the diverse topics which have resulted in the successful publishing of this book. They have passed on their knowledge of decades through this book. To expedite this challenging task, the publisher supported the team at every step. A small team of assistant editors was also appointed to further simplify the editing procedure and attain best results for the readers.

Our editorial team has been hand-picked from every corner of the world. Their multi-ethnicity adds dynamic inputs to the discussions which result in innovative outcomes. These outcomes are then further discussed with the researchers and contributors who give their valuable feedback and opinion regarding the same. The feedback is then collaborated with the researches and they are edited in a comprehensive manner to aid the understanding of the subject.

Apart from the editorial board, the designing team has also invested a significant amount of their time in understanding the subject and creating the most relevant covers. They scrutinized every image to scout for the most suitable representation of the subject and create an appropriate cover for the book.

The publishing team has been involved in this book since its early stages. They were actively engaged in every process, be it collecting the data, connecting with the contributors or procuring relevant information. The team has been an ardent support to the editorial, designing and production team. Their endless efforts to recruit the best for this project, has resulted in the accomplishment of this book. They are a veteran in the field of academics and their pool of knowledge is as vast as their experience in printing. Their expertise and guidance has proved useful at every step. Their uncompromising quality standards have made this book an exceptional effort. Their encouragement from time to time has been an inspiration for everyone.

The publisher and the editorial board hope that this book will prove to be a valuable piece of knowledge for researchers, students, practitioners and scholars across the globe.

List of Contributors

Silvia Giono-Cerezo
Departamento de Microbiología, Escuela Nacional de Ciencias Biológicas, IPN, México

Guadalupe Estrada-Gutiérrez
Departamento de Infectología, Instituto Nacional de Perinatología, México, D.F., México

José Antonio Rivera-Tapia and Jorge Antonio Yáñez-Santos
Benemérita Universidad Autónoma de Puebla, Puebla, México

Francisco Javier Díaz-García
Departamento de Salud Pública, Facultad de Medicina, UNAM, México

M.S. Paats, P.Th.W. van Hal, C.C. Baan, H.C. Hoogsteden, M.M. van der Eerden and R.W. Hendriks
Erasmus Medical Center, Rotterdam, The Netherlands

Pilar Morales
LungTrasplant Unit, Hospital Universitario La Fe, Valencia, Spain

Ana Gil-Brusola and María Santos
Microbiology Department, Hospital Universitario La Fe, Valencia, Spain

Tracey L. Bonfield
Inflammatory Mediator and Cystic Fibrosis Lung Disease Modeling CORE Center, Department of Pediatric Pulmonology, Case Western Reserve University, Cleveland, Ohio, USA

Damaris Lopera and Ángela Restrepo
Corporación para Investigaciones Biológicas (CIB), Medellín, Colombia

Luz E. Cano and Ángel González
Corporación para Investigaciones Biológicas (CIB), Medellín, Colombia
Escuela de Microbiología, Universidad de Antioquia (UdeA), Medellín, Colombia

Tonny W. Naranjo
Corporación para Investigaciones Biológicas (CIB), Medellín, Colombia
Escuela Ciencias de la Salud, Universidad Pontificia Bolivariana (UPB), Medellín, Colombia

Ayman M. Noreddin, Ghada Sawy, Walid Elkhatib, Ehab Noreddin and Atef Shibl
Hampton University, Hampton, VA, USA

Christian Peiser
Department for Pediatric Pneumology and Immunology, Charité, Medical University Berlin, Germany

Sachin Gupta
Division of Neonatology, Dept. of Ped., John Stroger Hospital of Cook County, USA

Shou-Yien Wu
Division of Neonatology, Dept. of Ped., John Stroger Hospital of Cook County, USA
Rosalind Franklin University of Medicine and Science, Chicago, Illinois, USA

Chung-Ming Chen
Dept. of Pediatrics, USA
Maternal Child Health Research Center, Taipei Medical University, Taipei, Taiwan

Tsu-Fuh Yeh
Dept. of Pediatrics, USA
Maternal Child Health Research Center, Taipei Medical University, Taipei, Taiwan
Dept. of Ped., China Medical University, Taichung, Taiwan

Jean-Claude Lavoie and Ibrahim Mohamed
Université de Montréal, Canada

Printed in the USA
CPSIA information can be obtained
at www.ICGtesting.com
JSHW011410221024
72173JS00003B/497

9 781632 411686